Orthopedic Treatment of Diseases and Fractures in Elderly

Orthopedic Treatment of Diseases and Fractures in Elderly

Editor

Gianluca Testa

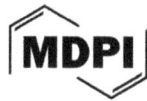

Basel • Beijing • Wuhan • Barcelona • Belgrade • Novi Sad • Cluj • Manchester

Editor
Gianluca Testa
Department of General Surgery and
Medical Surgical Specialties, Section of
Orthopaedics and Traumatology,
University of Catania
Catania, Italy

Editorial Office
MDPI
St. Alban-Anlage 66
4052 Basel, Switzerland

This is a reprint of articles from the Special Issue published online in the open access journal *Journal of Clinical Medicine* (ISSN 2077-0383) (available at: https://www.mdpi.com/journal/jcm/special_issues/Orthopedic_Treatment_Diseases_Fractures_Elderly).

For citation purposes, cite each article independently as indicated on the article page online and as indicated below:

Lastname, A.A.; Lastname, B.B. Article Title. *Journal Name* **Year**, *Volume Number*, Page Range.

ISBN 978-3-0365-9358-6 (Hbk)
ISBN 978-3-0365-9359-3 (PDF)
doi.org/10.3390/books978-3-0365-9359-3

© 2023 by the authors. Articles in this book are Open Access and distributed under the Creative Commons Attribution (CC BY) license. The book as a whole is distributed by MDPI under the terms and conditions of the Creative Commons Attribution-NonCommercial-NoDerivs (CC BY-NC-ND) license.

Contents

Eic Ju Lim, Won Uk Koh, Hyungtae Kim, Ha-Jung Kim, Hyun-Chul Shon and Ji Wan Kim
Regional Nerve Block Decreases the Incidence of Postoperative Delirium in Elderly Hip Fracture
Reprinted from: *Journal of Clinical Medicine* **2021**, *10*, 3586, doi:10.3390/jcm10163586 1

Valeska Hofmann, Christian Deininger, Stefan Döbele, Christian Konrads and Florian Wichlas
Mild Traumatic Brain Injury in Older Adults: Are Routine Second cCT Scans Necessary?
Reprinted from: *Journal of Clinical Medicine* **2021**, *10*, 3794, doi:10.3390/jcm10173794 11

Lisa Klute, Christian Pfeifer, Isabella Weiss, Agnes Mayr, Volker Alt and Maximilian Kerschbaum
Displacement of the Greater Tuberosity in Humeral Head Fractures Does Not only Depend on Rotator Cuff Status
Reprinted from: *Journal of Clinical Medicine* **2021**, *10*, 4136, doi:10.3390/jcm10184136 19

Jarosław Olech, Grzegorz Konieczny, Łukasz Tomczyk and Piotr Morasiewicz
A Randomized Trial Assessing the Muscle Strength and Range of Motion in Elderly Patients following Distal Radius Fractures Treated with 4- and 6-Week Cast Immobilization
Reprinted from: *Journal of Clinical Medicine* **2021**, *10*, 5774, doi:10.3390/jcm10245774 27

Norio Yamamoto, Hiroyuki Ohbe, Yosuke Tomita, Takashi Yorifuji, Mikio Nakajima, Yusuke Sasabuchi and et al.
Associations between Early Surgery and Postoperative Outcomes in Elderly Patients with Distal Femur Fracture: A Retrospective Cohort Study
Reprinted from: *Journal of Clinical Medicine* **2021**, *10*, 5800, doi:10.3390/jcm10245800 37

Patrocinio Ariza-Vega, Rafael Prieto-Moreno, Herminia Castillo-Pérez, Virginia Martínez-Ruiz, Dulce Romero-Ayuso and Maureen C. Ashe
Family Caregivers' Experiences with Tele-Rehabilitation for Older Adults with Hip Fracture
Reprinted from: *Journal of Clinical Medicine* **2021**, *10*, 5850, doi:10.3390/jcm10245850 49

Mario Herrera-Pérez, David González-Martín, Emilio J. Sanz and José L. Pais-Brito
Ethical Dilemmas with Regard to Elderly Patients with Hip Fracture: The Problem of Nonagenarians and Centenarians
Reprinted from: *Journal of Clinical Medicine* **2022**, *11*, 1851, doi:10.3390/jcm11071851 61

Leonardo Stramazzo, Giuseppe Rovere, Alessio Cioffi, Giulio Edoardo Vigni, Nicolò Galvano, Antonio D'Arienzo and et al.
Peri-Implant Distal Radius Fracture: Proposal of a New Classification
Reprinted from: *Journal of Clinical Medicine* **2022**, *11*, 2628, doi:10.3390/jcm11092628 69

Alejandro León-Andrino, David C. Noriega, Juan P. Lapuente, Daniel Pérez-Valdecantos, Alberto Caballero-García, Azael J. Herrero and et al.
Biological Approach in the Treatment of External Popliteal Sciatic Nerve (Epsn) Neurological Injury: Review
Reprinted from: *Journal of Clinical Medicine* **2022**, *11*, 2804, doi:10.3390/jcm11102804 75

Cheng-Hsun Chuang, Shun-Fa Yang, Pei-Lun Liao, Jing-Yang Huang, Man-Yee Chan and Chao-Bin Yeh
Association of Thiazide Use in Patients with Hypertension with Overall Fracture Risk: A Population-Based Cohort Study
Reprinted from: *Journal of Clinical Medicine* **2022**, *11*, 3304, doi:10.3390/jcm11123304 85

Gianluca Testa, Ludovico Lucenti, Salvatore D'Amato, Marco Sorrentino,
Pierluigi Cosentino, Andrea Vescio and et al.
Comparison between Vascular and Non-Vascular Bone Grafting in Scaphoid Nonunion: A Systematic Review
Reprinted from: *Journal of Clinical Medicine* 2022, *11*, 3402, doi:10.3390/jcm11123402 95

Gianluca Testa, Sara De Salvo, Silvia Boscaglia, Marco Montemagno, Antonio Longo, Andrea Russo and et al.
Hip Fractures and Visual Impairment: Is There a Cause–Consequence Mechanism?
Reprinted from: *Journal of Clinical Medicine* 2022, *11*, 3926, doi:10.3390/jcm11143926 109

Sara Dimartino, Vito Pavone, Michela Carnazza, Enrica Rosalia Cuffaro, Francesco Sergi and Gianluca Testa
Forearm Fracture Nonunion with and without Bone Loss: An Overview of Adult and Child Populations
Reprinted from: *Journal of Clinical Medicine* 2022, *11*, 4106, doi:10.3390/jcm11144106 115

Enrique González Marcos, Enrique González García, Josefa González-Santos,
Jerónimo J. González-Bernal, Adoración del Pilar Martín-Rodríguez and
Mirian Santamaría-Peláez
Determinants of Lack of Recovery from Dependency and Walking Ability Six Months after Hip Fracture in a Population of People Aged 65 Years and Over
Reprinted from: *Journal of Clinical Medicine* 2022, *11*, 4467, doi:10.3390/jcm11154467 125

Shira Lidar, Khalil Salame, Michelle Chua, Morsi Khashan, Dror Ofir, Alon Grundstein and et al.
Sarcopenia Is an Independent Risk Factor for Subsequent Osteoporotic Vertebral Fractures Following Percutaneous Cement Augmentation in Elderly Patients
Reprinted from: *Journal of Clinical Medicine* 2022, *11*, 5778, doi:10.3390/jcm11195778 141

Jihye Kim, Min Seong Kang and Tae-Hwan Kim
Prevalence of Sleep Disturbance and Its Risk Factors in Patients Who Undergo Surgical Treatment for Degenerative Spinal Disease: A Nationwide Study of 106,837 Patients
Reprinted from: *Journal of Clinical Medicine* 2022, *11*, 5932, doi:10.3390/jcm11195932 149

Manuel Enrique Suárez Rozo, Sara Trapero-Asenjo, Daniel Pecos-Martín,
Samuel Fernández-Carnero, Tomás Gallego-Izquierdo, José Jesús Jiménez Rejano and et al.
Reliability of the Spanish Version of the Movement Imagery Questionnaire-3 (MIQ-3) and Characteristics of Motor Imagery in Institutionalized Elderly People
Reprinted from: *Journal of Clinical Medicine* 2022, *11*, 6076, doi:10.3390/jcm11206076 165

Wen-Chien Wang, Yun-Che Wu, Yu-Hsien Lin, Yu-Tsung Lin, Kun-Hui Chen,
Chien-Chou Pan and et al.
Association of Body Mass Index with Long-Term All-Cause Mortality in Patients Who Had Undergone a Vertebroplasty for a Vertebral Compression Fracture
Reprinted from: *Journal of Clinical Medicine* 2022, *11*, 6519, doi:10.3390/jcm11216519 183

Michael Zyskowski, Markus Wurm, Frederik Greve, Philipp Zehnder, Patrick Pflüger,
Michael Müller and et al.
A Prospective Randomized Study Comparing Functional Outcome in Distal Fibula Fractures between Conventional AO Semitubular Plating and Minimal Invasive Intramedullary "Photodynamic Bone Stabilisation"
Reprinted from: *Journal of Clinical Medicine* 2022, *11*, 7178, doi:10.3390/jcm11237178 191

Jihye Kim, Jang Hyun Kim and Tae-Hwan Kim
Changes in Sleep Problems in Patients Who Underwent Surgical Treatment for Degenerative Spinal Disease with a Concurrent Sleep Disorder: A Nationwide Cohort Study in 3183 Patients during a Two-Year Perioperative Period
Reprinted from: *Journal of Clinical Medicine* **2022**, *11*, 7402, doi:10.3390/jcm11247402 . . . . **207**

Giulia Rita Agata Mangano, Marianna Avola, Chiara Blatti, Alessia Caldaci, Marco Sapienza, Rita Chiaramonte and et al.
Non-Adherence to Anti-Osteoporosis Medication: Factors Influencing and Strategies to Overcome It. A Narrative Review
Reprinted from: *Journal of Clinical Medicine* **2023**, *12*, 14, doi:10.3390/jcm12010014 . . . . **223**

Vito Pavone, Giacomo Papotto, Andrea Vescio, Gianfranco Longo, Salvatore D'Amato, Marco Ganci and et al.
Short and Middle Functional Outcome in the Static vs. Dynamic Fixation of Syndesmotic Injuries in Ankle Fractures: A Retrospective Case Series Study
Reprinted from: *Journal of Clinical Medicine* **2023**, *12*, 3637, doi:10.3390/jcm12113637 . . . . **237**

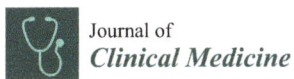

Article

Regional Nerve Block Decreases the Incidence of Postoperative Delirium in Elderly Hip Fracture

Eic Ju Lim [1], Won Uk Koh [2], Hyungtae Kim [2], Ha-Jung Kim [2], Hyun-Chul Shon [1] and Ji Wan Kim [3,*]

1. Department of Orthopedic Surgery, Chungbuk National University Hospital, Chungbuk National University College of Medicine, Cheongju 28644, Korea; limeicju@gmail.com (E.J.L.); hyunchuls@chungbuk.ac.kr (H.-C.S.)
2. Department of Anesthesiology and Pain Medicine, Asan Medical Center, University of Ulsan College of Medicine, Seoul 05505, Korea; koh9726@naver.com (W.U.K.); ingwei2475@gmail.com (H.K.); Alexakim06@gmail.com (H.-J.K.)
3. Department of Orthopedic Surgery, Asan Medical Center, University of Ulsan College of Medicine, Seoul 05505, Korea
* Correspondence: bakpaker@hanmail.net; Tel.: +82-2-3010-3530

Abstract: Postoperative delirium is common in elderly patients with hip fracture. Pain is a major risk factor for delirium, and regional nerve blocks (RNBs) effectively control pain in hip fractures. This study aimed to evaluate the effect of RNB on delirium after hip surgery in elderly patients. This retrospective comparative study was performed in a single institution, and the data were collected from medical records between March 2018 and April 2021. Patients aged ≥60 years who underwent proximal femoral fracture surgery were included, while those with previous psychiatric illness and cognitive impairment were excluded. Two hundred and fifty-two patients were enrolled and divided into an RNB or a control group according to RNB use. Delirium was assessed as the primary outcome and postoperative pain score, pain medication consumption, and rehabilitation assessment as the secondary outcomes. Between the RNB ($n = 129$) and control groups ($n = 123$), there was no significant difference in the baseline characteristics. The overall incidence of delirium was 21%; the rate was lower in the RNB group than in the control group (15 vs. 27%, respectively, $p = 0.027$). The average pain score at 6 h postoperatively was lower in the RNB group than in the control group (2.8 ± 1.5 vs. 3.3 ± 1.6, respectively, $p = 0.030$). There was no significant difference in the pain score at 12, 24, and 48 h postoperatively, amount of opioids consumed for 2 postoperative days, and time from injury to wheelchair ambulation. We recommend RNB as a standard procedure for elderly patients with hip fracture due to lower delirium incidence and more effective analgesia in the early postoperative period.

Keywords: hip fracture; nerve block; delirium; pain; opioids

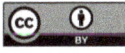

1. Introduction

Osteoporotic hip fracture is a major health problem because it is associated with high mortality, morbidity, and costs [1]. Although there are downward trends of mortality related to hip fracture, greater efforts are needed to achieve better outcomes [2]. The health status and health-related quality of life of elderly patients are seriously affected by the presence of hip fracture, and most patients cannot return to their performance status before injury [3].

Postoperative delirium is one of the most common complications in elderly patients with hip fracture and could result in cognitive impairment, short-term functional impairment, and increased mortality [4]. The known predisposing factors for delirium include advanced age, hip fracture surgery (in comparison to elective hip surgery), preoperative psychiatric illness, and preoperative cognitive impairment [5]. In addition, pain is a major risk factor for delirium; however, most elderly patients with hip fracture have a limited use of systemic opioid analgesics owing to side effects and their vulnerability in the drug metabolism process [6,7].

For this reason, comprehensive pain protocols have been suggested for elderly patients with hip fracture; these include evidence-based block use, timely repeated pain assessment, and multidisciplinary orthogeriatric care [8]. Regional nerve blocks (RNBs) have been proven to be effective in controlling pain in hip fractures, along with the advantages of few systemic effects [9]. Considering that pain control is essential for the reduction in delirium, we hypothesized that RNB use in hip fracture surgery would decrease postoperative pain and the incidence of delirium. This study aimed to evaluate the incidence of delirium according to RNB use in patients with hip fracture.

2. Materials and Methods

2.1. Study Population

This retrospective comparative study was performed in a single institution and approved by our institutional review board. The data were collected from medical records between March 2018 and April 2021. The inclusion criteria were as follows: (1) age of ≥60 years and (2) surgical treatment of proximal femoral fracture, which was defined as a femoral neck fracture, an intertrochanteric femoral fracture (AO/OTA 31) [10], and a subtrochanteric fracture (fracture extending 5 cm below the lower border of the lesser trochanter) [11]. Meanwhile, the exclusion criteria were as follows: (1) previous psychiatric illness, (2) previous cognitive impairment, (3) pathologic fracture, (4) prophylactic fixation, (5) revision of total hip replacement, (6) delayed surgery with neglected fracture, and (7) incomplete clinical data. Initially, 307 patients were included; ultimately, 252 patients were enrolled in this study. The patients who received general or spinal anesthesia followed by RNB were grouped into the RNB group. The patients who received only general or spinal anesthesia were grouped into the control group (Figure 1).

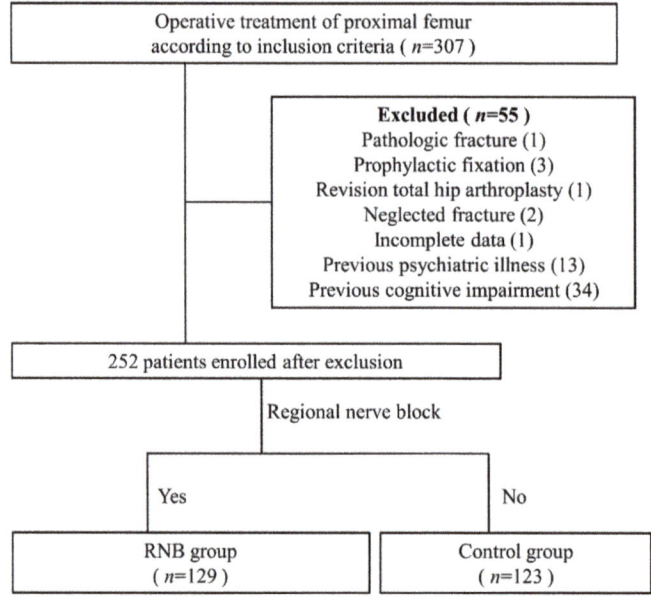

Figure 1. Flow diagram of patient enrollment and grouping.

2.2. Procedures

General or spinal anesthesia was performed according to the patients' overall health status, and RNB use was left to the discretion of the anesthesiologist. Under ultrasound guidance, a single shot of RNB, including fascia iliaca compartment block (FICB) [12], lumbar plexus block (LPB) [13], and pericapsular nerve group (PENG) block [14], was applied (Figure 2). For ultrasound-guided RNBs, a transportable ultrasound with 60 mm convex 2–5 MHz transducer for LPB and 25 mm linear 18–4 MHz transducer (Sonimage HS1TM, Konica Minolta Inc., Wayne, NJ, USA), and 21-gauge echoplex needle (Vygon, Ecouen, France) were used. After determining the insertion site, real-time ultrasound-guided perineural injection was conducted with the patient in supine or lateral position. Then, 30 mL of 0.3% ropivacaine was administered for LPB and FICB. Additionally, 20 mL of 0.3% ropivacaine was administered for PENG block.

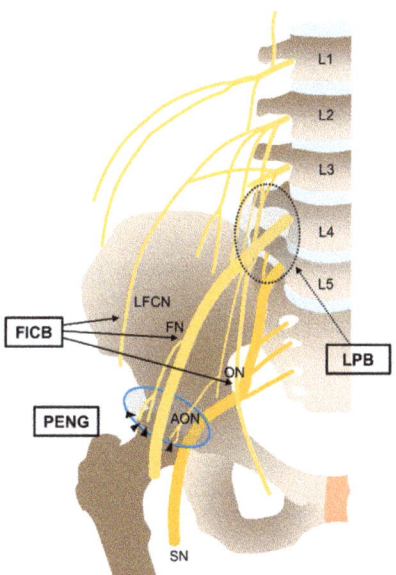

Figure 2. Illustration of the target nerves according to the type of regional nerve block. The fascia iliaca compartment block (FICB) targets the lateral femoral cutaneous (LFCN), femoral (FN), and obturator nerves (ON). The lumbar plexus block (LPB) targets the lumbar plexus (FN, ON, and LFCN) (dotted circle). The pericapsular nerve group (PENG) block mainly targets the articular branches (black arrowhead) of the FN and accessory obturator nerve (AON) (blue solid circle). SN: Sciatic nerve.

The patients with femoral neck fracture underwent bipolar hemiarthroplasty or internal fixation with multiple screws, while those with intertrochanteric and subtrochanteric fractures underwent intramedullary nailing. After surgery, intravenous patient-controlled analgesia (PCA) was applied in all patients. On the day of surgery, intravenous acetaminophen 1 g once a day was administered unless the patient had a contraindication. If the weight of the patient was less than 50 kg, the dose of acetaminophen was controlled at 15 mg/kg. The day after surgery, oral pain medications included a tramadol 37.5 mg/acetaminophen 325 mg tablet given twice daily and tapentadol 100 mg given twice daily. Rescue analgesia during postoperative period was intravenous tramadol 50 mg or hydromorphone 0.5 or 1.0 mg. Periarticular injection was not performed. We encouraged wheelchair ambulation as soon as possible from the day after surgery, and tolerable weight-bearing ambulation started on 2 days postoperatively.

2.3. Data Collection

Demographic data were collected from the patients' medical records, including age, sex, body mass index (BMI), age-adjusted Charlson comorbidity index (ACCI), Koval score before injury, injury mechanism, anesthesia method, fracture type, time from injury to surgery, time from admission to surgery, and type of surgery. The Charlson comorbidity index (CCI) was calculated by adding the coefficient assigned to comorbidities when injured. The ACCI was calculated by adding 1 point for each decade after the age of 40 years to the CCI value [15]. Falls from heights of 1 m or less were defined as "low-energy mechanism of injury" [16].

Delirium was recorded and defined using the confusion assessment method on any postoperative day or night of their hospital stay following surgery as the primary outcome [17]. Postoperative pain score, pain medication consumption, and rehabilitation assessment were evaluated as the secondary outcomes. The pain scores at 6, 12, 24, and 48 h postoperatively were assessed using the visual analog scale pain score. The consumption of pain medication for 2 postoperative days was examined. The amount of analgesics was calculated into milligrams of oral morphine according to the equianalgesic table [18–20]. A rehabilitation assessment was performed on the basis of the time (days) from surgery to wheelchair ambulation. All these parameters (pain score, incidence of delirium, pain medication consumption, and rehabilitation assessment) were included in the standardized protocol of our hospital.

The primary and secondary outcomes were compared between the RNB and control groups. A subgroup analysis for incidence of postoperative delirium between general and spinal anesthesia was performed. A subgroup analysis between FICB, LPB, and PENG block was performed to evaluate the differences between the blocks.

A multivariable analysis was performed to assess which variables were associated with incidence of delirium and clinically significant parameters were included in the model such as age, gender, CCI, RNB, and anesthesia type [21–23]. Nerve block-related complications, such as falls within 48 h after surgery and nerve injury, were assessed from the medical records. Postoperative medical complications, including deep vein thrombosis, pulmonary embolism, pneumonia, angina, myocardial infarction, and urinary tract infection, were evaluated.

2.4. Statistical Analysis

Categorical variables (e.g., sex, injury mechanism, method of anesthesia, fracture type, type of surgery, and incidence of delirium) were analyzed using the chi-square or Fisher's exact test. Continuous variables (e.g., age, BMI, ACCI, Koval score, time from injury to surgery, pain score, amount of analgesics consumed, and time to wheelchair ambulation) were analyzed using an independent t-test or the Mann–Whitney test. The Shapiro–Wilk test was used to check if the data distribution was normal. The Kruskal–Wallis test was used when compare more than two continuous variables. A logistic regression analysis was conducted for multivariable analysis. All continuous data are described as means and standard deviations. Statistical significance was accepted for p-values of <0.05 using SPSS version 23.0 (IBM Corp., Armonk, NY, USA).

3. Results

The RNB group consisted of 129 patients, while the control group consisted of 123 patients. The baseline characteristics of the two study groups are presented in Table 1. There was no significant difference found in the average age, BMI, ACCI, Koval score before injury, injury mechanism, method of anesthesia, fracture type, time from injury to surgery, time from admission to surgery, and type of surgery. The methods of RNB are summarized in Table 2.

Table 1. Baseline characteristics of the RNB and control groups.

	RNB Group (n = 129)	Control Group (n = 123)	p-Value
Age (years)	78.1 ± 8.3	77.6 ± 8.8	0.646
Sex			
Male	32 (25%)	40 (32%)	0.175
Female	97 (75%)	83 (68%)	
BMI	22.4 ± 3.7	22.7 ± 3.8	0.560
ACCI	6.3 ± 2.0	5.9 ± 1.8	0.108
Koval score before injury *	1.9 ± 1.5	2.1 ± 1.7	0.238
Injury mechanism			
Low energy	125 (97%)	117 (95%)	0.532
High energy	4 (3%)	6 (5%)	
Anesthesia method			
General	60 (46%)	58 (47%)	1.000
Spinal	69 (54%)	65 (53%)	
Fracture type			
Femoral neck fracture	53 (41%)	58 (47%)	0.611
Pertrochanteric fracture	63 (49%)	53 (43%)	
Subtrochanteric fracture	13 (10%)	12 (10%)	
Time from injury to surgery (hour) †	89.7 ± 99.4	111.0 ± 164.1	0.197
Time from admission to surgery (hour)	59.4 ± 68.7	62.6 ± 96.7	0.757
Type of surgery			
Osteosynthesis	88 (68%)	76 (62%)	0.285
Arthroplasty	41 (32%)	47 (38%)	

RNB, regional nerve block; BMI, body mass index; ACCI, age-adjusted Charlson comorbidity index; * calculated from 249 patients who had clinical records on the preoperative Koval score; † calculated from 246 patients who had clinical records on the time from injury to surgery.

Table 2. Type of RNB for hip fracture.

Type of RNB	
Fascia iliaca compartment block	78 (60%)
Lumbar plexus block	29 (23%)
Pericapsular nerve group block	22 (17%)

RNB, regional nerve block.

The overall incidence of delirium was 21%; the rate in the RNB group was lower than that in the control group (15 vs. 27%, $p = 0.027$). There were no nerve block-related complications, including falls within 48 h after surgery and nerve injury.

The average pain score at 6 h postoperatively in the RNB group was lower than that in the control group (2.8 ± 1.5 vs. 3.3 ± 1.6, respectively, $p = 0.030$) (Table 3). There was no significant difference in the pain score at 12 (RNB group: 2.8 ± 1.6 vs. control group: 2.7 ± 1.5, $p = 0.432$), 24 (RNB group: 2.5 ± 1.3 vs. control group: 2.4 ± 1.4, $p = 0.154$), and 48 (RNB group: 2.2 ± 1.1 vs. control group: 2.0 ± 1.1, $p = 0.083$) hours postoperatively. There was also no significant difference in the amount of opioids consumed for 2 postoperative days (oral morphine; RNB group: 36.2 ± 25.4 mg vs. control group: 33.5 ± 28.0 mg, $p = 0.322$) and time from injury to wheelchair ambulation (RNB group: 1.8 ± 2.4 days vs. control group: 1.7 ± 1.1 days, $p = 0.407$).

In the subgroup analysis between general and spinal anesthesia, there was no significant difference in the incidence of postoperative delirium (Table 4). In the subgroup analysis between FICB, LPB, and PENG block, there was no significant difference in the incidence of postoperative delirium, pain score, and amount of opioids consumed, but time to wheelchair ambulation presented a significant difference for PENG block compared with FICB and LPB (Table 5).

Table 3. Comparison of the postoperative pain score, incidence of delirium, amount of opioids consumed, and time to wheelchair ambulation.

	RNB Group (n = 129)	Control Group (n = 123)	p-Value
Incidence of postoperative delirium	20 (15%)	33 (27%)	0.027
Postoperative pain score			
6 h postoperatively	2.8 ± 1.5	3.3 ± 1.6	0.030
12 h postoperatively	2.8 ± 1.6	2.7 ± 1.5	0.432
24 h postoperatively	2.5 ± 1.3	2.4 ± 1.4	0.154
48 h postoperatively	2.2 ± 1.1	2.0 ± 1.1	0.083
Amount of opioids consumed (mg) *	36.2 ± 25.4	33.5 ± 28.0	0.322
Time to wheelchair ambulation (days) †	1.8 ± 2.4	1.7 ± 1.1	0.407

RNB, regional nerve block; * expressed as milligrams of oral morphine by equianalgesic conversion; † calculated from 247 patients who had clinical records on the time to wheelchair ambulation.

Table 4. Subgroup analysis for the incidence of delirium between general and spinal anesthesia.

Incidence of Postoperative Delirium	General Anesthesia	Spinal Anesthesia	p-Value
RNB group	9/60 (15.0%)	11/69 (15.9%)	0.883
Control group	15/58 (25.9%)	18/65 (27.7%)	0.819
Total	24/118 (20.3%)	29/134 (21.6%)	0.800

RNB, regional nerve block.

Table 5. Subgroup analysis for the postoperative pain score, incidence of delirium, amount of opioids consumed, and time to wheelchair ambulation between FICB, LPB and PENG block.

	FICB (n = 78)	LPB (n = 29)	PENG Block (n = 22)	p-Value
Incidence of postoperative delirium	13 (17%)	5 (17%)	2 (9.1%)	0.786
Postoperative pain score				
6 h postoperatively	3.0 ± 1.5	2.4 ± 1.6	2.9 ± 1.5	0.215
12 h postoperatively	2.7 ± 1.6	2.7 ± 1.7	3.3 ± 1.4	0.264
24 h postoperatively	2.5 ± 1.3	2.4 ± 1.4	3.0 ± 1.0	0.161
48 h postoperatively	2.1 ± 1.1	2.3 ± 1.4	2.6 ± 0.9	0.118
Amount of opioids consumed (mg) *	35.7 ± 24.4	33.6 ± 29.2	41.6 ± 24.9	0.372
Time to wheelchair ambulation (days) †	1.7 ± 1.2	2.5 ± 4.5	1.0 ± 0.2	0.020

FICB, fascia iliaca compartment block; LPB, lumbar plexus block; PENG block, pericapsular nerve group block; * expressed as milligrams of oral morphine by equianalgesic conversion; † calculated from 106 patients who had clinical records on the time to wheelchair ambulation.

In the multivariable analysis, age and RNB were significantly associated with the incidence of postoperative delirium (Table 6). There was also no significant difference in the postoperative medical complications between them (Table 7).

Table 6. Bivariate and multivariable logistic regression analysis for the risk factors of postoperative delirium.

	Incidence of Postoperative Delirium			
	Bivariate Analysis		Multivariable Logistic Regression *	
	Odds Ratio (95% CI)	p-Value	Odds Ratio (95% CI)	p-Value
Age	1.060 (1.020–1.101)	0.003	1.062 (1.022–1.104)	0.002
Female sex	0.906 (0.467–1.757)	0.769		
CCI	1.091 (0.934–1.275)	0.270		
RNB	0.500 (0.269–0.932)	0.029	0.476 (0.252–0.898)	0.022
Spinal anesthesia	1.082 (0.589–1.978)	0.800		

* The results of multivariable logistic regression analysis were presented only for the variables which were remained in the final model.

Table 7. Postoperative complications.

	RNB Group (n = 129)	Control Group (n = 123)	p-Value
Deep vein thrombosis	1 (1%)	1 (1%)	>0.999
Pulmonary embolism	1 (1%)	1 (1%)	>0.999
Pneumonia	5 (4%)	4 (3%)	>0.999
Angina or myocardial infarction	1 (1%)	3 (2%)	0.360
Urinary tract infection	4 (3%)	3 (2%)	>0.999

RNB, regional nerve block.

4. Discussion

4.1. Incidence of Delirium

In this study, RNB reduced the incidence of delirium. It is widely accepted that pain reduction is important for the prevention of delirium [6], and we hypothesized that postoperative pain control could prevent delirium after hip fracture surgery. Our study results proved the effect of RNB on the incidence of postoperative delirium after hip fracture surgery. Herein, we excluded patients with a high risk of developing delirium, including those with psychiatric illness and cognitive impairment, which was based on a study by Mouzopoulos et al. [22]. They classified patients into intermediate or high risk for postoperative delirium, and FICB did not affect the incidence of delirium in patients with high risk after hip fracture surgery. In contrast, a significant reduction in the incidence of delirium (FICB group vs. placebo group: 2.4 vs. 16.9%) was observed among patients with an intermediate in their study.

The results of RNB and delirium in patients with hip fracture are inconsistent. RNB was reported to be associated with less postoperative analgesia, a lower incidence of delirium, and shorter inpatient stay [24,25]. In contrast, Guay et al. presented that there were no differences in the incidence of acute confusional state in their Cochrane review based on seven trials with 676 participants [26]. However, the study has a limitation of heterogeneity and lack of risk stratification. Unneby et al. reported that femoral nerve block (FNB) did not reduce the incidence of postoperative delirium in patients with hip fracture [27]. They focused on patients with dementia, and a large proportion developed delirium (FNB group vs. placebo group: 50/52 vs. 55/57) regardless of FNB use. This suggests that patients with major risk factors, such as cognitive and psychiatric disorders, are highly prone to developing delirium regardless of pain control. In the present study, we could prove the effect of RNB on the incidence of delirium by excluding high risk patients with the inclusion of a relatively large number of patients as a single study. Additionally, we performed a multivariable analysis with other known risk factors of delirium [21–23]. Age and RNB were presented to be associated with postoperative delirium, which means an appropriate risk stratification of present study. Therefore, we believe the RNB helps to prevent postoperative delirium after hip fracture surgery except in high risk elderly patients.

4.2. Effect on Pain Intensity and Opioid Consumption

Opioids are useful in reducing pain after surgery but have limitations regarding side effects and drug poisoning [28]. Elderly patients are known to be vulnerable to the side effects of opioids, with reductions in renal and hepatic blood flow [29]; in our study, one of our purposes was the reduction in opioid consumption with the effect of nerve block. Thompson et al. reported that preoperative fascia iliaca block significantly decreased postoperative opioid consumption [30]. They reduced the amount of tramadol by 43% and morphine by 98% with fascia iliaca block. However, contrary to our expectations, there was no significant difference in the amount of opioids consumed despite early pain reduction in our study. The first possible reason is that diverse types of opioids were prescribed with a retrospective feature. Although we calculated the equianalgesic dose of each opioid into milligrams of oral morphine [18–20], the results could be influenced by the diversity of the opioid types prescribed. The second possible reason is that all patients received intravenous PCA because it is a customary procedure desired by patients. In addition to additional opioids injected by nurses, rescue opioids were also administered through PCA, which were not included in the calculation of the quantity of opioids consumed. These reasons may have influenced the outcome for the quantity of opioids.

4.3. Functional Recovery

Based on the results reported by Marino et al., who demonstrated that continuous lumbar plexus block provided pain reduction during physical therapy [31], we expected that functional recovery could be encouraged with nerve block. However, there was no significant difference observed in the time to wheelchair ambulation between the two groups, which can be explained by some reasons. A consistent rehabilitation protocol was applied to the patients in both groups. In addition, Kim et al. demonstrated that the postoperative ambulatory capacity after hip fracture surgery is decided not by only a single factor but by multiple factors, including age, sex, preoperative ambulatory capacity, and combined medical diseases [32]. Since the postoperative ambulatory capacity is significantly associated with preoperative factors, it is possible that the reduction in pain itself could not affect the short-term functional recovery.

4.4. Subgroup Analysis According to Type of RNB and Anesthesia Method

In clinical practice, we usually perform LPB after induction of general anesthesia because it should be conducted in the lateral decubitus position. In contrast, FICB is usually performed before induction of spinal anesthesia because it could be conducted in the supine position, which could reduce pain for positioning of spinal anesthesia. Since LPB and FICB could block both anterior innervations of the hip joint and some surgical incision site, similar pain reduction and delirium prevention could be expected in both blocks (Figure 2). In our study, the subgroup analysis between RNBs did not demonstrate significant differences in the postoperative pain score and amount of opioids consumed, but time to wheelchair ambulation of PENG block presented significant differences compared to that of FICB and LPB. The possible reason for these results was that PENG block was introduced as a potential motor sparing analgesic block [14,33], which could encourage patients to ambulate early. However, investigation for PENG block is very limited, and validation to propose motor sparing and analgesic benefit is needed [33]. Additionally, with a relatively small number of patients included in each RNBs in the present study, detailed analysis according to block type requires careful interpretation.

There could be concerns regarding anesthesia method. Previous studies showed controversial results. Choi et al. reported general anesthesia was an independent predictor of immediate delirium [23]. In contrast, Patel et al. concluded that there was no evidence to suggest that anesthesia type influence postoperative delirium in their systematic review [34]. In the present study, there were no significant differences in the incidence of delirium between general and spinal anesthesia in subgroup analysis, and multivariate analysis showed no effect on postoperative delirium according to anesthesia method.

4.5. Procedure-Related Complications

Falls and procedure-related nerve injuries are important complications of RNB in patients with hip fracture [35,36]; in our study, no complication was observed. While wheelchair ambulation was encouraged from the day after surgery, the protocol of our institution was to involve at least three individuals (nurse, caregiver, and paramedics) in the transfer of a patient to a wheelchair. At 2 days postoperatively, the patients were permitted to bear weight as tolerable. Considering that the duration of a single shot of bupivacaine 0.5% (20 mL) is 22 (range, 15–32) hours [37], it is unlikely that a fall would occur during ambulation owing to RNB. Further, all RNBs were performed by experienced anesthesiologists under ultrasound guidance. We believe that our rehabilitation protocol and technique for RNB could ensure the safeness of RNB in patients with hip fracture.

4.6. Study Limitations

There were some limitations in this study. First, our study had a selection bias in relation to the retrospectively evaluated characteristics. RNB use was decided by the anesthesiologists, and there was no clear criterion. Future prospective studies with randomization are needed. Second, the types of nerve block used varied. FICB, LSPB, and PENG block were used herein, which might have confounded the results. Third, the severity of delirium was not considered. Some patients only demonstrated temporary inattention; however, other patients demonstrated irritability that needed restraint. We classified these demonstrations as delirium. Subgroup analyses according to the severity of delirium will be helpful in the evaluation of the effects of RNB. Despite these limitations, our study provided evidence that RNB can reduce the incidence of delirium, and we believe that its use can help improve the prognosis of elderly patients with hip fracture.

5. Conclusions

RNB reduced the occurrence of delirium in elderly patients with hip fracture and relieved acute pain after surgery without complications. Therefore, we recommend RNB as a standard procedure for elderly patients with hip fracture due to lower delirium incidence and more effective analgesia in the early postoperative period.

Author Contributions: Writing—original draft, formal analysis, visualization, E.J.L.; Investigation and resources, data curation, W.U.K.; Investigation and resources, H.K.; Validation, project administration, H.-J.K.; Methodology, supervision, H.-C.S.; Conceptualization, investigation and resources, writing—review and editing, J.W.K. All authors have read and agreed to the published version of the manuscript.

Funding: This research was supported by the Technology Innovation Program (20000397, Development of Two Track Customized 3D Printing Implant Manufacturing and Commercializing Techniques for Complex Bone Fractures) funded by the Ministry of Trade, Industry and Energy (MOTIE, Korea).

Institutional Review Board Statement: The study was conducted according to the guidelines of the Declaration of Helsinki and approved by the Institutional Review Board of ASAN MEDICAL CENTER (protocol no. 2019-0267; December, 2019).

Informed Consent Statement: Patient consent was waived owing to the retrospective nature of this study.

Data Availability Statement: The data presented in this study are available on request from the corresponding author. The data are not publicly available due to conditions of the ethics committee of our university.

Conflicts of Interest: The authors declare no conflict of interest.

References

1. Braithwaite, R.S.; Col, N.F.; Wong, J.B. Estimating hip fracture morbidity, mortality and costs. *J. Am. Geriatr. Soc.* **2003**, *51*, 364–370. [CrossRef]
2. Orces, C.H. Hip Fracture-Related Mortality among Older Adults in the United States: Analysis of the CDC WONDER Multiple Cause of Death Data, 1999–2013. *Epidemiol. Res. Int.* **2016**, *2016*, 8970259. [CrossRef]
3. Alexiou, K.I.; Roushias, A.; Varitimidis, S.E.; Malizos, K.N. Quality of life and psychological consequences in elderly patients after a hip fracture: A review. *Clin. Interv. Aging* **2018**, *13*, 143–150. [CrossRef]
4. Lee, H.B.; Oldham, M.A.; Sieber, F.E.; Oh, E.S. Impact of Delirium After Hip Fracture Surgery on One-Year Mortality in Patients With or Without Dementia: A Case of Effect Modification. *Am. J. Geriatr. Psychiatry* **2017**, *25*, 308–315. [CrossRef]
5. Rizk, P.; Morris, W.; Oladeji, P.; Huo, M. Review of Postoperative Delirium in Geriatric Patients Undergoing Hip Surgery. *Geriatr. Orthop. Surg. Rehabil.* **2016**, *7*, 100–105. [CrossRef] [PubMed]
6. Morrison, R.S.; Magaziner, J.; Gilbert, M.; Koval, K.J.; McLaughlin, M.A.; Orosz, G.; Strauss, E.; Siu, A.L. Relationship between pain and opioid analgesics on the development of delirium following hip fracture. *J. Gerontol. Ser. A Biol. Sci. Med. Sci.* **2003**, *58*, 76–81. [CrossRef]
7. Nie, H.; Zhao, B.; Zhang, Y.Q.; Jiang, Y.H.; Yang, Y.X. Pain and cognitive dysfunction are the risk factors of delirium in elderly hip fracture Chinese patients. *Arch. Gerontol. Geriatr.* **2012**, *54*, e172–e174. [CrossRef] [PubMed]
8. Scurrah, A.; Shiner, C.T.; Stevens, J.A.; Faux, S.G. Regional nerve blockade for early analgesic management of elderly patients with hip fracture—a narrative review. *Anaesthesia* **2018**, *73*, 769–783. [CrossRef] [PubMed]
9. Godoy Monzón, D.; Vazquez, J.; Jauregui, J.R.; Iserson, K.V. Pain treatment in post-traumatic hip fracture in the elderly: Regional block vs. systemic non-steroidal analgesics. *Int. J. Emerg. Med.* **2010**, *3*, 321–325. [CrossRef]

10. Meinberg, E.G.; Agel, J.; Roberts, C.S.; Karam, M.D.; Kellam, J.F. Fracture and Dislocation Classification Compendium-2018. *J. Orthop. Trauma* **2018**, *32* (Suppl. 1), S1–S170. [CrossRef] [PubMed]
11. Loizou, C.L.; McNamara, I.; Ahmed, K.; Pryor, G.A.; Parker, M.J. Classification of subtrochanteric femoral fractures. *Injury* **2010**, *41*, 739–745. [CrossRef]
12. Godoy Monzon, D.; Iserson, K.V.; Vazquez, J.A. Single fascia iliaca compartment block for post-hip fracture pain relief. *J. Emerg. Med.* **2007**, *32*, 257–262. [CrossRef]
13. Amiri, H.R.; Zamani, M.M.; Safari, S. Lumbar plexus block for management of hip surgeries. *Anesth Pain Med.* **2014**, *4*, e19407. [CrossRef]
14. Girón-Arango, L.; Peng, P.W.H.; Chin, K.J.; Brull, R.; Perlas, A. Pericapsular Nerve Group (PENG) Block for Hip Fracture. *Reg. Anesth. Pain Med.* **2018**, *43*, 859. [CrossRef] [PubMed]
15. Charlson, M.; Szatrowski, T.P.; Peterson, J.; Gold, J. Validation of a combined comorbidity index. *J. Clin. Epidemiol.* **1994**, *47*, 1245–1251. [CrossRef]
16. Bergstrom, U.; Bjornstig, U.; Stenlund, H.; Jonsson, H.; Svensson, O. Fracture mechanisms and fracture pattern in men and women aged 50 years and older: A study of a 12-year population-based injury register, Umea, Sweden. *Osteoporos. Int.* **2008**, *19*, 1267–1273. [CrossRef] [PubMed]
17. Inouye, S.K.; van Dyck, C.H.; Alessi, C.A.; Balkin, S.; Siegal, A.P.; Horwitz, R.I. Clarifying confusion: The confusion assessment method. A new method for detection of delirium. *Ann. Intern. Med.* **1990**, *113*, 941–948. [CrossRef]
18. Farrington, C.; Palliative Care Expert Group. *Therapeutic Guidelines: Palliative Care*, 3rd ed.; Therapeutic Guidelines Limited: Melbourne, Australia, 2010. [CrossRef]
19. Twycross, R.; Wilcock, A. *PCF3: Palliative Care Formulary*; Russell House Publishing: Nottingham, UK, 2007.
20. Gippsland Region Palliative Care Consortium. *Opioid Conversion Guidelines*; GRPCC: Melbourne, Australia, 2011.
21. Yang, Y.; Zhao, X.; Dong, T.; Yang, Z.; Zhang, Q.; Zhang, Y. Risk factors for postoperative delirium following hip fracture repair in elderly patients: A systematic review and meta-analysis. *Aging Clin. Exp. Res.* **2017**, *29*, 115–126. [CrossRef]
22. Mouzopoulos, G.; Vasiliadis, G.; Lasanianos, N.; Nikolaras, G.; Morakis, E.; Kaminaris, M. Fascia iliaca block prophylaxis for hip fracture patients at risk for delirium: A randomized placebo-controlled study. *J. Orthop. Traumatol.* **2009**, *10*, 127–133. [CrossRef] [PubMed]
23. Choi, Y.H.; Kim, D.H.; Kim, T.Y.; Lim, T.W.; Kim, S.W.; Yoo, J.H. Early postoperative delirium after hemiarthroplasty in elderly patients aged over 70 years with displaced femoral neck fracture. *Clin. Interv. Aging* **2017**, *12*, 1835–1842. [CrossRef]
24. Callear, J.; Shah, K. Analgesia in hip fractures. Do fascia-iliac blocks make any difference? *BMJ Qual. Improv. Rep.* **2016**, *5*, u210130.w214147. [CrossRef]
25. Del Rosario, E.; Esteve, N.; Sernandez, M.J.; Batet, C.; Aguilar, J.L. Does femoral nerve analgesia impact the development of postoperative delirium in the elderly? A retrospective investigation. *Acute Pain* **2008**, *10*, 59–64. [CrossRef]
26. Guay, J.; Parker, M.J.; Griffiths, R.; Kopp, S.L. Peripheral Nerve Blocks for Hip Fractures: A Cochrane Review. *Anesth. Analg.* **2018**, *126*, 1695–1704. [CrossRef]
27. Unneby, A.; Svensson, P.O.; Gustafson, P.Y.; Lindgren, A.P.B.; Bergström, U.; Olofsson, P.B. Complications with focus on delirium during hospital stay related to femoral nerve block compared to conventional pain management among patients with hip fracture—A randomised controlled trial. *Injury* **2020**, *51*, 1634–1641. [CrossRef] [PubMed]
28. Helmerhorst, G.T.; Teunis, T.; Janssen, S.J.; Ring, D. An epidemic of the use, misuse and overdose of opioids and deaths due to overdose, in the United States and Canada: Is Europe next? *Bone Jt. J.* **2017**, *99-b*, 856–864. [CrossRef]
29. Chau, D.L.; Walker, V.; Pai, L.; Cho, L.M. Opiates and elderly: Use and side effects. *Clin. Interv. Aging* **2008**, *3*, 273–278. [CrossRef] [PubMed]
30. Thompson, J.; Long, M.; Rogers, E.; Pesso, R.; Galos, D.; Dengenis, R.C.; Ruotolo, C. Fascia Iliaca Block Decreases Hip Fracture Postoperative Opioid Consumption: A Prospective Randomized Controlled Trial. *J. Orthop. Trauma* **2020**, *34*, 49–54. [CrossRef] [PubMed]
31. Marino, J.; Russo, J.; Kenny, M.; Herenstein, R.; Livote, E.; Chelly, J.E. Continuous lumbar plexus block for postoperative pain control after total hip arthroplasty. A randomized controlled trial. *J. Bone Jt. Surg. Am. Vol.* **2009**, *91*, 29–37. [CrossRef]
32. Kim, J.L.; Jung, J.S.; Kim, S.J. Prediction of Ambulatory Status After Hip Fracture Surgery in Patients Over 60 Years Old. *Ann. Rehabil. Med.* **2016**, *40*, 666–674. [CrossRef]
33. Kim, D.H.; Kim, S.J.; Liu, J.; Beathe, J.; Memtsoudis, S.G. Fascial plane blocks: A narrative review of the literature. *Reg. Anesth. Pain Med.* **2021**, *46*, 600–617. [CrossRef]
34. Patel, V.; Champaneria, R.; Dretzke, J.; Yeung, J. Effect of regional versus general anaesthesia on postoperative delirium in elderly patients undergoing surgery for hip fracture: A systematic review. *BMJ Open* **2018**, *8*, e020757. [CrossRef] [PubMed]
35. Johnson, R.L.; Kopp, S.L.; Hebl, J.R.; Erwin, P.J.; Mantilla, C.B. Falls and major orthopaedic surgery with peripheral nerve blockade: A systematic review and meta-analysis. *Br. J. Anaesth* **2013**, *110*, 518–528. [CrossRef] [PubMed]
36. Borgeat, A. Neurologic deficit after peripheral nerve block: What to do? *Minerva Anestesiol.* **2005**, *71*, 353–355.
37. Cuvillon, P.; Nouvellon, E.; Ripart, J.; Boyer, J.C.; Dehour, L.; Mahamat, A.; L'Hermite, J.; Boisson, C.; Vialles, N.; Lefrant, J.Y.; et al. A comparison of the pharmacodynamics and pharmacokinetics of bupivacaine, ropivacaine (with epinephrine) and their equal volume mixtures with lidocaine used for femoral and sciatic nerve blocks: A double-blind randomized study. *Anesth. Analg.* **2009**, *108*, 641–649. [CrossRef] [PubMed]

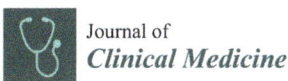

Article

Mild Traumatic Brain Injury in Older Adults: Are Routine Second cCT Scans Necessary?

Valeska Hofmann [1,*], Christian Deininger [2], Stefan Döbele [1], Christian Konrads [1] and Florian Wichlas [2]

[1] BG Trauma Centre, Department of Trauma and Reconstructive Surgery, University of Tübingen, 72076 Tübingen, Germany; sdoebele@bgu-tuebingen.de (S.D.); ckonrads@bgu-tuebingen.de (C.K.)

[2] Department of Orthopedics and Traumatology, University Hospital Salzburg, 5020 Salzburg, Austria; christian.deininger@hotmail.com (C.D.); fwichlas@icloud.com (F.W.)

* Correspondence: hofmann_valeska@gmx.net

Abstract: Fall-related hospitalizations among older adults have been increasing in recent decades. One of the most common reasons for this is minimal or mild traumatic brain injury (mTBI) in older individuals taking anticoagulant medication. In this study, we analyzed all inpatient stays from January 2017 to December 2019 of patients aged > 75 years with a mTBI on anticoagulant therapy who received at least two cranial computer tomography (cCT) scans. Of 1477 inpatient stays, 39 had primary cranial bleeding, and in 1438 the results of initial scans were negative for cranial bleeding. Of these 1438 cases, 6 suffered secondary bleeding from the control cCT scan. There was no significance for bleeding related to the type of anticoagulation. We conclude that geriatric patients under anticoagulant medication don't need a second cCT scan if the primary cCT was negative for intracranial bleeding and the patient shows no clinical signs of bleeding. These patients can be dismissed but require an evaluation for need of home care or protective measures to prevent recurrent falls. The type of anticoagulant medication does not affect the risk of bleeding.

Keywords: anticoagulation; concussion; geriatric trauma; overdiagnosis

1. Introduction

Older populations are growing continuously in high income countries (HIC) [1]. In addition to the increasing number of comorbidities and medications, musculoskeletal decay has become relevant for this part among the population [2]. Osteopenia, sarcopenia, and dementia impede musculoskeletal coordination and lead to recurrent falls of geriatric patients [3–5]. As a result of the aging process, these patients have difficulty performing daily tasks; a fall represents an early symptom of coping-failure [6]. These patients are likely to require care by family or nursing professionals sooner or later. A fall is the main reason for orthopaedic-traumatological admissions for older patients [7,8]. Frequent reasons for hospital admission include fractures of the proximal femur, the spine, the proximal humerus, and the distal radius [9]. Besides these fractures, traumatic brain injury (TBI) caused by a fall is an increasing reason for hospitalization in older patients [10]. In older patients, a fall is the main reason for a traumatic brain injury (51%), followed by car accidents (9%) [11].

The first goal in the treatment of TBI in older adults is to diagnose and exclude intracranial bleeding. A cranial computer tomography (cCT) scan is the imaging technique of choice for the diagnosis of intracranial bleeding. Guidelines for its indication are well established and validated [12,13]. Patient's age greater than 65 has been recognized as being a factor towards the indication for a cCT.

As comorbidities and medications for geriatric patients increase, the use of oral anticoagulants and antiplatelets (ACAP) has increased significantly [14]. The risk for bleeding complications after trauma for patients under ACAP-treatment has been widely described [15,16]. Furthermore, the use of ACAP has also been implemented as a risk factor in the guidelines for primary cCT for TBI. Most clinical departments have already established a protocol for diagnosing delayed secondary bleeding, but no guidelines for the detection of such intracranial bleeding has been described.

The aim of this study was to investigate the risk for a delayed intracranial bleeding in older patients taking ACAP after a fall with minimal or mild TBI (mTBI). The definition of minimal or mild TBI was based on the GCS interval of the Head Injury Severity Score (HISS) [17]. We evaluated the incidence of a delayed intracranial bleeding after primary negative cCT of older patients admitted to the hospital. Additionally, we determined the rate of readmission to the hospital, the duration of hospital stay, the ACAP taken, and the primary bleeding.

The incidence of the delayed intracranial bleeding should determine the need for a second cCT control and for a hospital stay. The number of readmissions and the duration of the hospital stay should show the necessity for caregiving. The ACAP taken and the number of primary bleeding should estimate the risk for intracranial bleeding.

2. Materials and Methods

We retrospectively analyzed data from 1477 inpatient stays of 1129 patients with mTBI admitted to a level-one-trauma center of a university hospital from January 2017 to December 2019, in Salzburg, Austria.

Inclusion criteria were:
- mTBI.
- Age > 75 years.
- Taking ACAP at time of injury.
- Low impact trauma mechanism by fall.
- Two or more cCT scans.

Exclusion criteria were:
- Other concomitant injuries that would indicate inpatient treatment.
- High impact trauma.
- One cCT Scan only.

Demographic data of the study population are shown in Table 1.

Table 1. Patient demographics.

Parameter	Males	Females	Σ	$\varnothing$
N	440	689	1129	
Age				85.56 (75–105)

On the 1477 inpatient stays, 3021 cCT scans were performed; in 1437 cases 2 cCT scans, in 27 cases 3, in 7 cases 4, in 2 cases 5, in 2 cases 6, in 1 case 7, and in 1 case 9 cCTs were conducted. The first cCT scan was conducted on the day of admission and the second 24 h later.

The CT scanner was a 16-slice scanner (Siemens Somatom Emotion 16, Siemens, Erlangen/Germany). The scans were evaluated by an on-call radiological and trauma consultant and the authors of the study. Scans that could not be diagnosed sufficiently due to artifacts were excluded.

Primary negative cCT scans for an intracranial bleed were recorded if they were positive on the control scan. When the cCT control scan was positive for intracranial bleeding, we evaluated the bleeding on the cCT control scans and the resulting hospital stay.

The number of readmission and the duration of the hospital stay of all patients was evaluated. The intake of antiplatelet or anticoagulant medication was noted and possible association of such a medication with the incidence of primary and secondary bleeding was analyzed.

3. Results

3.1. Readmission and Duration of Stay

Inpatient admission occurred in 1129 patients; in 931 (83%) patients once; and in 198 (17%) multiple times. This resulted in 1477 admissions in total (Table 2).

Table 2. Number of hospital admissions of geriatric patients with mTBI due to a fall.

Hospital Admissions	Patients (n)
1	931
2	123
3	42
4	16
5	8
6	4
7	0
8	1
9	2
10	2

The duration of inpatient stays ranged from 1 to 37 days. The regular stay was 2 days in 1271 cases. Of the remaining, 25 patients could not be mobilized and dismissed at home, 21 had elevated infection parameters and were treated anti-infectively, and 12 needed more than traumatological consultation. For the rest, the reason for prolonged hospitalization could not be determined retrospectively.

3.2. cCT Control Scans, Hospital Stay

Of 1477 inpatient stays, 39 (2.64%) cases had a primary bleeding and 1438 (97.36%) had an initial negative scan. Secondary intracranial bleeding was present in 6 of these 1438 cases, as shown in Table 3.

Table 3. Distribution of cCT findings with "bleeding" and "no bleeding" among all patients.

cCT	Bleeding	No Bleeding	Total Number
Primary	39 (2.64%)	1438 (97.36%)	1477 (100%)
Secondary	6 (0.42%)	1432 (99.58%)	1438 (100%)

In the cases with an initial negative scan and no secondary bleeding (n = 1432), a total of 2852 cCT scans were performed. In these cases, the mean stay was 1.7 days.

In the six patients with a secondary bleeding, two had one cCT control, three had two, and one had three after the initial cCT scan. The intracranial bleeding was an intraparenchymal hemorrhage in four cases, a subdural hematoma in one case, and a combination of both in one case. All six were treated conservatively and five were dismissed home without any further therapy. They had no symptoms or their bleeding was decreasing in the cCT control. The patient with the combined intraparenchymal hemorrhage and subdural hematoma had symptoms with an increasing unconsciousness. He had increasing bleeding on cCT scans and died seven days after admission at the age of eighty-nine. The mean hospital stay of these six patients was four days.

In the cases with a primary bleeding (n = 39), 134 cCT scans were performed. Most patients received three cCT scans, and one of them nine scans (Table 4). In these cases, the mean in-hospital stay was 6.3 days.

Table 4. Number of cCT-scans of patients with primary bleeding.

Number of cCT-Scans	Cases (n)
2	9
3	18
4	6
5	2
6	2
7	1
8	0
9	1

3.3. Oral Anticoagulants and Antiplatelet Medication

Of 1477 cases, 1443 patients were taking one ACAP, 33 were taking a dual medication, and 1 patient was taking a triple combination. Every double medication was a combination of an oral anticoagulants with an antiplatelet agent.

Every patient with a primary (39) or secondary (6) bleeding has been taking one ACAP. In the cases where bleeding did not occur (1398), they were taking an ACAP. Table 5 shows the intake of one ACAP in every case.

Table 5. ACAPs taken by patients admitted to in-hospital stay due to mTBI.

	n	Percent
Acetylsalicylic Acid (100 mg)	661	46%
Clopidogrel	88	6%
Apixaban	192	13%
Dabigatran	95	7%
Rivaroxaban	206	14%
Phenprocoumon	74	5%
Acenocoumarol	111	8%
Others	16	1%
	1443	100.00

Two patients with a secondary intracranial bleeding had been taking acetylsalicylic acid, two clopidogrel, one apixaban, and one acenocoumarol. The comparison of patients with a secondary bleeding and without intracranial bleeding regarding the intake of antiplatelet (4/720) or anticoagulant medication (2/678) was statistically not significant (Chi-square statistic is 0.5548, $p = 0.456367$; not significant at $p > 0.05$).

In 39 cases with a primary bleeding, the difference between antiplatelet and anticoagulant intake (Table 6) was also statistically not significant in comparison with the cases without bleeding (Chi-square statistic is 1.9976, $p = 0.157549$; not significant at $p > 0.05$).

Table 6. ACAP of patients with primary bleeding.

	n	Percent
Acetylsalicylic Acid (100 mg)	21	54%
Clopidogrel	4	10%
Apixaban	4	10%
Dabigatran	2	5%
Rivaroxaban	1	3%
Phenprocoumon	2	5%
Acenocoumarol	5	13%
Others	0	0%
	39	100.00%

Two patients were treated surgically by craniotomy, one of them died after 8 days. Another patient died without any surgical therapy. The other patients were treated conservatively and left the hospital after the bleeding subsided.

4. Discussion

Of 1477 admitted cases aged above 75 years and taking ACAP, 39 had a primary intracranial bleeding and only 6 developed a delayed intracranial bleeding after 24 h. Although guidelines for cCT scans exist, every patient with anamnestic fall resulting in a mTBI and anticoagulating medication received a cCT scan. The Canadian head CT rule explicitly excludes bleeding disorders but indicates a cCT scan for minor head injury for patients older than 64 years [18]. The New Orleans Criteria indicate the cCT scan for patients who are older than 59 years with minor head trauma and loss of consciousness and are neurologically normal [19]. They do not consider bleeding disorders. The Scandinavian guidelines consider patients age > 64 and coagulation disorders [13]. They differentiate between patients > 64 years taking antiplatelet and patients of any age taking a therapeutic anticoagulation. The first group is recommended to undergo a cCT scan, or 12 h observation, and discharge if the cCT scan is negative. The second group is recommended to undergo a cCT scan and admission > 24 h independent of the findings. In our collective, the difference of these bleeding disorders was not significant (although the number of patients with intracranial bleeding was low). The number of patients taking antiplatelet and those taking other anticoagulant medication were almost the same. Nevertheless, we couldn't find any statistical significance.

The patients of this study fulfill the guidelines for a primary cCT scan according to the Scandinavian guidelines [13]. Although no guidelines for cCT scan control after mTBI exist, each patient received a cCT control 24 h after the initial scan. A meta-analysis of studies identified 0.60% of secondary intracranial bleeding and 0.13% of neurosurgical intervention for patients ($n = 1494$) with mild traumatic brain injury, negative primary cCT scan, and anticoagulation using vitamin K antagonists [20]. The authors of this study therefore do not recommend cCT controls as part of a standard procedure. The patients of this study showed 0.42% risk for secondary intracranial bleeding and none for neurosurgical intervention. We demonstrated that for these patients the cCT control had no therapeutic consequence besides the longer hospital stay (4 days). The need for a cCT control is at least to be doubted, especially when the consequence is two additional days of hospital stay. The second cCT scan means that the criteria for over-diagnosis have been attained [21]. Based on the data of this study, we recommend that if the primary cCT scan is negative for a traumatic bleeding and the patient has no clinical symptoms, a possible cCT control in an outpatient setting would be sufficient. Even the outpatient control can be discussed since it has no therapeutic consequence but it takes an effort for the older patient. Geriatric patients do not tolerate a change in their surroundings or an interruption in their daily routine well [22].

The primary intracranial bleeding in the study population taking ACAP was 2.64%. The role of cCT controls in these patients is to detect the development of bleeding in order to make decisions regarding further therapy. Guidelines for surgery exist and they mainly consist in craniotomy [23].

In the study population, more than 60% of patients with primary bleeding have been taking antiplatelet medication. Contrary to the Scandinavian guidelines, we could not find a difference in bleeding risk between antiplatelet medication and anticoagulation. We did not find a higher risk of intracerebral bleeding for patients on anticoagulation.

The admission of older patients in traumatological-orthopedic departments has been increasing dramatically during the last decade [24]. Mild traumatic brain injury is one of the most common reasons for emergency department admission and falls are often related to medical conditions (e.g., syncope) [25]. In our study cohort, 17% of the patients were admitted more than once for the same reason (mTBI after a fall). In our opinion, patients represent a lack of preventive measures for falls among geriatrics and care of the older adults. Although it is well known that a fall in older adults is a major reason for hospitalization, 17% of the patients in our study cohort were not taken care of after the first fall. A fall in the older patient should always alert every treating discipline as it probably is a sign for physiologic deterioration and the loss of the ability to handle daily tasks. This seems to be underlined by another fact that in 25 cases of 1432 (1.7%) without bleeding, the patients cannot be dismissed back home because they cannot be mobilized adequately. The fall of these patients seems to be a final surrender for living alone. Most falls in older adults have only minor injury consequences. However, the resulting pain and discomfort often leads to a loss of self-confidence and independence [26]. These patients can't be returned injudiciously to their homes without questioning the surrounding care. In another 21 cases (1.4%), patients couldn't be dismissed after mTBI since they had elevated infection parameters. This could be the result of a rapid deterioration of health of the older adults due to infection. Secondarily, this can lead to a faster reduction of independence at home. However, we believe that a fall for an older person is more than just an accident; it marks the initiation of inability to deal with daily living activities.

The main limitation of this study is its retrospective design. Although it was a single-institution study we were able to include a large sample. It is comparable to existing systematic reviews on this topic.

5. Conclusions

In conclusion, the results of this study suggest that after initial cCT in geriatric patients without primary intracranial bleeding under anticoagulant medication, a secondary control cCT is not necessary if no clinical signs of intracranial bleeding are apparent. For patients without relevant concomitant injuries requiring inpatient treatment, the inpatient stay can be shortened or outpatient treatment can be provided. In geriatric patients, the focus should be on home care and fall prevention.

Author Contributions: Conceptualization, V.H. and F.W.; methodology, V.H.; software, C.D. and S.D.; validation, C.K., formal analysis, C.D.; investigation, V.H. and C.D.; writing—original draft preparation, V.H.; writing—review and editing, F.W. and C.K.; visualization, S.D.; supervision, F.W.; project administration, F.W. All authors have read and agreed to the published version of the manuscript.

Funding: This research received no external funding.

Institutional Review Board Statement: The study was conducted according to the guidelines of the Declaration of Helsinki, and approved by the Ethics Committee of Salzburg (protocol code EK Nr:1071/2021 and 09.06.2021).

Informed Consent Statement: Not applicable due to the retrospective study design.

Data Availability Statement: The data presented in this study are available on request from the corresponding author. The data are not publicly available due to privacy.

Acknowledgments: We acknowledge support from the Open Access Publishing Fund of University of Tübingen.

Conflicts of Interest: The authors declare no conflict of interest.

References

1. Klenk, J.; Keil, U.; Jaensch, A.; Christiansen, M.C.; Nagel, G. Changes in Life Expectancy 1950–2010: Contributions from Age-and Disease-Specific Mortality in Selected Countries. *Popul. Health Metr.* **2016**, *14*, 20. [CrossRef]
2. Keller, J.M.; Sciadini, M.F.; Sinclair, E.; O'Toole, R.V. Geriatric Trauma: Demographics, Injuries, and Mortality. *J. Orthop. Trauma* **2012**, *26*, 5. [CrossRef] [PubMed]
3. Walter, J.; Unterberg, A. Das Schädel-Hirn-Trauma beim Älteren. *Geriatr. Up2date* **2019**, *1*, 55–65. [CrossRef]
4. Hollis, S.; Lecky, F.; Yates, D.W.; Woodford, M. The Effect of Pre-Existing Medical Conditions and Age on Mortality After Injury. *J. Trauma Inj. Infect. Crit. Care* **2006**, *61*, 1255–1260. [CrossRef] [PubMed]
5. McGwin, G.; MacLennan, P.A.; Fife, J.B.; Davis, G.G.; Rue, L.W. Preexisting Conditions and Mortality in Older Trauma Patients. *J. Trauma Inj. Infect. Crit. Care* **2004**, *56*, 1291–1296. [CrossRef] [PubMed]

6. Boyé, N.D.A.; Mattace-Raso, F.U.S.; Van der Velde, N.; Lieshout, E.M.M.V.; De Vries, O.J.; Hartholt, K.A.; Kerver, A.J.H.; Bruijninckx, M.M.M.; Van der Cammen, T.J.M.; Patka, P.; et al. Circumstances Leading to Injurious Falls in Older Men and Women in the Netherlands. *Injury* **2014**, *45*, 1224–1230. [CrossRef] [PubMed]
7. Samaras, N.; Chevalley, T.; Samaras, D.; Gold, G. Older Patients in the Emergency Department: A Review. *Ann. Emerg. Med.* **2010**, *56*, 261–269. [CrossRef] [PubMed]
8. Zhao, R.; Bu, W.; Chen, X. The Efficacy and Safety of Exercise for Prevention of Fall-Related Injuries in Older People with Different Health Conditions, and Differing Intervention Protocols: A Meta-Analysis of Randomized Controlled Trials. *BMC Geriatr.* **2019**, *19*, 341. [CrossRef] [PubMed]
9. Peel, N.M. Population Based Study of Hospitalised Fall Related Injuries in Older People. *Inj. Prev.* **2002**, *8*, 280–283. [CrossRef]
10. Haring, R.S.; Narang, K.; Canner, J.K.; Asemota, A.O.; George, B.P.; Selvarajah, S.; Haider, A.H.; Schneider, E.B. Traumatic Brain Injury in the Elderly: Morbidity and Mortality Trends and Risk Factors. *J. Surg. Res.* **2015**, *195*, 1–9. [CrossRef]
11. Thompson, H.J.; McCormick, W.C.; Kagan, S.H. Traumatic Brain Injury in Older Adults: Epidemiology, Outcomes, and Future Implications: Traumatic brain injury and older adults. *J. Am. Geriatr. Soc.* **2006**, *54*, 1590–1595. [CrossRef] [PubMed]
12. Mata-Mbemba, D.; Mugikura, S.; Nakagawa, A.; Murata, T.; Kato, Y.; Tatewaki, Y.; Takase, K.; Kushimoto, S.; Tominaga, T.; Takahashi, S. Canadian CT Head Rule and New Orleans Criteria in Mild Traumatic Brain Injury: Comparison at a Tertiary Referral Hospital in Japan. *SpringerPlus* **2016**, *5*, 176. [CrossRef] [PubMed]
13. Undén, J.; Ingebrigtsen, T.; Romner, B. Scandinavian Guidelines for Initial Management of Minimal, Mild and Moderate Head Injuries in Adults: An Evidence and Consensus-Based Update. *BMC Med.* **2013**, *11*, 50. [CrossRef] [PubMed]
14. Peck, K.A.; Calvo, R.Y.; Schechter, M.S.; Sise, C.B.; Kahl, J.E.; Shackford, M.C.; Shackford, S.R.; Sise, M.J.; Blaskiewicz, D.J. The Impact of Preinjury Anticoagulants and Prescription Antiplatelet Agents on Outcomes in Older Patients with Traumatic Brain Injury. *J. Trauma Acute Care Surg.* **2014**, *76*, 431–436. [CrossRef]
15. Pieracci, F.M.; Eachempati, S.R.; Shou, J.; Hydo, L.J.; Barie, P.S. Use of Long-Term Anticoagulation Is Associated With Traumatic Intracranial Hemorrhage and Subsequent Mortality in Elderly Patients Hospitalized After Falls: Analysis of the New York State Administrative Database. *J. Trauma Inj. Infect. Crit. Care* **2007**, *63*, 519–524. [CrossRef]
16. Rosand, J.; Eckman, M.H.; Knudsen, K.A.; Singer, D.E.; Greenberg, S.M. The Effect of Warfarin and Intensity of Anticoagulation on Outcome of Intracerebral Hemorrhage. *Arch. Intern. Med.* **2004**, *164*, 880. [CrossRef]
17. Stein, S.C.; Spettell, C. The Head Injury Severity Scale (HISS): A Practical Classification of Closed-Head Injury. *Brain Inj.* **1995**, *9*, 437–444. [CrossRef]
18. Stiell, I.G.; Wells, G.A.; Vandemheen, K.; Clement, C.; Lesiuk, H.; Laupacis, A.; McKnight, R.D.; Verbeek, R.; Brison, R.; Cass, D.; et al. The Canadian CT Head Rule for Patients with Minor Head Injury. *Lancet* **2001**, *357*, 1391–1396. [CrossRef]
19. Haydel, M.J.; Blaudeau, E. Indications for Computed Tomography in Patients with Minor Head Injury. *N. Engl. J. Med.* **2000**, *343*, 100–105. [CrossRef]
20. Chauny, J.-M.; Marquis, M.; Bernard, F.; Williamson, D.; Albert, M.; Laroche, M.; Daoust, R. Risk of Delayed Intracranial Hemorrhage in Anticoagulated Patients with Mild Traumatic Brain Injury: Systematic Review and Meta-Analysis. *J. Emerg. Med.* **2016**, *51*, 519–528. [CrossRef]
21. Singh, H.; Dickinson, J.A.; Thériault, G.; Grad, R.; Groulx, S.; Wilson, B.J.; Szafran, O.; Bell, N.R. Overdiagnosis: Causes and Consequences in Primary Health Care. *Can. Fam. Physician* **2018**, *64*, 654–659. [PubMed]
22. Kirchen-Peters, S. Menschen mit Demenz im Akutkrankenhaus. In *Pflege-Report 2017: Schwerpunkt: Die Versorgung der Pflegebedürftigen*; Schattauer: Stuttgart, Germany, 2017; pp. 153–161. ISBN 978-3-7945-3244-5.
23. Sahuquillo, J.; Dennis, J.A. Decompressive Craniectomy for the Treatment of High Intracranial Pressure in Closed Traumatic Brain Injury. *Cochrane Database Syst. Rev.* **2019**, *12*, CD003983. [CrossRef] [PubMed]
24. Pfortmueller, C.A.; Kunz, M.; Lindner, G.; Zisakis, A.; Puig, S.; Exadaktylos, A.K. Fall-Related Emergency Department Admission: Fall Environment and Settings and Related Injury Patterns in 6357 Patients with Special Emphasis on the Elderly. Available online: https://www.hindawi.com/journals/tswj/2014/256519/ (accessed on 6 March 2021).
25. Watson, W.L.; Mitchell, R. Conflicting Trends in Fall-Related Injury Hospitalisations among Older People: Variations by Injury Type. *Osteoporos. Int.* **2011**, *22*, 2623–2631. [CrossRef] [PubMed]
26. Hopewell, S.; Adedire, O.; Copsey, B.J.; Boniface, G.J.; Sherrington, C.; Clemson, L.; Close, J.C.; Lamb, S.E. Multifactorial and Multiple Component Interventions for Preventing Falls in Older People Living in the Community. *Cochrane Database Syst. Rev.* **2018**, *7*, CD012221. [CrossRef]

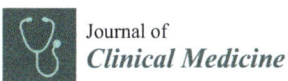

Article

Displacement of the Greater Tuberosity in Humeral Head Fractures Does Not only Depend on Rotator Cuff Status

Lisa Klute *, Christian Pfeifer, Isabella Weiss, Agnes Mayr, Volker Alt and Maximilian Kerschbaum

Clinic of Trauma Surgery, University Medical Center Regensburg, Franz-Josef-Strauss-Allee 11, 93053 Regensburg, Germany; christian.pfeifer@ukr.de (C.P.); weiss.isabella@t-online.de (I.W.); agnes-mayr@t-online.de (A.M.); volker.alt@ukr.de (V.A.); maximilian.kerschbaum@ukr.de (M.K.)
* Correspondence: Lisa.Klute@ukr.de; Tel.: +49-941-944-6841

Citation: Klute, L.; Pfeifer, C.; Weiss, I.; Mayr, A.; Alt, V.; Kerschbaum, M. Displacement of the Greater Tuberosity in Humeral Head Fractures Does Not only Depend on Rotator Cuff Status. *J. Clin. Med.* **2021**, *10*, 4136. https://doi.org/10.3390/jcm10184136

Academic Editor: Gianluca Testa

Received: 27 July 2021
Accepted: 10 September 2021
Published: 14 September 2021

Publisher's Note: MDPI stays neutral with regard to jurisdictional claims in published maps and institutional affiliations.

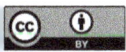

Copyright: © 2021 by the authors. Licensee MDPI, Basel, Switzerland. This article is an open access article distributed under the terms and conditions of the Creative Commons Attribution (CC BY) license (https://creativecommons.org/licenses/by/4.0/).

Abstract: It is assumed that dorsocranial displacement of the greater tuberosity in humeral head fractures is caused by rotator cuff traction. The purpose of this study was to investigate the association between rotator cuff status and displacement characteristics of the greater tuberosity in four-part humeral head fractures. Computed tomography scans of 121 patients with Neer type 4 fractures were analyzed. Fatty infiltration of the supra- and infraspinatus muscles was classified according to Goutallier. Position determination of the greater tuberosity fragment was performed in both coronary and axial planes to assess the extent of dorsocranial displacement. Considering non-varus displaced fractures, the extent of the dorsocranial displacement was significantly higher in patients with mostly inconspicuous posterosuperior rotator cuff status compared to advanced fatty degenerated cuffs (cranial displacement: Goutallier 0–1: 6.4 mm ± 4.6 mm vs. Goutallier 2–4: 4.2 mm ± 3.5 mm, $p = 0.020$; dorsal displacement: Goutallier 0–1: 28.4° ± 32.3° vs. Goutallier 2–4: 13.1° ± 16.1°, $p = 0.010$). In varus displaced humeral head fractures, no correlation between the displacement of the greater tuberosity and the condition of the posterosuperior rotator cuff could be detected ($p \geq 0.05$). The commonly accepted theory of greater tuberosity displacement in humeral head fractures by rotator cuff traction cannot be applied to all fracture types.

Keywords: humeral head fracture; greater tuberosity; rotator cuff; fatty degeneration

1. Introduction

In 1970, Neer established a new classification system for proximal humeral fractures that is still widely used in clinical practice today [1]. This classification system is based on the four main fracture fragments (humeral shaft, calotte, and greater and lesser tuberosity), firstly described by Codman in 1934 [2]. Neer assumed that traction of the rotator cuff is responsible for the characteristic fragment displacement, especially of the greater tuberosity. The supraspinatus and infraspinatus tendons are known to be responsible for the dorsocranial displacement of this key fragment [1]. In elderly patients with humeral head fractures, concomitant chronic degenerative rotator cuff pathologies are common [3,4]. Milgrom et al., for example, found rotator cuff lesions in 80% of asymptomatic patients 80 years of age and older [5].

Corresponding to the coexistent pattern of rotator cuff degeneration and humeral head fractures, it would be desirable to identify reciprocal influences between these pathologies [6]. The hypothesis was that patients with chronic degenerative changes of the posterosuperior rotator cuff do not show the typical dorsocranial displacement of the greater tuberosity, as described by Neer [1]. The aim of the present study was to evaluate whether the integrity of the posterosuperior rotator cuff influences the displacement characteristics of the greater tuberosity in proximal humeral fractures [7].

2. Materials and Methods

Patients with humeral head fractures diagnosed in our trauma department between 2008 and 2018 were identified. Patients with computed tomography (CT) scans of the affected shoulder were included. CT scans with low image quality or missing medial slices to assess the rotator cuff were excluded. All fractures were categorized according to Neer's classification system (Table 1) [1]. Two- and Three-Part fractures, as well as fracture-dislocations and head-split fractures, were also excluded in order to generate a homogenous study population of four-Part fractures without fracture-dislocation (Figure 1). The study has been approved by the Ethics Committee at the University of Regensburg (20-1848-104).

Table 1. Schematic overview of Neer's modified classification system [1].

Fracture Type	Number of Fragments		
	2	3	4
I			
II	anatomical neck		
III	surgical neck		
IV		greater tuberosity	
V		lesser tuberosity	
VI		anterior or posterior luxation	

I: minimal dislocation, under 1 cm and less angulation than 45°.

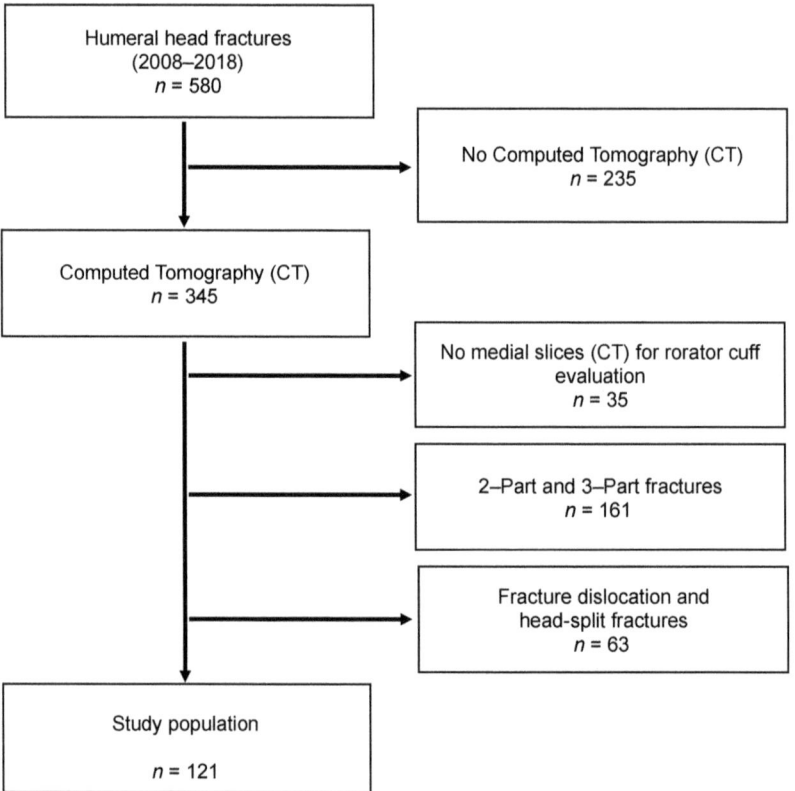

Figure 1. Flowchart of case inclusion/exclusion. The study population consists only of four-Part fractures of the humeral head.

2.1. Radiological Evaluation

The radiological evaluation was carried out on the basis of CT scans of the affected shoulder. Next to axial slices, parasagittal and coronal reconstructions were used for the radiological measurements. All measurements were performed digitally using the software package OsiriX MD Version 6.5 (Pixmeo, Berne, Switzerland).

2.2. Head-Shaft Angle (HSA)

The head–shaft angle is created by a line parallel to the axis of the humeral shaft and perpendicular to the anatomical neck plane. We measured every head–shaft angle of the 121 included patients in the coronal plane to distinguish between varus (HSA < 125°) and non-varus fractures (HSA > 125°) (Figure 2A).

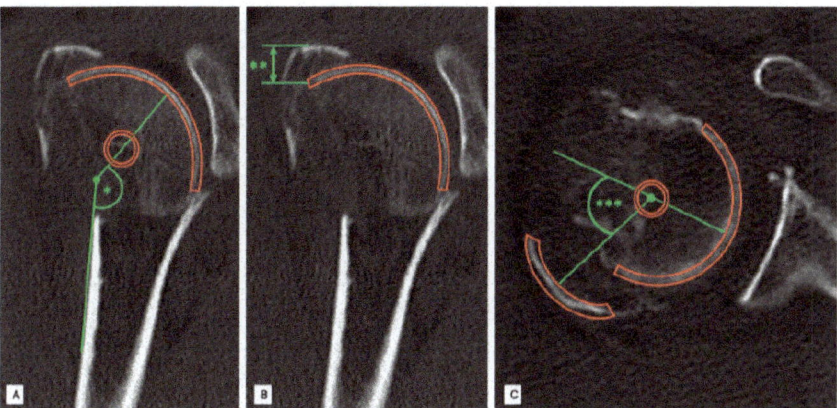

Figure 2. Standardized radiological measurements in a patient with a Neer type 4 fracture injury of the right proximal humerus. (**A**) Standardized radiological measurement (*) of the head-shaft angle [°] in coronal slices. (**B**) Standardized radiological measurement (**) of the greater tuberosity displacement [mm] in vertical plane in coronal slices. (**C**) Standardized radiological measurement (***) of dorsal displacement [°] angle of the greater tuberosity in axial slices.

2.3. Position Determination of the Greater Tuberosity in the Vertical Plane (Cranial Displacement)

The displacement of the greater tuberosity in the vertical plane was measured using coronary reconstructions. Firstly, the most distant part of the fragment and the initial attachment of this fragment were identified and the distance between these two was quantified [mm] (Figure 2B).

2.4. Position Determination of the Greater Tuberosity in the Horizontal Plane (Dorsal Displacement)

The position of the greater tuberosity in the horizontal plane was evaluated by analyzing axial CT slices. Therefore, determination of dorsal displacement of the greater tuberosity was measured using an angle [°] formed by a line that passes the original insertion of the greater tuberosity and a line through the center of the greater tuberosity fragment (Figure 2C).

2.5. Classification of Fatty Degeneration of Rotator Cuff

The posterosuperior rotator cuff was evaluated using the CT-based classification system described by Goutallier [8]. Medial parasagittal slices were set in a typical "Y-shaped-position". Thus, the supraspinous fossa could be displayed since the plane perpendicular to the scapula runs through the medial border of the coracoid process [9]. Muscular state of the supra- and infraspinatus muscle was then assessed according to Gouttallier's classification system of fatty degeneration (grade 0 = no fatty infiltration; grade 1 = low fatty infiltration; grade 2 = less muscular fat than muscle mass; grade 3 = fatty degeneration identical with muscle mass; grade 4 = increased fatty degeneration compared to muscle mass). The patients were then divided into two groups: No or minimal fatty infiltration (Goutallier grade 0–1) (Figure 3A) and advanced fatty degeneration of the rotator cuff (Goutallier grade 2–4) (Figure 3B).

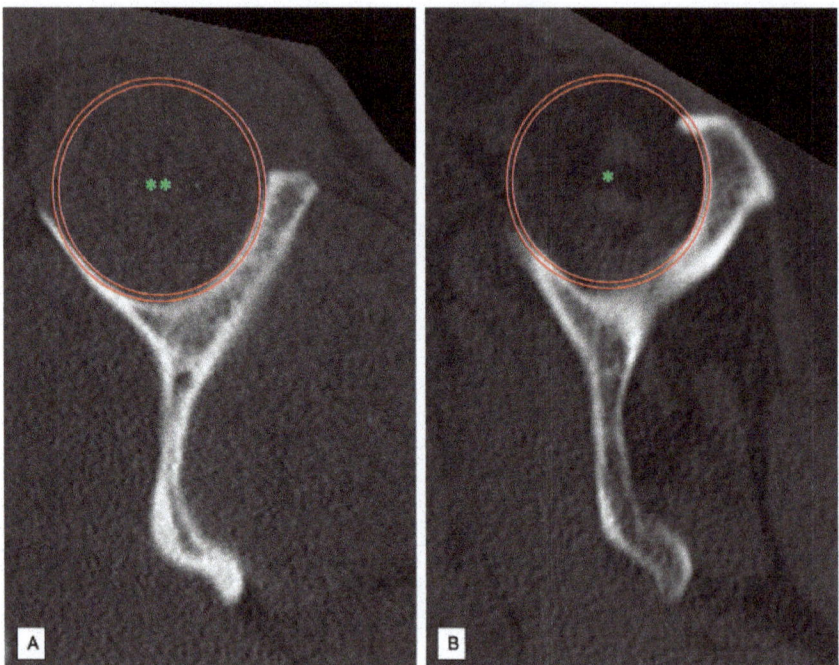

Figure 3. Analysis of the fatty degeneration of the supraspinatus muscle using the Goutallier classification system in parasagittal slices; Red Circle: Supraspinous fossa. (**A**) Goutallier grade 0: No fatty degeneration of the supraspinatus muscle (**). (**B**) Goutallier grade 3–4: Advanced fatty infiltration of the supraspinatus muscle (*).

2.6. Statistical Analysis

Statistical analysis was carried out using SPSS software package version 25 (SPSS Inc., Chicago, IL, USA). The independent t-test was used to compare continuous variables after determining that all variables were normally distributed (Kolmogorov–Smirnov normality test). *p*-values < 0.05 were considered significant. All graphs are displayed with mean value and 95% confidence interval.

3. Results

A total of 121 patients (86 female, 35 male) with a mean age of 67.7 years (female Ø71.7 ± 11.9 and male Ø57.9 ± 14.8) met the inclusion/exclusion criteria. Age and sex distribution in our population was normal ($p < 0.000$). 38% (46/121) showed an HSA of less than 125° (mean age 71.4 years), and 62% (75/121) of the patients had an HSA of more than 125° (mean age 65.5 years). In 86 patients (71%; mean age 69.5 years), high-grade fatty degeneration of the posterosuperior rotator cuff was observed (Goutallier 2–4). Statistical analysis revealed that patients with varus displaced humeral head fractures (HSA < 125°) and patients with advanced signs of rotator cuff degeneration (Goutallier 2–4 of the posterosuperior cuff) were older compared to the others (HSA: $p = 0.026$; Fatty degeneration: $p = 0.027$). Figure 4 displays the age distribution of the study collective with regard to the HSA and the fatty degeneration of the posterosuperior rotator cuff.

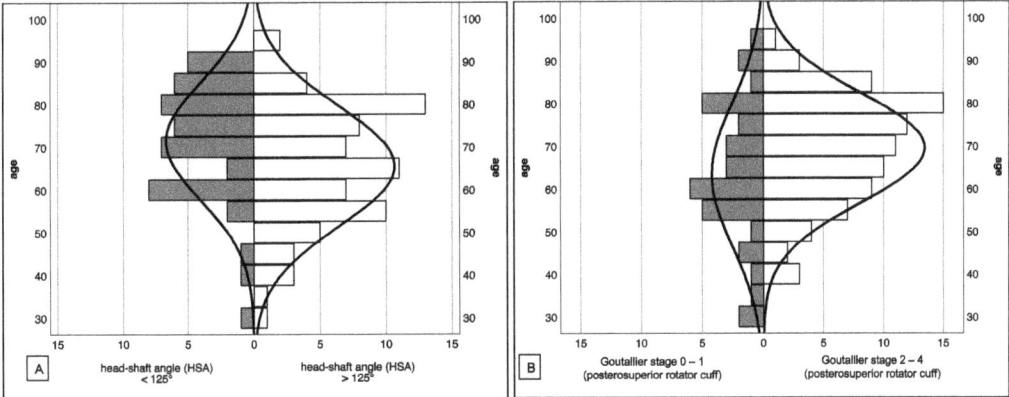

Figure 4. Age distribution of the study collective with regard to the head-shaft angle (**A**) and the posterosuperior rotator cuff (**B**) Patients with varus-displaced fractures and advanced signs of fatty degeneration of the posterosuperior rotator cuff are significantly older compared to the others ($p \leq 0.05$).

3.1. Cranial Displacement of the Greater Tuberosity

Analyzing the entire collective ($n = 121$) cranial displacement of the greater tuberosity of 4.5 mm ± 3.8 mm (0–15 mm) was observed. No significant difference between the displacement height and the condition of the supraspinatus muscle could be detected (Goutallier 0–1: 4.9 mm + 4.4 mm vs. Goutallier 2–4: 4.3 ± 3.5 mm; $p = 0.428$).

For those fractures with a head–shaft angle of more than 125° a significantly increased cranial displacement of the greater tuberosity was measured in patients with no or minimal signs of supraspinatus muscle degeneration (Goutallier 0–1) compared to those with advanced signs of fatty infiltration (Goutallier 2–4; $p = 0.020$; Figure 5A).

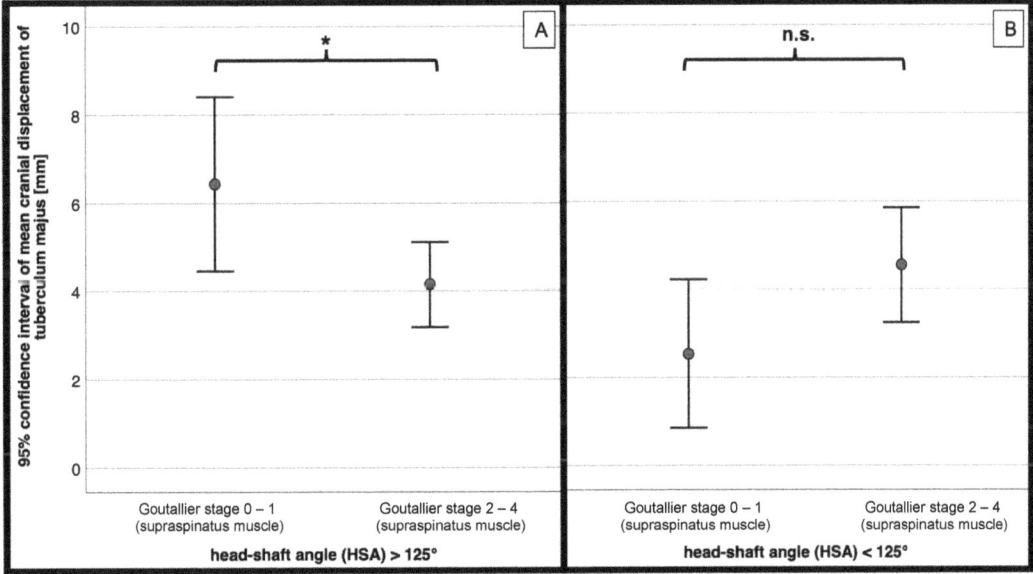

Figure 5. Mean cranial displacement [mm] of greater tuberosity depending on the Goutallier stage of the supraspinatus muscle. (**A**) Head-shaft angle > 125° ($n = 75$), (**B**) head-shaft angle < 125° ($n = 46$). * = significant, n.s. = not significant.

In varus dislocated proximal humeral fractures, the cranial displacement tended to be lower in patients with Goutallier grade 0–1 compared to high-grade degenerated supraspinatus muscles (Goutallier 2–4) without significant differences ($p = 0.467$; Figure 5B).

3.2. Dorsal Displacement of the Greater Tuberosity

Within the entire study collective ($n = 121$), a dorsal displacement of the greater tuberosity of 25.8° ± 28.7° was measured. Comparing the dorsal displacement grade in patients with largely intact infraspinatus muscles (Goutallier 0–1) to those with advanced signs of fatty degeneration (Goutallier 2–4), no significant differences could be detected (Goutallier 0–I: 27.3° ± 30.8° vs. Goutallier II–IV: 21.5° ± 21.2°; $p = 0.332$).

For non-varus displaced fractures with a head-shaft angle of more than 125°, significant less dorsal displacement of the greater tuberosity fragment was noticed for higher grades of infraspinatus muscle degeneration (Goutallier 2–4) compared to patients with less fatty infiltration (Goutallier 0–1; $p = 0.010$; Figure 6A).

Varus displaced fractures in patients with no or minimal signs of fatty infiltration of the infraspinatus muscle (Goutallier 0–1) tended to have less dorsal displacement of the greater tuberosity compared to those with high-grade degenerated infraspinatus muscles (Goutallier 2–4; $p = 0.467$; Figure 6B).

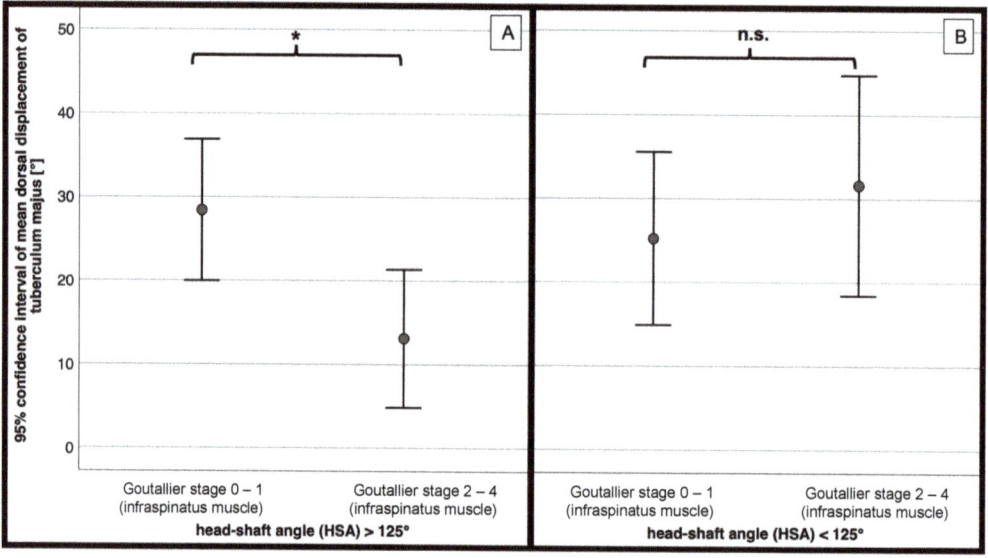

Figure 6. Mean dorsal displacement [°] of greater tuberosity depending on the Goutallier stage of the infraspinatus muscle. (**A**) Head-shaft angle > 125° ($n = 75$). (**B**) head-shaft angle < 125° ($n = 46$). * = significant, n.s. = not significant.

4. Discussion

The key findings of the present study are:

- In non-varus four-part humeral head fractures, cranial and dorsal displacement of the greater tuberosity depends on the status of the posterosuperior rotator cuff.
- In varus displaced humeral head fractures, no correlation between displacement of the greater tuberosity and the condition of the posterosuperior rotator cuff could be detected.

In clinical practice, dorsocranial displacement of the greater tuberosity in humeral head fractures is frequently seen. Neer postulated that displacement of this key fragment is caused by traction of the posterosuperior rotator cuff [1]. Although this theory still acts as an explanatory model, this assumption has not yet been sufficiently investigated [10]. Accordingly, there should be differences in the displacement of the greater tuberosity in patients with a sufficient rotator cuff and patients with an insufficient cuff, e.g., caused by rupture.

In the present study, we assessed the condition of the posterosuperior rotator cuff by evaluating the supraspinatus and infraspinatus muscles according to Goutallier on CT scans [8]. Barry et al. showed that the degree of fatty infiltration, especially of the supra- and infraspinatus muscles, are related to the tear severity [11]. This study demonstrated that in the case of an advanced fatty infiltration (Goutallier $\geq$ 2), only 6.5% had no supraspinatus tendon tears, while the majority of patients suffered from partial or complete ruptures [11].

Overall, demographic change in western countries has led to an increased number of dislocated proximal humeral fractures in elderly patients [12]. These patients often show preexisting rotator cuff tears [4,5,13]. In the present patient population, the incidence of degenerative rotator cuff pathologies in older patients was also higher than in younger patients. In addition, varus displaced humeral head fractures were more frequent in elderly patients, similar to previously published studies [14].

Interestingly, we found differences in the displacement mode of the greater tuberosity in patients with varus displaced fractures compared to others. In fractures with a head–shaft angle of more than 125°, we detected a significantly higher displacement grade of the greater tuberosity in patients without or with minimal degenerative changes of the posterosuperior cuff compared to patients with high-grade degeneration. These results support the theory that the displacement of this fragment is merely caused by force vectors of the cuff, as described by Neer [1].

In varus displaced fractures, we have made contrary observations. In patients with high-grade degeneration of the posterosuperior cuff, the greater tuberosity tended to be more displaced than in patients with inconspicuous rotator cuff status.

A possible explanation could be that in varus impacted fractures, an impression injury caused by the acromion is more likely than fracture displacement due to rotator cuff traction. The intact supra- and infraspinatus tendons can then possibly act as a placeholder in these fractures and thus partially prevent a fragment displacement of the greater tuberosity.

Several limitations of the present study have to be discussed. Only CTs were used to assess the rotator cuff. Although we have only used scans with existing medial slices and computed tomography is a proven diagnostic modality to classify fatty infiltration of the rotator cuff [15,16], some limitations of CT for assessing the rotator cuff status are obvious.

It is also possible that advanced fatty infiltrated rotator cuff parts insert at the greater tuberosity and contribute a part to the displacement by residual activity. In addition, it is possible that acute complete ruptures, without relevant fatty infiltration of the cuff but without any mechanical possibility to contribute to fragment displacement, are included in the study collective. Nevertheless, a fatty degeneration of the musculature is already detectable 6 weeks after a complete rupture, which is why the number of missed complete ruptures should be limited [8,17]. Additionally, this study is a radiological study without evaluation of clinical parameters. Nevertheless, clinical data could not help answering the questions of the present study. One important point is that there is a risk of measurement inaccuracy, although scans with low image quality have been excluded. A certain deviation due to different measurements of the displacement cannot be denied.

Despite the limitations mentioned above, this study is the first to show that in some humeral head fractures, the displacement of the greater tuberosity occurs particularly in intact posterosuperior rotator cuffs, thus supporting Neer's theory that fragment displacement is due to rotator cuff traction [1]. However, in some fractures (varus displaced fractures), fragment displacement follows a different pathophysiological pattern.

To what impact these results may influence treatment strategies for such injuries, or whether it may be useful as a prognostic tool of such fracture patterns must be clarified in further studies.

5. Conclusions

The present study demonstrates that in non-varus four-part humeral head fractures, cranial and dorsal displacement of the greater tuberosity depends on the status of the posterosuperior rotator cuff, whereas in varus displaced humeral head fractures, no correlation between the displacement of the greater tuberosity and the condition of the posterosuperior rotator cuff could be detected. These results imply that the commonly accepted theory of greater tuberosity displacement in humeral head fractures by rotator cuff traction cannot be applied to all fracture types.

Author Contributions: Conceptualization: M.K. and L.K.; methodology: M.K. and C.P.; formal analysis and investigation: L.K., A.M. and I.W.; writing—original draft preparation: L.K.; writing—review and editing: M.K.; resources: M.K. and L.K.; supervision: V.A. and C.P. All authors have read and agreed to the published version of the manuscript.

Funding: This research received no external funding.

Institutional Review Board Statement: Due to the Ethics Committee at the University of Regensburg there are no professional ethical or legal objections to the implementation of this research project.

Data Availability Statement: Data is available.

Conflicts of Interest: The authors have no potential conflict of interest to declare that are relevant to the content of this article.

References

1. Neer, C.S. Displaced proximal humeral fractures: Part, I. Classification and evaluation, 1970. *Clin. Orthop. Relat. Res.* **2006**, *442*, 77–82. [CrossRef] [PubMed]
2. Codman, E. Rupture of the supraspinatus tendon and other lesions in or about the subacromial bursa. *Shoulder Thomas Todd* **1934**, *45*, 612–616.
3. Yamamoto, A.; Takagishi, K.; Osawa, T.; Yanagawa, T.; Nakajima, D.; Shitara, H.; Kobayashi, T. Prevalence and risk factors of a rotator cuff tear in the general population. *J. Shoulder Elb. Surg.* **2010**, *19*, 116–120. [CrossRef] [PubMed]
4. Sher, J.S.; Uribe, J.W.; Posada, A.; Murphy, B.J.; Zlatkin, M.B. Abnormal findings on magnetic resonance images of asymptomatic shoulders. *J. Bone Jt. Surg. Am. Vol.* **1995**, *77*, 10–15. [CrossRef]
5. Milgrom, C.; Schaffler, M.; Gilbert, S.; van Holsbeeck, M. Rotator-cuff changes in asymptomatic adults. The effect of age, hand dominance and gender. *J. Bone Jt. Surg. Br. Vol.* **1995**, *77*, 296–298. [CrossRef]
6. Scheibel, M. Humeral head fracture and cuff. *Unfallchirurg* **2011**, *114*, 1075–1078, 1081–1082. [CrossRef]
7. Bahrs, C.; Rolauffs, B.; Stuby, F.; Dietz, K.; Weise, K.; Helwig, P. Effect of Proximal Humeral Fractures on the Age-Specific Prevalence of Rotator Cuff Tears. *J. Trauma Inj. Infect. Crit. Care* **2010**, *69*, 901–906. [CrossRef] [PubMed]
8. Goutallier, D.; Postel, J.M.; Bernageau, J.; Lavau, L.; Voisin, M.C. Fatty muscle degeneration in cuff ruptures. Pre- and postoperative evaluation by CT scan. *Clin. Orthop. Relat. Res.* **1994**, *304*, 78–83.
9. Thomazeau, H.; Duval, J.M.; Darnault, P.; Dréano, T. Anatomical relationships and scapular attachments of the supraspinatus muscle. *Surg. Radiol. Anat.* **1996**, *18*, 221–225. [CrossRef] [PubMed]
10. Bahrs, C.; Lingenfelter, E.; Fischer, F.; Walters, E.M.; Schnabel, M. Mechanism of injury and morphology of the greater tuberosity fracture. *J. Shoulder Elb. Surg.* **2006**, *15*, 140–147. [CrossRef]
11. Barry, J.J.; Lansdown, D.A.; Cheung, S.; Feeley, B.T.; Ma, C.B. The relationship between tear severity, fatty infiltration, and muscle atrophy in the supraspinatus. *J. Shoulder Elb. Surg.* **2013**, *22*, 18–25. [CrossRef] [PubMed]
12. Bahrs, C.; Bauer, M.; Blumenstock, G.; Eingartner, C.; Bahrs, S.D.; Tepass, A.; Weise, K.; Rolauffs, B. The complexity of proximal humeral fractures is age and gender specific. *J. Orthop. Sci.* **2013**, *18*, 465–470. [CrossRef]
13. Yamaguchi, K.; Ditsios, K.; Middleton, W.D.; Hildebolt, C.F.; Galatz, L.M.; Teefey, S.A. The Demographic and Morphological Features of Rotator Cuff Disease. A Comparison of Asymptomatic and Symptomatic Shoulders. *J. Bone Jt. Surg. Am. Vol.* **2006**, *88*, 1699–1704. [CrossRef]
14. Robinson, C.M.; Stirling, P.H.; Goudie, E.B.; MacDonald, D.J.; Strelzow, J.A. Complications and Long-Term Outcomes of Open Reduction and Plate Fixation of Proximal Humeral Fractures. *J. Bone Jt. Surg. Am. Vol.* **2019**, *101*, 2129–2139. [CrossRef] [PubMed]
15. Fuchs, B.; Weishaupt, D.; Zanetti, M.; Hodler, J.; Gerber, C. Fatty degeneration of the muscles of the rotator cuff: Assessment by computed tomography versus magnetic resonance imaging. *J Shoulder Elb. Surg.* **1999**, *8*, 599–605. [CrossRef]
16. Nardo, L.; Karampinos, D.C.; Lansdown, D.A.; Carballido-Gamio, J.; Lee, S.; Maroldi, R.; Ma, C.B.; Link, T.M.; Krug, R. Quantitative assessment of fat infiltration in the rotator cuff muscles using water-fat MRI. *J. Magn. Reson. Imaging* **2013**, *39*, 1178–1185. [CrossRef] [PubMed]
17. Frich, L.H.; Fernandes, L.R.; Schrøder, H.D.; Hejbøl, E.K.; Nielsen, P.V.; Jørgensen, P.H.; Stensballe, A.; Lambertsen, K.L. The inflammatory response of the supraspinatus muscle in rotator cuff tear conditions. *J. Shoulder Elb. Surg.* **2021**, *30*, e261–e275. [CrossRef] [PubMed]

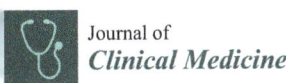

Article

A Randomized Trial Assessing the Muscle Strength and Range of Motion in Elderly Patients following Distal Radius Fractures Treated with 4- and 6-Week Cast Immobilization

Jarosław Olech [1], Grzegorz Konieczny [2], Łukasz Tomczyk [3] and Piotr Morasiewicz [4,*]

[1] Provincial Specialist Hospital in Legnica, Orthopedic Surgery Department, Iwaszkiewicza 5, 59-220 Legnica, Poland; o.jaroslaw@yahoo.com
[2] Faculty of Health Sciences and Physical Education, Witelon State University of Applied Sciences, Sejmowa 5A Street, 59-220 Legnica, Poland; gkonieczny@wp.pl
[3] Department of Food Safety and Quality Management, Poznan University of Life Sciences, 60-624 Poznan, Poland; lukasz.tomczyk@up.poznan.pl
[4] Department of Orthopaedic and Trauma Surgery, University Hospital in Opole, Institute of Medical Sciences, University of Opole, al. Witosa 26, 45-401 Opole, Poland
* Correspondence: morasp@poczta.onet.pl

Abstract: Background: There is no consensus among orthopedic surgeons as to the required period of cast immobilization in distal radius fractures in elderly patients. The purpose of this study was to assess muscle strength and range of motion symmetry in elderly patients after distal radius fractures with different periods of cast immobilization. Methods: This study evaluated 50 patients (33 women and 17 men), aged over 65 years, after cast immobilization treatment for distal radius fracture. The mean age at the beginning of treatment was 71 years. The mean duration of follow-up was 1 year and 3 months. The first subgroup ($n = 24$) comprised the patients whose fractures had been immobilized in a cast for 6 weeks, another subgroup ($n = 26$) comprised the patients with 4-week cast immobilization. We assessed: (1) muscle strength, (2) range of motion. Results: The mean grip strength in the treated limb was 71% and 81% of that in the healthy limb in the groups with 4-week and 6-week cast immobilization, respectively ($p = 0.0432$). The study groups showed no differences in the mean grip strength in the treated limbs or the mean grip strength in the healthy limbs. The mean treated limb flexion was 62° and 75° in the 4-week and 6-week immobilization groups, respectively ($p = 0.025$). The evaluated groups showed no differences in terms of any other range of motion parameters. The grip strength and range of motion values were significantly lower in the treated limb than in the healthy limb in both evaluated groups. Only the values of wrist radial deviation in the 6-week cast immobilization group showed no differences between the treated and healthy limbs. Conclusion: Higher values of injured limb muscle strength and greater mean range of wrist flexion were achieved in the 6-week subgroup. Neither of the evaluated groups achieved a symmetry of muscle strength or range of motion after treatment. Full limb function did not return in any of the elderly distal radius fracture patients irrespective of cast immobilization duration.

Keywords: distal radius; fracture; muscle strength; grip strength; range of motion; aging

1. Introduction

Distal radius fractures (DRFs) pose a serious problem due to their high incidence [1–15]. The risk of DRF has been reported as 9–139/10,000 people per year [3,4,8,11,12,15]. These fractures most commonly involve the distal radial epiphysis, which is estimated to be the site of 15–21% of all fractures. This is also the third most common location of osteoporotic fractures [1–12,14].

In elderly patients with poor bone quality and poor condition of the adjacent soft tissues, with only slight radial deformity and shortening and a fracture morphology that justifies conservative treatment, the preferred treatment method is closed reduction with cast immobilization [11,13,15–17]. In elderly patients Kilic prefers treatment via immobilization in a cast [16]. Moreover, elderly patients have shown good clinical and functional outcomes with cast immobilization [11].

One aspect of DFR treatment regarding which there is no consensus is the duration of cast immobilization [9,13,15–18], with some orthopedic surgeons advocating for 4 weeks [9,16], some for 5 weeks [13,16,18], and some for up to 6 weeks [9,17] of immobilization. The issue of muscle strength and range of motion in elderly patients with DRF treated via cast immobilization for different lengths of time has not been fully evaluated.

Long-term cast immobilization after DRF adversely affects muscle strength, range of motion, and limb function [14,15,18,19]. Thus, on the one hand, shortening the period of cast immobilization after DRF should be beneficial, on the other hand, a shorter period of cast immobilization may lead to nonunion and bone fragment displacement.

Arora et al. compared range of motion and muscle strength in patients aged over 65 years with DRF treated with a cast and those treated with a volar locking plate [13]. Those authors reported a lack of difference between the groups in terms of range of motion, whereas muscle strength was greater in the volar locking plate group [13]. Egol reported greater muscle strength in elderly patients with DRF treated surgically, in comparison with that in patients treated with a cast, and a greater degree of supination in patients treated with cast immobilization [20]. Zengin observed greater muscle strength in elderly patients with DRF treated with plate fixation than that in cast-immobilized patients, with no difference between the groups in terms of range of motion [17]. None of those authors evaluated muscle strength and range of motion in elderly patients following cast immobilization of varied duration.

We hypothesized that the duration of limb immobilization in a cast affects the symmetry of both muscle strength and range of motion in elderly patients following DRF treatment.

Due to the lack of a broader analysis of this important issue, the purpose of our study was to assess the symmetry of functional parameters following DRF treatment with two different cast immobilization periods.

2. Materials and Methods

This was a prospective study. Over the period from June 2020 to November 2020, there were 117 patients treated at our center for DRFs. The study inclusion criteria were: a DRF treated with closed reduction and cast immobilization; age of 65 years or older; follow-up of at least 1 year after treatment completion; available complete medical records regarding the treatment; and complete data on range of motion and grip strength assessment. The exclusion criteria were: a compound fracture; treatment with other methods, such as external fixation, plate fixation, or K-wire fixation; age under 65 years; incomplete treatment records (i.e., patients who continued their treatment elsewhere); and incomplete data on range of motion or grip strength. All patients had been informed that study participation was completely voluntary. The study had been approved by the local review board.

The study inclusion criteria were met by 50 patients (33 women and 17 men). The mean age at the beginning of treatment was 71 years (ranging from 65 to 86 years). The mean duration of follow-up was 1 year and 3 months (ranging from 1 year to 1 year and 6 months).

Once the diagnoses had been established and written informed consent obtained, the patients were randomized into two groups (cast immobilization for 4 or 6 weeks) with the use of sequentially numbered, closed envelopes.

The patients, who were stratified by the period of DRF cast immobilization, formed two study subgroups. One subgroup ($n = 24$) were the patients treated with cast immobilization for 6 weeks, and the other subgroup ($n = 26$) were the patients who underwent closed reduction and cast immobilization for 4 weeks.

All patients included in the study underwent emergency room closed reduction and immobilization in a below-elbow cast. In the entire study group there were no cases of a secondary bone fragment displacement that would require surgical correction.

All patients underwent outpatient radiographic follow-up after 5–7 days, 4–6 weeks, and in 3-month intervals thereafter. Outpatient clinical and radiographic follow-up visits were scheduled in 2–6-week intervals.

The plaster casts were removed after 4 or 6 weeks, depending on the study group. For the first 3–6 weeks following cast removal, the patients were advised to use the limb sparingly and were assigned finger and wrist exercises. Limb loading was increased gradually, based on the progress of bone remodeling at the fracture site, as assessed radiographically, as well as based on clinical symptoms. Wrist and finger strengthening exercises were introduced at 3–6 weeks.

The following functional parameters were assessed: (1) muscle strength, (2) range of motion.

Muscle strength (grip strength), expressed in kilograms, was assessed with a Smedley Hand Dynamometer (GIMA). The grip strength in the uninjured (healthy) hand was compared with that in the treated limb, with the result expressed as the percentage of the grip strength measured in the healthy limb [7,9,17].

Range of motion was measured with a goniometer and included: wrist flexion, extension, abduction (radial deviation), and adduction (ulnar deviation), with the results expressed in degrees [7,9,17].

All these parameters were evaluated at a follow-up visit at least 1 year after treatment completion. One experienced orthopedist performed dynamometer and goniometer measurements.

The study subgroups (representing different cast immobilization periods) were compared in terms of the individual functional parameters.

The data were analyzed statistically using Statistica 13.1. The Shapiro–Wilk test was used to check for normality of distribution. Student's t-test was used to compare variables assuming a normal distribution. The Mann–Whitney test was used in the case of variables assuming a different order than the normal one. The level of statistical significance was set at $p < 0.05$.

3. Results

The individual subgroups did not differ in terms of mean patient age ($p = 0.5628$) (Table 1).

Table 1. Detailed results of the grip power and range of motion of individual subgroups.

Analyzed Variable (Mean ± Standard Deviation)	4-Week Group $n = 26$	6-Week Group $n = 24$	p Value
age of patients (years)	71.34 ± 4.99	72.20 ± 5.46	0.5628 *
grip power (%)	71.12 ± 14.24	81.07 ± 12.59	0.0321 **
grip power treated limb (kg)	25.45 ± 12.53	27.6 ± 11.46	0.5317 *
grip power healthy limb (kg)	34.48 ± 11.92	31.17 ± 9.69	0.2893 *
flexion treated limb (degrees)	61.53 ± 9.1	74.87 ± 10.66	0.025 *
flexion healthy limb (degrees)	84.46 ± 13.1	84.37 ± 13.7	0.9818 *
extension treated limb (degrees)	50.17 ± 17.47	57.02 ± 17.34	0.1711 *
extension healthy limb (degrees)	66.38 ± 14.92	58.6 ± 12.47	0.0521 *
ulnar deviation treated limb (degrees)	33.25 ± 13.22	39.54 ± 15.41	0.127 *
ulnar deviation healthy limb (degrees)	45.38 ± 13.93	46.7 ± 11.47	0.7167 *
radial deviation treated limb (degrees)	18.59 ± 11.7	21.18 ± 15.31	0.5026 *
radial deviation healthy limb (degrees)	27.76 ± 16.67	22.56 ± 14.3	0.2436 *

* student's t-test. ** Mann–Whitney U test.

Our study showed the mean grip strength following DRFs in all patients to be approximately 76% of that in the healthy limb. The mean relative grip strength values in the 4-week and 6-week subgroups were 71% and 81%, respectively. These differences were statistically significant ($p = 0.0432$) (Table 1, Figure 1).

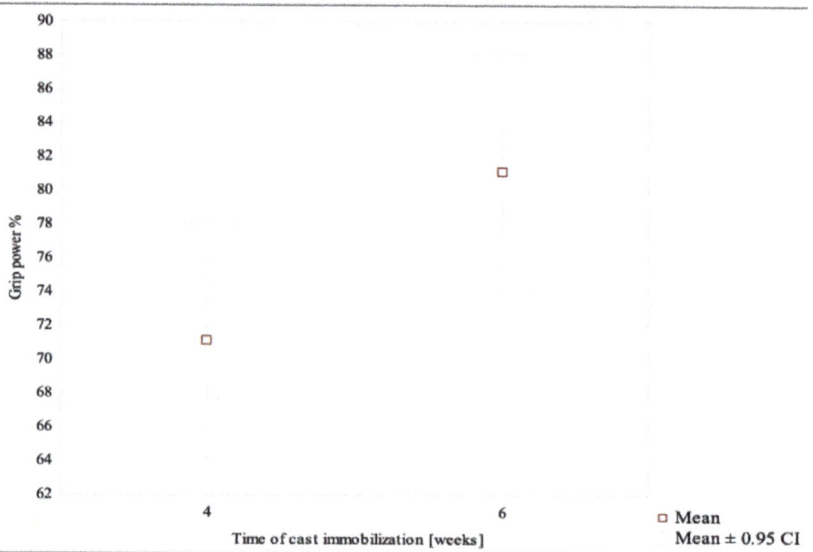

Figure 1. The mean relative grip strength values in the 4-week and 6-week subgroups.

The 4-week cast immobilization subgroup showed a lack of grip strength symmetry between the healthy and treated limb ($p = 0.01047$) (Table 2, Figure 2). The patients from the 6-week subgroup also showed a lack of grip strength symmetry between the uninjured and injured limb ($p = 0.06218$) (Table 2, Figure 3).

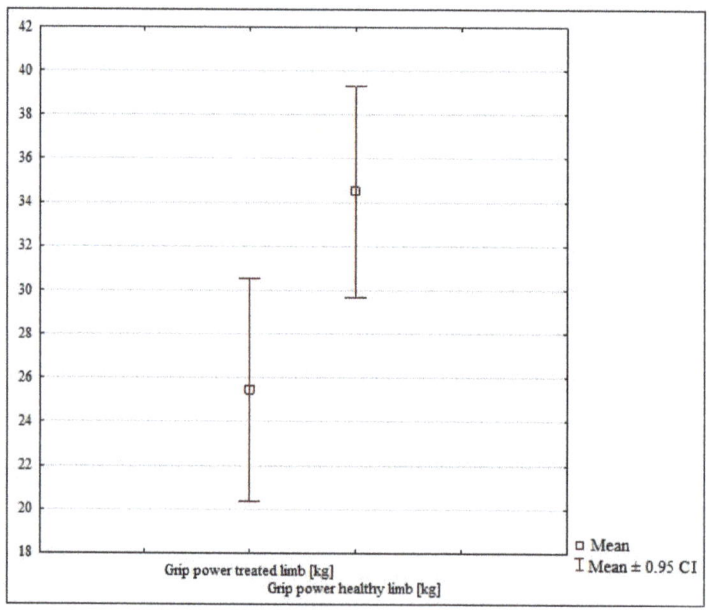

Figure 2. The grip strength in the healthy and treated limb in the 4-week subgroup.

Table 2. The grip power and range of motion symmetry in the 4-week group and 6-week group.

Analyzed Variable (Mean ± Standard Deviation)	Treated Limb	Healthy Limb	p Value
	4-Week Group		
grip power (kg)	25.45 ± 8.53	34.48 ± 9.32	0.01124 **
flexion (degrees)	61.53 ± 14.1	84.46 ± 13.1	0.00001 *
extension (degrees)	50.17 ± 12.47	66.38 ± 14.92	0.00073 *
ulnar deviation (degrees)	33.25 ± 13.21	45.38 ± 12.63	0.00224 *
radial deviation (degrees)	18.59 ± 9.12	27.76 ± 10.32	0.0258 *
Analyzed Variable (Mean ± Standard Deviation)	**Treated Limb**	**Healthy Limb**	***p* Value**
	6-Week Group		
grip power (kg)	26.48 ± 9.96	32.89 ± 8.92	0.005213 **
flexion (degrees)	67.94 ± 15.21	84.42 ± 12.32	0.00002 *
extension (degrees)	53.46 ± 12.58	62.65 ± 10.21	0.004961 *
ulnar deviation (degrees)	36.27 ± 11.52	46.02 ± 10.69	0.000547 *
radial deviation (degrees)	19.84 ± 13.47	25.27 ± 15.64	0.06597 *

* student's *t*-test. ** Mann–Whitney U test.

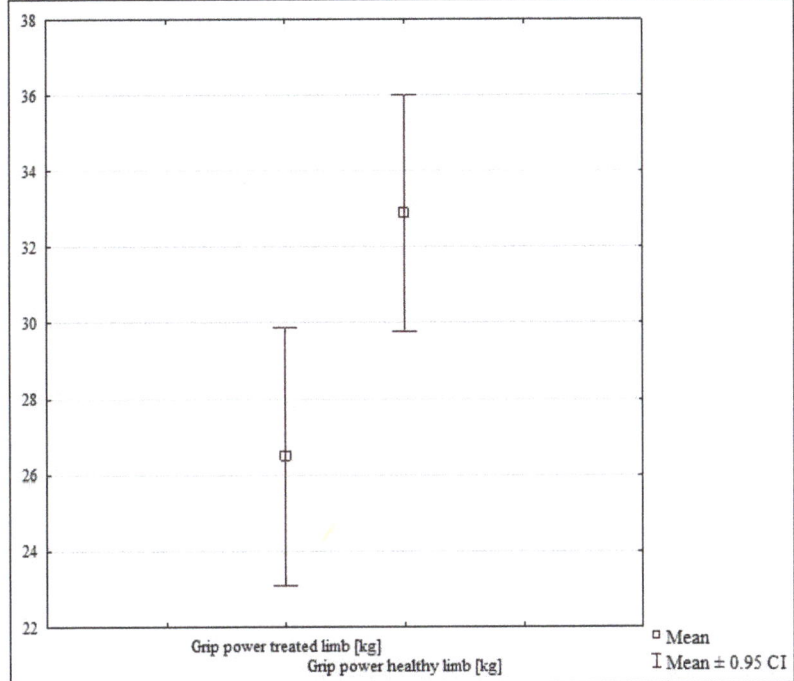

Figure 3. The grip strength in the healthy and treated limb in 6-week subgroup.

The mean wrist flexion measured in all study subjects was 67.9° in the treated limb and 84.4° in the healthy limb. The best range of flexion (74.9°) was achieved in the 6-week subgroup, and the most limited flexion (61.5°) was observed in the 4-week subgroup. These differences were significant ($p = 0.025$) (Table 1, Figure 4). The 4-week immobilization subgroup exhibited significant differences in wrist flexion between the healthy and treated limb ($p = 0.00001$) (Table 2). The 6-week immobilization subgroup also showed significant differences in wrist flexion between the healthy and treated limb ($p = 0.00002$) (Table 2).

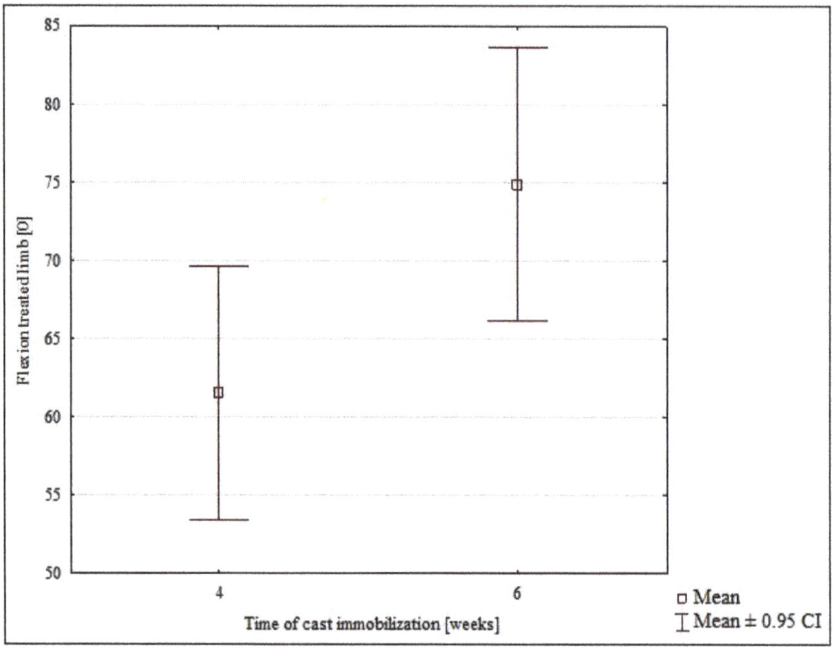

Figure 4. The range of flexion in the 4-weeks and 6-week subgroups.

The mean wrist extension in the 4-week subgroup was 50.1°, whereas in the 6-week subgroup it was 57°; the difference was not statistically significant (Table 1). Wrist extension asymmetry was observed in the 4-week subgroup ($p = 0.00073$) (Table 2). The range of wrist extension in the healthy and treated limb was also asymmetrical in the 6-week subgroup ($p = 0.004961$) (Table 2).

The mean radial deviation was 18.6° and 21.2° in the patients whose fractures were immobilized in a cast for 4 weeks and 6 weeks, respectively; this difference was not statistically significant (Table 1). The 4-week subgroup showed significant differences in terms of mean radial deviation between the uninjured and injured limb ($p = 0.0258$) (Table 2). Conversely, there were no significant differences in terms of mean radial deviation in the healthy and treated limbs in patients treated with a cast for 6 weeks ($p = 0.06597$) (Table 2).

The mean ulnar deviation in the 4-week subgroup was 33.3°, whereas in the 6-week subgroup it was 39.5°; this difference was not statistically significant (Table 1). However, there was a significant difference in terms of mean ulnar deviation between the healthy and treated limb of patients who had worn a cast for 4 weeks, which demonstrates an asymmetry of this parameter ($p = 0.00224$) (Table 2). The 6-week subgroup showed differences in the mean ulnar deviation between the healthy and treated limb ($p = 0.000547$) (Table 2). There were no differences in complications in the two assessed groups. There was no need for changing casts in any of the evaluated patients.

4. Discussion

This study aimed to verify whether a shorter period of cast immobilization (4 weeks) in elderly DRF patients would help them complete the treatment and resume their normal activities earlier than those treated with 6 weeks of cast immobilization. So far, there have been no studies assessing the functional outcomes of cast immobilization treatment of varied duration in elderly DRF patients. We observed a significantly greater grip strength in the treated limb (81% of the grip strength in the healthy limb, on average) and a greater range of flexion in the treated limb (75° on average) in our 6-week subgroup than in the 4-week subgroup. Our study groups showed no differences in terms of any other evaluated parameters. Thus, the results of our study support our hypothesis only to some extent.

The distal radial epiphysis is one of the most common fracture locations [1–15], and the treatment of these fractures is an important part of patient management in any trauma/orthopedic ward. Stable extra-articular fractures, particularly those in elderly patients, can be treated via closed reduction with immobilization in a plaster cast [11,13,15–17,19].

Assessing multiple parameters following orthopedic treatment is important from the point of view of orthopedic and rehabilitation specialists and the patients themselves [7–9,13–15,17,20]. Apart from the radiographic and biomechanical assessment, functional assessment seems to be of great significance, as it is the post-treatment limb function that is of crucial importance to patients, doctors, and rehabilitation specialists alike. Some authors have demonstrated good functional outcomes, despite worse radiographic outcomes, in DRF patients treated with cast immobilization, in comparison with those treated surgically [9,11,17]. Conversely, some authors reported a relationship between good radiographic and good clinical outcomes following DRF treatment [5,21,22].

There is no consensus among orthopedic surgeons as to the required period of cast immobilization in DRF [9,13,15–18]. Various authors prefer an immobilization period of 4 weeks [9,16], 5 weeks [13,16,18], or 6 weeks [9,17]. A long period of cast immobilization may reduce the post-treatment range of motion and muscle strength in the limb [14,15,18,19]. A shorter period of cast immobilization, provided bone union has been achieved, may allow for earlier rehabilitation as well as earlier use and resumed function of the limb [14,15,17,18]. Theoretically, muscle strength and range of motion should be comparable (symmetrical) in both upper limbs [15,17,19]. Achieving statistically similar (i.e., symmetrical) values of muscle strength and range of motion in the treated and healthy limbs following DRF treatment indicates good clinical and functional outcomes [15,19].

Katayama et al. reported a mean grip strength of 84.6% of that in the healthy limb in patients with osteoarthritis following DRF treatment with volar plate fixation [7]. Lameijer et al. reported a mean grip strength of 79% of that measured in the uninjured limb [8]. Toon et al. observed a mean grip strength of 83.29% of that in the unaffected limb in patients who underwent DRF internal fixation with a volar plate and 81.26% in patients treated with a plaster cast [9]. Kilic reported a mean grip strength of 57.3% of that in the healthy limb in DRF patients managed with plaster cast immobilization [16]. In a study by Zengin et al. the patients treated with a volar locking plate and those treated with a plaster cast exhibited a mean grip strength of 67.7% and 57.5% of that in the uninjured limb, respectively [17]. Arora et al. assessed muscle strength in patients over 65 years of age with DRF treated with cast immobilization or volar locking plate fixation [13]. Twelve months after the fracture, those authors observed a greater muscle strength in the volar locking plate subgroup (22.2 kg) in comparison with that in the plaster cast subgroup (18.8 kg) [13]. Egol reported a greater muscle strength in elderly DRF patients treated surgically (17.7 kg) than in those treated with cast immobilization (12.7 kg), whereas the range of supination was greater in the plaster cast subgroup [20]. Other authors reported a mean grip strength of 19 kg in 67 treated DRF patients [14]. In our study, there were no differences in grip strength between the study groups. Our study results are similar to those reported in the literature [7–9,13,14,16,17]. We observed a lack of symmetry between the healthy and treated limb in terms of grip strength in both groups of patients. This indicates incomplete return of pre-fracture limb function after DRF in elderly patients irrespective of the duration of cast immobilization. The pain or discomfort that persisted following treatment completion may have additionally reduced post-treatment muscle strength and intensified grip strength asymmetry.

The mean range of wrist extension reported by Lameijer et al. was 53° [8]. Toon et al. observed a mean wrist extension of 67.5° in their group of DRF patients managed with volar plate fixation and 72.9° in their plaster cast group [9]. Arora et al. compared range of motion in 73 patients over 65 years of age with DRF treated with cast immobilization or volar locking plate fixation [13]. Those authors reported a lack of differences in terms of range of motion between these two groups [13]. Zengin observed no differences in range of motion between the elderly patients with DRF treated with plate fixation and those treated with a plaster cast [17]. The range of wrist extension in our patients was similar in both evaluated subgroups; these results are consistent with those reported in the literature [8,9,13]. In our study, we observed wrist extension asymmetry between the healthy and treated limb in both evaluated groups. In terms of wrist flexion, the mean range reported by Lameijer et al., was 52° [8]. Toon et al. reported mean wrist flexion of 63.1° in their DRF patients managed with a volar plate and 64.1° in the group managed with a plaster cast [9]. Arora et al. reported a mean wrist flexion of 57° in elderly patients following 5 weeks of cast immobilization [13]. In our study, the greatest significant difference between treated subgroups was in the range of wrist flexion with the 6-week subgroup (74.9°) compared with the 4-week subgroup (61.5°); these results are consistent with those reported in the literature [8,9,13]. We noted a wrist flexion asymmetry between the healthy and treated limb in both groups of patients. Lameijer et al. observed a mean radial deviation of 14° [8]. Toon et al. reported a mean radial deviation of 15.6° in their DRF group managed with a volar plate and 15.7° in patients immobilized with a plaster cast [9]. Our results were consistent with those reported in the literature [8,9,13]. In our study, the range of radial deviation in the healthy limb was comparable with that in the treated limb in patients treated with cast immobilization for 6 weeks. A study by Lameijer et al. demonstrated a mean ulnar deviation of 23° [8]. Toon et al., reported a mean ulnar deviation of 22.8° in DRF patients treated with a volar plate and 17.9° in the cast immobilization group [9]. In our study there were no differences in the range of ulnar deviation between the two evaluated subgroups. We observed an ulnar deviation range asymmetry between the healthy and treated limb in both evaluated subgroups. Range of motion limitations and range of motion asymmetry between the healthy and treated limb suggest incomplete return of limb function in elderly DRF patients. Longer rehabilitation protocols should be considered particularly in patients treated with 4-week cast immobilization. The observed asymmetry in the evaluated parameter values may have been associated with a certain level of pain persisting after treatment completion.

The shorter cast immobilization period in the elderly may have produced incomplete bone remodeling at the fracture site. This, in turn, may have increased pain and worsened limb function in comparison with those parameters in the 6-week subgroup.

The greatest muscle strength and greatest mean range of wrist flexion in the 6-week immobilization subgroup may be due to the fact that the patients from this subgroup resumed their daily activities earlier, while the patients from the other (4 week-) subgroup were inhibited by fears of destabilizing their fracture, and to the fact that the proportion of patients who resumed exposing the fractured limb to normal load bearing was the highest in the 6-week immobilization subgroup. Well-chosen, intensive, individualized, and long-lasting rehabilitation may improve upper limb function following DRF treatment in elderly patients.

Our study has several limitations. Firstly, the sample size was relatively small. Nevertheless, other authors have also conducted their studies in similar-sized or even smaller groups of patients [7,9,14,16–18]. Secondly, the study did not have control participants who did not have a DRF. In the future, we plan to study with control participants who did not have a DRF. The strengths of our study include a uniform rehabilitation protocol, patient randomization, the individual groups showing no differences in terms of patient age, examinations being conducted by one surgeon following a single protocol.

5. Conclusions

We observed incomplete return of full limb function after DRF in elderly patients, irrespective of the duration of cast immobilization.

We observed an asymmetry in terms of grip strength and range of motion between the affected and unaffected limb in both evaluated subgroups.

Greater muscle strength in the affected limb (though not quite equal to that in the uninjured limb) and greater mean range of wrist flexion was achieved in the 6-week subgroup.

Our study indicates that elderly patients with DRF managed with cast immobilization should undergo longer and more intensive rehabilitation regimens.

Author Contributions: Conceptualization, J.O. and P.M.; methodology, J.O., G.K., Ł.T. and P.M.; software, J.O. and Ł.T.; validation, J.O., Ł.T. and P.M; formal analysis, J.O. and P.M.; investigation, J.O. and G.K.; resources, J.O., G.K. and Ł.T.; data curation, J.O., G.K. and P.M.; writing—original draft preparation, J.O., G.K., Ł.T. and P.M.; writing—review and editing, J.O., G.K., Ł.T. and P.M.; visualization, J.O., G.K., Ł.T. and P.M.; supervision, J.O. and P.M.; project administration, J.O. and P.M. All authors have read and agreed to the published version of the manuscript.

Funding: This research received no external funding.

Institutional Review Board Statement: The study was conducted according to the guidelines of the Declaration of Helsinki, and approved by the Bioethics Committee at the Lower Silesian Medical Chamber in Wrocław (protocol code 2/PNDR/2020, date of approval 10 June 2020).

Informed Consent Statement: Informed consent was obtained from all subjects involved in the study.

Data Availability Statement: The data presented in this study are available on request from the corresponding author. The data are not publicly available due to privacy.

Conflicts of Interest: The authors declare no conflict of interest.

References

1. Kwon, H.Y.; Kim, H.H.; Sung, Y.K.; Ha, Y.C. Incidence and Mortality of Osteoporotic Fracture in Rheumatoid Arthritis in South Korea Using Nationwide Claims Data. *J. Bone Metab.* **2019**, *26*, 97–104. [CrossRef] [PubMed]
2. Ogunleye, A.A.; Mullner, D.F.; Skochdopole, A.; Armstrong, M.; Herrera, F.A. Remote Injuries and Outcomes After Distal Radius Fracture Management. *Hand* **2019**, *14*, 102–106. [CrossRef] [PubMed]
3. Ochi, K.; Go, Y.; Furuya, T.; Ikari, K.; Taniguchi, A.; Yamanaka, H.; Momohara, S. Risk factors associated with the occurrence of distal radius fractures in Japanese patients with rheumatoid arthritis: A prospective observational cohort study. *Clin. Rheumatol.* **2014**, *33*, 477–483. [CrossRef] [PubMed]
4. Ali, M.; Eiriksdottir, A.; Murtadha, M.; Åkesson, A.; Atroshi, I. Incidence of distal radius fracture in a general population in southern Sweden in 2016 compared with 2001. *Osteoporos. Int.* **2020**, *31*, 715–720. [CrossRef]
5. Talmaç, M.A.; Görgel, M.A.; Kanar, M.; Tok, O.; Özdemir, H.M. Comparison of three surgical methods in the treatment of intraarticular comminuted distal radius fractures: Volar locking plate, non-bridging external fixator, and bridging external fixator. *Eklem Hastalik. Cerrahisi* **2019**, *30*, 224–232. [CrossRef] [PubMed]
6. Chung, K.C.; Malay, S.; Shauver, M.J.; Kim, H.M. WRIST Group. Assessment of Distal Radius Fracture Complications Among Adults 60 Years or Older: A Secondary Analysis of the WRIST Randomized Clinical Trial. *JAMA Netw. Open* **2019**, *4*, e187053. [CrossRef] [PubMed]
7. Katayama, T.; Ono, H.; Omokawa, S. Comparison of Five Years Clinical and Radiological Outcomes between Progressive and Non-Progressive Wrist Osteoarthritis after Volar Locking Plate Fixation of Distal Radius Fractures. *J. Hand Surg. Asian Pac.* **2019**, *24*, 30–35. [CrossRef] [PubMed]
8. Lameijer, C.M.; Ten Duis, H.J.; Dusseldorp, I.V.; Dijkstra, P.U.; van der Sluis, C.K. Prevalence of posttraumatic arthritis and the association with outcome measures following distal radius fractures in non-osteoporotic patients: A systematic review. *Arch. Orthop. Trauma Surg.* **2017**, *137*, 1499–1513. [CrossRef] [PubMed]
9. Toon, D.H.; Premchand, R.A.X.; Sim, J.; Vaikunthan, R. Outcomes and financial implications of intra-articular distal radius fractures: A comparative study of open reduction internal fixation (ORIF) with volar locking plates versus nonoperative management. *J. Orthop. Traumatol.* **2017**, *18*, 229–234. [CrossRef]
10. Rundgren, J.; Bojan, A.; Navarro, C.M.; Enocson, A. Epidemiology, classification, treatment and mortality of distal radius fractures in adults: An observational study of 23,394 fractures from the national Swedish fracture register. *BMC Musculoskelet. Disord.* **2020**, *21*, 88. [CrossRef]
11. Hevonkorpi, T.P.; Launonen, A.P.; Huttunen, T.T.; Kannus, P.; Niemi, S.; Mattila, V.M. Incidence of distal radius fracture surgery in Finns aged 50 years or more between 1998 and 2016—Too many patients are yet operated on? *BMC Musculoskelet. Disord.* **2018**, *19*, 70. [CrossRef] [PubMed]
12. Kelsey, J.L.; Samelson, E.J. Variation in Risk Factors for Fractures at Different Sites. *Curr. Osteoporos. Rep.* **2007**, *7*, 127–133. [CrossRef]

13. Arora, R.; Lutz, M.; Deml, C.; Krappinger, D.; Haug, L.; Gabl, M. A Prospective Randomized Trial Comparing Nonoperative Treatment with Volar Locking Plate Fixation for Displaced and Unstable Distal Radial Fractures in Patients Sixty-five Years of Age and Older. *J. Bone Jt. Surg. Am.* **2011**, *93*, 2146–2153. [CrossRef]
14. Reid, S.A.; Andersen, J.M.; Vicenzino, B. Adding mobilisation with movement to exercise and advice hastens the improvement in range, pain and function after non-operative cast immobilisation for distal radius fracture: A multicentre, randomised trial. *J. Physiother.* **2020**, *66*, 105–112. [CrossRef] [PubMed]
15. Filipova, V.; Lonzarić, D.; Jesenšek Papež, B. Efficacy of combined physical and occupational therapy in patients with conservatively treated distal radius fracture: Randomized controlled trial. *Wien. Klin. Wochenschr.* **2015**, *127*, 282–287. [CrossRef] [PubMed]
16. Kilic, A.; Ozkaya, U.; Kabukcuoglu, Y.; Sokucu, S.; Basilgan, S. The results of non-surgical treatment for unstable distal radius fractures in elderly patients. *Acta Orthop. Traumatol. Turc.* **2009**, *43*, 229–234. [CrossRef]
17. Zengin, E.C.; Ozcan, C.; Aslan, C.; Bulut, T.; Sener, M. Cast immobilization versus volar locking plate fixation of AO type C distal radial fractures in patients aged 60 years and older. *Acta Orthop. Traumatol. Turc.* **2019**, *53*, 15–18. [CrossRef] [PubMed]
18. Christensen, O.M.; Kunov, A.; Hansen, F.F.; Christiansen, T.C.; Krasheninnikoff, M. Occupational therapy and Colles' fractures. *Int. Orthop.* **2001**, *25*, 43–45. [CrossRef]
19. Jakob, M.; Mielke, S.; Keller, H.; Metzger, U. Results of therapy after primary conservative management of distal radius fractures in patients over 65 years of age. *Handchir. Mikrochir. Plast. Chir.* **1999**, *31*, 241–245. [CrossRef] [PubMed]
20. Egol, K.A.; Walsh, M.; Romo-Cardoso, S.; Dorsky, S.; Paksima, N. Distal radial fractures in the elderly: Operative compared with nonoperative treatment. *J. Bone Jt. Surg. Am.* **2011**, *92*, 1851–1857. [CrossRef] [PubMed]
21. Leung, F.; Tu, Y.K.; Chew, W.Y.; Chow, S.P. Comparison of external and percutaneous pin fixation with plate fixation for intra-articular distal radial fractures. A randomized study. *J. Bone Jt. Surg. Am.* **2008**, *90*, 16–22. [CrossRef] [PubMed]
22. Mulders, M.A.M.; Detering, R.; Rikli, D.A.; Rosenwasser, M.P.; Goslings, J.C.; Schep, N.W.L. Association Between Radiological and Patient-Reported Outcome in Adults With a Displaced Distal Radius Fracture: A Systematic Review and Meta-Analysis. *J. Hand Surg. Am.* **2018**, *43*, 710–719. [CrossRef] [PubMed]

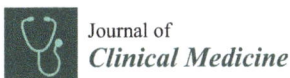

Article

Associations between Early Surgery and Postoperative Outcomes in Elderly Patients with Distal Femur Fracture: A Retrospective Cohort Study

Norio Yamamoto [1,2,3], Hiroyuki Ohbe [4,*], Yosuke Tomita [5], Takashi Yorifuji [2], Mikio Nakajima [4,6], Yusuke Sasabuchi [7], Yuki Miyamoto [4,8], Hiroki Matsui [4], Tomoyuki Noda [9] and Hideo Yasunaga [4]

1. Department of Orthopedic Surgery, Miyamoto Orthopedic Hospital, Okayama 773-8236, Japan; norio-yamamoto@umin.ac.jp
2. Department of Epidemiology, Graduate School of Medicine, Dentistry and Pharmaceutical Sciences, Okayama University, Okayama 700-8558, Japan; yorichan@md.okayama-u.ac.jp
3. Systematic Review Workshop Peer Support Group (SRWS-PSG), Osaka 541-0043, Japan
4. Department of Clinical Epidemiology and Health Economics, School of Public Health, The University of Tokyo, Tokyo 113-0033, Japan; mikioh@ks.kyorin-u.ac.jp (M.N.); mimonism@yahoo.co.jp (Y.M.); ptmatsui-tky@umin.ac.jp (H.M.); yasunagah-tky@umin.ac.jp (H.Y.)
5. Department of Physical Therapy, Faculty of Health Care, Takasaki University of Health and Welfare, Takasaki 370-0033, Japan; tomita-y@takasaki-u.ac.jp
6. Emergency Life-Saving Technique Academy of Tokyo, Foundation for Ambulance Service Development, Tokyo 192-0364, Japan
7. Data Science Center, Jichi Medical University, Tochigi 329-0498, Japan; rhapsody77777@gmail.com
8. Department of Emergency Medicine, Kyoto Prefectural University of Medicine, Kyoto 602-8566, Japan
9. Department of Orthopaedic Surgery and Traumatology, Kawasaki Medical School General Medical Center, Okayama 700-8505, Japan; tnoda@med.kawasaki-m.ac.jp
* Correspondence: hohbey@gmail.com

Abstract: Previous literature has provided conflicting results regarding the associations between early surgery and postoperative outcomes in elderly patients with distal femur fractures. Using data from the Japanese Diagnosis Procedure Combination inpatient database from April 2014 to March 2019, we identified elderly patients who underwent surgery for distal femur fracture within two days of hospital admission (early surgery group) or at three or more days after hospital admission (delayed surgery group). Of 9678 eligible patients, 1384 (14.3%) were assigned to the early surgery group. One-to-one propensity score matched analyses showed no significant difference in 30-day mortality between the early and delayed groups (0.5% versus 0.5%; risk difference, 0.0%; 95% confidence interval, −0.7% to 0.7%). Patients in the early surgery group had significantly lower proportions of the composite outcome (death or postoperative complications), shorter hospital stays, and lower total hospitalization costs than patients in the delayed surgery group. Our results showed that early surgery within two days of hospital admission for geriatric distal femur fracture was not associated with a reduction in 30-day mortality but was associated with reductions in postoperative complications and total hospitalization costs.

Keywords: distal femur fracture; surgical timing; mortality; complications; length of hospital stay; medical costs; database

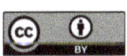

1. Introduction

The incidence of distal femur fracture increases markedly with age [1]. Elderly patients with distal femur fracture were reported to have similar demographic characteristics and outcomes to elderly patients with hip fracture [2]. Elderly patients with distal femur fracture have poor postoperative outcomes because of their many perioperative complications caused by preoperative immobilization [2,3], which is similar to the case for elderly patients with hip fracture [4]. In elderly patients with hip fracture, systematic reviews have demonstrated the beneficial effects of early surgery on postoperative outcomes, including mortality and postoperative complications [5,6].

However, prior studies have provided mixed results regarding the association between the timing of surgery and postoperative mortality in elderly patients with distal femur fracture. Several observational studies found that early surgery was associated with reduced mortality [7–9], while other studies showed no such association [10–13]. One of the reasons for these conflicting results may be small patient numbers used in previous studies (n = 88 to 392) [2,3,7–12]. In addition, confounding factors may not have been sufficiently adjusted for because of the small numbers of patients.

The purpose of the present study was to examine the associations between early surgery and postoperative outcomes in elderly patients with distal femur fractures using data from a nationwide inpatient database. We hypothesized that early surgery is associated with a lower in-hospital mortality, a lower proportion of postoperative complications, and lower medical costs. By clarifying these associations, we suggest a better treatment strategy for geriatric distal femur fracture that will improve patient outcomes and the social economy of healthcare.

2. Materials and Methods

This study was a retrospective cohort study using a national administrative inpatient database under the REporting of studies Conducted using Observational Routinely-collected Data (RECORD) statement reporting guidelines [14]. This study was conducted in accordance with the Declaration of Helsinki and was approved by the Institutional Review Board of The University of Tokyo (approval number: 3501-(3); 25 December 2017). The requirement for informed consent was waived because of the anonymous nature of the data.

2.1. Data Source

We used the Japanese Diagnosis Procedure Combination inpatient database under the management of the Ministry of Health, Labour, and Welfare, which includes administrative claims data and discharge abstracts from more than 1600 acute-care hospitals and covers approximately 90% of all tertiary emergency hospitals in Japan [15]. The database includes information on age, sex, body weight, body height, smoking history, level of consciousness at admission, home medical care use, location before hospital admission, ambulance use, diagnoses recorded with International Classification of Diseases Tenth Revision (ICD-10) codes, treatments recorded with Japanese medical procedure codes, medications administered, discharge status, and hospitalization costs [15]. The diagnoses at admission, comorbidities at admission, and complications during hospitalization are recorded in the database. The attending physicians are required to report objective evidence for their diagnoses for the purpose of cost reimbursement because the diagnostic records are linked to a payment system [15]. In a validation study of the database, the recorded procedures had a high sensitivity and specificity, while the recorded diagnoses had a high specificity and moderate sensitivity [16]. We also used facility information and statistics data from the Survey of Medical Institutions 2015 [17]. We combined these data with the data from the Japanese Diagnosis Procedure Combination inpatient database using specific hospital identifiers. The Survey of Medical Institutions data included the hospital type (academic hospital, teaching hospital, or tertiary emergency hospital) and the number of hospital beds.

2.2. Patient Selection

We searched the database and included patients who: (i) were admitted for distal femur fracture (ICD-10 code, S724), (ii) underwent surgery for distal femur fracture during hospitalization, and (iii) were discharged between April 2014 and March 2019. We excluded patients who: (i) were less than 60 years of age, (ii) were transferred from another hospital, (iii) had subsequent admission for distal femur fracture during the study period, (iv) were admitted to hospitals that could not be linked with data from the Survey of Medical Institutions 2015, (v) were admitted for open distal femur fracture (ICD-10 code, S7241), (vi) were treated with external fixation, (vii) had non-union, (viii) had bone tumor, and (ix) underwent surgery beyond 12 days after hospital admission.

2.3. Main Exposure

The main exposure was timing to surgery after hospital admission. We divided the eligible patients into an early surgery group (surgery within two days of hospital admission) and a delayed surgery group (surgery at three or more days after hospital admission). We defined the timing for early surgery as within two days of hospital admission, because this was considered representative timing for surgery in previous studies on distal femur fracture and hip fracture [7,8,10,18].

2.4. Outcomes

The primary outcome was the all-cause 30-day in-hospital mortality. Patients discharged alive within 30 days of hospital admission were considered alive at 30 days. The 30-day observation period was the common follow-up period used in previous studies [2,19]. The secondary outcomes were all-cause in-hospital mortality, composite outcome of death or postoperative complications during hospitalization, length of hospital stay, length of time from surgery to discharge, and total hospitalization costs [19]. The composite outcome was defined as death during hospitalization or at least one postoperative complication in the post-admission complication diagnoses detected by relevant ICD-10 codes (listed in Supplementary Materials Table S1) [20]. Length of hospital stay was defined as the duration of hospital admission to hospital discharge. The exchange rate for total hospitalization costs was set at 1 US dollar to 110 Japanese yen.

2.5. Covariates

The covariates were age; sex; body mass index at admission; smoking history; level of consciousness at admission using the Japan Coma Scale, which is well correlated with the Glasgow Coma Scale [21]; home medical care use; admission from nursing home; ambulance use, admission on a weekend (Friday to Sunday); calendar year; comorbidities according to the ICD-10 codes (listed in Supplementary Materials Table S2), Charlson comorbidity index [22]; ICD-10-based trauma mortality prediction score [23]; intensive care unit or high care unit use at admission; fracture type of periprosthetic fracture; operative method used for distal femur fracture; and hospital characteristics. We comprehensively selected these covariates as confounders based on existing literature with clinical judgment [18,19].

Body mass index (kg/m^2) was categorized as <18.5, 18.5–24.9, 25.0–29.9, ≥30.0, and missing data. An ICD-10-based trauma mortality prediction score was developed and validated by Wada et al. [23]; it has achieved a high accuracy for mortality prediction in the Japanese Diagnosis Procedure Combination inpatient database. Patients were considered to have severe medical conditions at admission if they were admitted to an intensive care unit or a high care unit on the day of admission [18]. We defined hospital volume as the number of operations for distal femur fracture during the study period.

2.6. Statistical Analysis

A propensity score matching method was applied to compare the outcomes between the early and delayed surgery groups. First, we performed a multivariable logistic regression analysis to estimate the propensity scores for patients receiving early surgery using all covariates listed in Table 1. Briefly, we performed one-to-one nearest-neighbor matching without replacement using a caliper width set at 20% of the standard deviation for the estimated propensity scores [24]. Absolute standardized differences were calculated for all covariates in the unmatched and matched cohorts to confirm the balance of the covariate distributions between the early and delayed surgery groups. The imbalance in the covariate distributions was considered negligible when the absolute standardized differences between the two groups were less than 10% [24]. The propensity score matching was performed using the PSMATCH2 module of STATA (Edwin Leuven and Barbara Sianesi) [25]. We calculated risk differences and their 95% confidence intervals for the outcomes using a generalized linear model with the identity link function and with cluster-robust standard errors for individual hospitals as clusters.

Subsequently, we performed the following four subgroup analyses to estimate the heterogeneity of the treatment effect on the primary outcome in the propensity score-matched cohort: patients with admission on the weekend, patients with a Charlson comorbidity index ≥ 1, patients with a hospital size < 400 beds, and patients with a hospital volume <4.

Categorical variables were presented as numbers and percentages, while continuous variables were presented as means and standard deviations (SDs). All p-values were two-sided and values of $p < 0.05$ were considered statistically significant. All analyses were performed using the STATA/MP 16.0 software (StataCorp, College Station, TX, USA).

Table 1. Patient characteristics before and after propensity score matching.

	Unmatched Cohort			Matched Cohort		
	Early Surgery (≤2 Days) n = 1384	Delayed Surgery (≥3 Days) n = 8294	ASD	Early Surgery (≤2 Days) n = 1382	Delayed Surgery (≥3 Days) n = 1382	ASD
Age (years), mean (SD)	81.3 (9.4)	81.1 (9.3)	2.3	81.3 (9.4)	81.4 (9.5)	0.7
Female sex, n (%)	1227 (88.7)	7515 (90.6)	6.4	1225 (88.6)	1214 (87.8)	2.6
Body mass index (kg/m^2), n (%)						
<18.5	264 (19.1)	1495 (18.0)	2.7	264 (19.1)	262 (19.0)	0.4
18.5–24.9	718 (51.9)	4384 (52.9)	2	716 (51.8)	701 (50.7)	2.2
25.0–29.9	235 (17.0)	1478 (17.8)	2.2	235 (17.0)	252 (18.2)	3.2
≥30	64 (4.6)	399 (4.8)	0.9	64 (4.6)	69 (5.0)	1.7
Missing	103 (7.4)	538 (6.5)	3.8	103 (7.5)	98 (7.1)	1.4
Smoking history, n (%)						
Non-smoker	1189 (85.9)	7080 (85.4)	1.6	1187 (85.9)	1182 (85.5)	1.0
Current/past smoker	96 (6.9)	602 (7.3)	1.3	96 (6.9)	99 (7.2)	0.8
Missing	99 (7.2)	612 (7.4)	0.9	99 (7.2)	101 (7.3)	0.6
Unconscious at admission, n (%)	186 (13.4)	979 (11.8)	4.9	184 (13.3)	180 (13.0)	0.9
Home medical care use, n (%)	107 (7.7)	693 (8.4)	2.3	107 (7.7)	106 (7.7)	0.3
Admission from nursing home, n (%)	246 (17.8)	1281 (15.4)	6.3	245 (17.7)	232 (16.8)	2.5
Ambulance use, n (%)	796 (57.5)	5129 (61.8)	8.8	795 (57.5)	794 (57.5)	0.1
Admission on weekend, n (%)	182 (13.2)	3444 (41.5)	67.1	182 (13.2)	183 (13.2)	0.2
Calendar year, n (%)						
2014	282 (20.4)	1862 (22.4)	5.1	282 (20.4)	274 (19.8)	1.4
2015	284 (20.5)	1750 (21.1)	1.4	284 (20.5)	311 (22.5)	4.8
2016	280 (20.2)	1633 (19.7)	1.4	280 (20.3)	250 (18.1)	5.5
2017	278 (20.1)	1595 (19.2)	2.2	276 (20.0)	291 (21.1)	2.7
2018	260 (18.8)	1454 (17.5)	3.3	260 (18.8)	256 (18.5)	0.7
Comorbidities, n (%)						
Dementia						
Absent	861 (62.2)	5239 (63.2)	2	860 (62.2)	855 (61.9)	0.7
Mild	261 (18.9)	1702 (20.5)	4.2	260 (18.8)	273 (19.8)	2.4
Moderate/severe	262 (18.9)	1353 (16.3)	6.9	262 (19.0)	254 (18.4)	1.5

Table 1. Cont.

		Unmatched Cohort			Matched Cohort		
		Early Surgery (≤2 Days) n = 1384	Delayed Surgery (≥3 Days) n = 8294	ASD	Early Surgery (≤2 Days) n = 1382	Delayed Surgery (≥3 Days) n = 1382	ASD
Myocardial infarction		4 (0.3)	80 (1.0)	8.6	4 (0.3)	5 (0.4)	0.9
Chronic heart failure		69 (5.0)	609 (7.3)	9.8	69 (5.0)	68 (4.9)	0.3
Peripheral vascular disease		11 (0.8)	98 (1.2)	3.9	11 (0.8)	14 (1.0)	2.2
Cerebrovascular disease		120 (8.7)	783 (9.4)	2.7	120 (8.7)	115 (8.3)	1.3
Chronic pulmonary disease		39 (2.8)	286 (3.4)	3.6	39 (2.8)	38 (2.7)	0.4
Rheumatic disease		44 (3.2)	436 (5.3)	10.3	44 (3.2)	37 (2.7)	2.5
Peptic ulcer		40 (2.9)	264 (3.2)	1.7	40 (2.9)	41 (3.0)	0.4
Mild liver dysfunction		46 (3.3)	389 (4.7)	7	46 (3.3)	40 (2.9)	2.2
Diabetes mellitus without complications		225 (16.3)	1571 (18.9)	7.1	224 (16.2)	197 (14.3)	5.1
Diabetes mellitus with complications		21 (1.5)	239 (2.9)	9.3	21 (1.5)	23 (1.7)	1
Hemiplegia		14 (1.0)	57 (0.7)	3.5	14 (1.0)	15 (1.1)	0.8
Renal dysfunction		28 (2.0)	307 (3.7)	10.1	28 (2.0)	41 (3.0)	5.6
Malignancy		37 (2.7)	277 (3.3)	3.9	37 (2.7)	35 (2.5)	0.8
Severe liver dysfunction		3 (0.2)	9 (0.1)	2.7	3 (0.2)	4 (0.3)	1.8
Charlson comorbidity index		0.7 (1.0)	0.9 (1.1)	17.9	0.7 (1.0)	0.7 (0.9)	1.1
Trauma mortality prediction score, mean (SD)		3.6 (1.5)	3.5 (1.5)	4.5	3.6 (1.5)	3.6 (1.7)	1.1
ICU/HCU at admission, n (%)		59 (4.3)	195 (2.4)	10.7	57 (4.1)	56 (4.1)	0.4
Periprosthetic fracture, n (%)		92 (6.6)	672 (8.1)	5.6	92 (6.7)	94 (6.8)	0.6
Operation, n (%)							
Treatment with plating		772 (55.8)	4813 (58.0)	4.5	772 (55.9)	799 (57.8)	3.9
Treatment with nailing		462 (33.4)	2684 (32.4)	2.2	460 (33.3)	429 (31.0)	4.8
Treatment with arthroplasty		9 (0.7)	36 (0.4)	2.9	9 (0.7)	6 (0.4)	3
Treatment unknown		141 (10.2)	761 (9.2)	3.4	141 (10.2)	148 (10.7)	1.7
Academic hospital, n (%)		219 (15.8)	1206 (14.5)	3.6	219 (15.8)	216 (15.6)	0.6
Teaching hospital, n (%)		1064 (76.9)	6298 (75.9)	2.2	1062 (76.8)	1047 (75.8)	2.6
Tertiary hospital, n (%)		447 (32.3)	2226 (26.8)	12	445 (32.2)	457 (33.1)	1.9
Hospital beds, n (%)							
<200		196 (14.2)	1307 (15.8)	4.5	196 (14.2)	202 (14.6)	1.2
200–399		528 (38.2)	3335 (40.2)	4.2	527 (38.1)	532 (38.5)	0.7
400–599		463 (33.5)	2398 (28.9)	9.8	462 (33.4)	458 (33.1)	0.6
600–799		160 (11.6)	900 (10.9)	??	160 (11.6)	152 (11.0)	1.8
>800		37 (2.7)	354 (4.3)	8.7	37 (2.7)	38 (2.7)	0.4
Hospital volume, n (%)		5.0 (2.4)	4.5 (2.4)	19.1	5.0 (2.4)	5.0 (2.6)	1.0

ASD, absolute standardized difference; ICU, intensive care unit; HCU, high care unit. Body mass index was calculated as weight in kilograms divided by height in meters squared.

3. Results

After the application of the exclusion criteria, a total of 9678 patients were eligible for the study (Figure 1). The mean (SD) age was 81.1 (9.3) years, and 90.3% were women. Among the eligible patients, 1384 (14.3%) were assigned to the early surgery group and 8294 (85.7%) were assigned to the delayed surgery group. Surgery on day 4 after hospital admission (15.4%) was the most common timing (Figure 2). The mean (SD) timing for surgery after hospital admission was 1.8 (0.4) days in the early surgery group and 5.9 (2.3) days in the delayed surgery group.

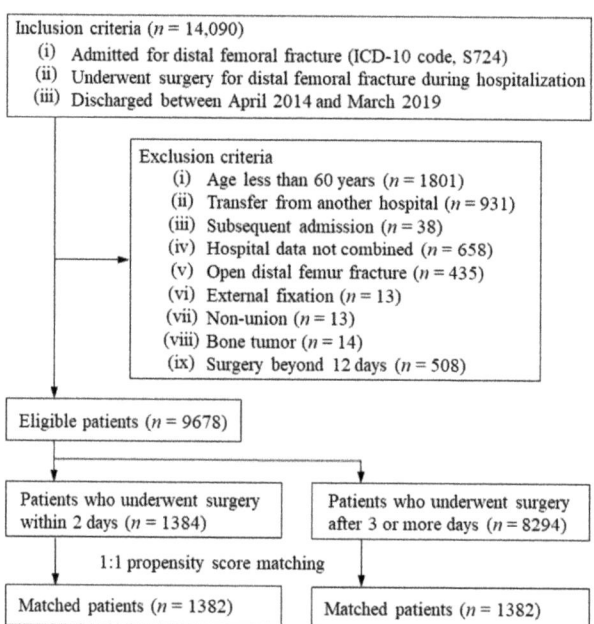

Figure 1. Flow chart for patient inclusion and exclusion.

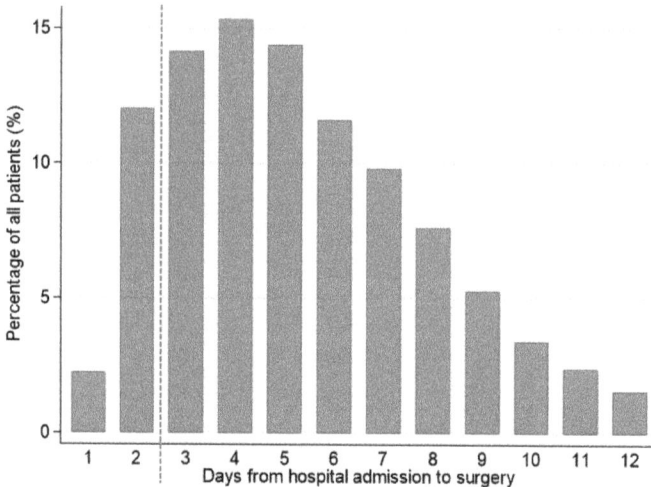

Figure 2. Days from hospital admission to surgery. The dotted line shows the border between the early and delayed surgery groups.

Table 1 shows the patient characteristics in the two groups before and after propensity score matching. Before propensity score matching, patients in the early surgery group tended to have intensive care unit or high care unit use at admission and be admitted to a hospital with a high hospital volume, while patients in the delayed surgery group tended to have admission on the weekend, comorbidities of rheumatic diseases and renal dysfunction, and a higher Charlson comorbidity index. The proportions of periprosthetic fracture were 6.6% in the early surgery group and 8.1% in the delayed surgery group. After propensity score matching, the patient characteristics were found to be well-balanced between the two groups (Supplementary Materials Figure S1). The propensity score distributions before and after propensity score matching are shown in Supplementary Materials Figures S2 and S3.

Table 2 shows the outcomes before and after propensity score matching. Before propensity score matching, 30-day mortality in the early and delayed surgery groups was 0.9% and 0.5%, respectively. After propensity score matching, there was no significant difference in 30-day mortality between the two groups (risk difference, 0.0%; 95% CI, −0.7% to 0.7%). There was no significant difference in in-hospital mortality between the two groups. The composite outcome was significantly less common in the early surgery group compared with the delayed surgery group (13.5% versus 17.1%; risk difference, −3.7%; 95% CI, −6.5% to −0.9%). Regarding postoperative complications, acute coronary syndrome was significantly less frequent in the early surgery group compared with the delayed surgery group (Supplementary Materials Table S3). Patients in the early surgery group had a significantly shorter length of hospital stay (risk difference, −8.4 days; 95% CI, −11.8 to −5.0 days), a shorter length of time from surgery to discharge (risk difference, −4.5 days; 95% CI, −7.9 to −1.0 days), and lower total hospitalization costs (risk difference, −2101 US dollars; 95% CI, −2991 to −1212 US dollars) than patients in the delayed surgery group.

Table 2. Outcomes in the original unmatched cohort and matched cohort.

	Unmatched Cohort		Matched Cohort			
	Early Surgery (≤2 Days) n = 1384	Delayed Surgery (≥3 Days) n = 8294	Early Surgery (≤2 Days) n = 1382	Delayed Surgery (≥3 Days) n = 1382	Risk Difference (95% CI)	p-Value
Primary outcome						
30-day mortality, n (%)	12 (0.9)	41 (0.5)	12 (0.9)	12 (0.9)	0.0 (−0.7 to 0.7)	>0.999
Secondary outcomes						
In-hospital mortality, n (%)	21 (1.5)	106 (1.3)	21 (1.5)	21 (1.5)	0.0 (−0.9 to 0.9)	>0.999
Composite outcome, n (%)	187 (13.5)	1383 (16.7)	186 (13.5)	237 (17.1)	−3.7 (−6.5 to −0.9)	0.007
Length of hospital stay (days), mean (SD)	42 (42)	53 (36)	42 (42)	50 (36)	−8.4 (−11.8 to −5.0)	<0.001
Length of time from surgery to discharge (days), mean (SD)	41 (42)	48 (36)	41 (42)	45 (36)	−4.5 (−7.9 to −1.0)	0.011
In-hospital costs (US dollars), mean (SD)	16,099 (10,721)	18,844 (10,803)	16,101 (10,729)	18,202 (9859)	−2101 (−2991 to −1212)	<0.001

Hospital costs were calculated using the exchange rate of 1 US dollar = 110 Japanese yen.

The four subgroup analyses showed no significant differences in 30-day mortality between the two groups and the results were consistent with those in the main analysis (Table 3).

Table 3. Subgroup analyses for 30-day mortality in the propensity score-matched cohort.

	Early Surgery	Delayed Surgery	Risk Difference (95% CI)	p-Value
Admission on weekend				
30-day mortality, n (%)	1/182 (0.5)	2/183 (1.1)	−0.5 (−2.4 to 1.3)	0.571
Charlson comorbidity index ≥ 1				
30-day mortality, n (%)	4/652 (0.6)	6/670 (0.9)	−0.3 (−1.2 to 0.7)	0.552
Hospital size < 400 beds				
30-day mortality, n (%)	5/723 (0.7)	8/734 (1.1)	−0.4 (−1.4 to 0.6)	0.415
Hospital volume < 4				
30-day mortality, n (%)	5/548 (0.9)	5/578 (0.9)	−0.0 (−1.1 to 1.2)	0.933

4. Discussion

The present study was a large-scale investigation of the effectiveness of early surgery for distal femur fracture in elderly patients using data from a nationwide inpatient database in Japan. The results showed that early surgery within two days of hospital admission was not associated with a reduction in 30-day mortality but was significantly associated with reductions in postoperative complications, length of hospital stay, and total hospitalization costs.

Early surgery did not have clinical effectiveness in reducing 30-day mortality. This finding was consistent with that of previous studies on geriatric distal femur fracture that assessed outcomes with covariate adjustment using a multivariable logistic regression model [10,12]. However, the finding that early surgery in elderly patients with distal femur fracture did not reduce 30-day mortality differed from results gained in elderly patients with hip fracture [19].

Regardless of the timing of surgery, the 30-day mortality in the present study was less than 1% and much lower than the rates of 3% to 8% seen in previous studies on geriatric distal femur fracture [2,7,10,11]. However, the low 30-day mortality was consistent with the 30-day mortality rates in geriatric hip fracture studies that used data from large databases (0.6% to 1.0% in Japan; 5.8% to 6.5% in Canada; 6.3% in Sweden) [3,18–20]. In our cohort with a very low 30-day mortality, early surgery did not have clinical effectiveness for 30-day mortality.

Early surgery was associated with better clinical outcomes and lower costs, as demonstrated by the lower frequency of the composite outcome, shorter length of hospital stay, and lower total hospitalization costs. Early surgery was associated with fewer postoperative complications, consistent with a previous study [8]. Elderly patients are vulnerable and the prevention of postoperative complications may be associated with favorable functional outcomes and improved quality of life [26]. Similar to the case for geriatric hip fracture patients, this may have arisen because early surgery in geriatric distal femur fracture patients enabled the early initiation of rehabilitation, increasing the chance for better functional recovery, resulting in fewer postoperative complications, and having positive impacts on hospital stay and total hospitalization costs [18,27]. The mechanism for the benefits of early surgery on functional outcomes should be addressed in future studies.

The present study had several strengths. To the best of our knowledge, this was the first large-scale study to demonstrate the effectiveness of early surgery for distal femur fracture in elderly patients on in-hospital mortality, postoperative complications, length of hospital stay, and total hospitalization costs. The study was able to compensate for limitations of previous studies that arose from their small sample sizes and low external validity due to the use of single-center data. Targeting the performance of surgery within two days of admission represents a significant change in practice, because 85.7% of the patients in the study did not receive surgery within two days. The early timing of surgery in hip fracture is already recognized worldwide as a quality indicator for the assessment of hospital performance; therefore, the results of the present study may inform existing distal femur fracture care guidelines and policies.

This study also has some limitations. First, this study may have immortal time biases for the two time points—namely, the time from hospital admission to surgery and time after early discharge [28]. In this study, time from hospital admission to surgery was considered immortal because the performance of surgery implied that the patients survived until surgery. Therefore, the delayed surgery group had a guaranteed survival advantage over the early surgery group because of the immortal time from hospital admission to surgery. Meanwhile, time after early discharge was considered immortal because patients who were discharged alive were considered to remain alive at 30 days in this study. Therefore, the early surgery group had a guaranteed survival advantage over the delayed surgery group because of the immortal time after early discharge. Second, this observational study using a real-world database unmeasured confounding variables. Thus, individual surgeons decided the timing of surgery according to the criteria in their own settings, which would lead to confounding by indication. We attempted to control for possible confounding factors described in previous reports, including covariates of patient and surgeon-hospital characteristics. However, we were unable to obtain detailed data on the distal femur fracture type and the time from injury to admission. We assumed that the day of injury was the same as the day of hospital admission. The appropriate timing for surgery needs to be further investigated with better time resolution, such as hours, instead of number of days from admission to surgery in future studies. Third, the Japanese Diagnosis Procedure Combination inpatient database does not contain links to data after discharge. Therefore, we could not evaluate the outcomes after longer follow-up (90 or 365 days). Previous studies showed that delayed surgery by more than two days in geriatric distal femur fracture patients was significantly associated with increased 1-year mortality [7,8]. In addition, the assumption that patients who were discharged alive within 30 days of hospital admission remained alive at 30 days could lead to misclassification for 30-day in-hospital mortality. Therefore, further studies are needed to examine the effectiveness of early surgery on mortality with longer follow-up periods. Fourth, there is a lack of external validity because all the data were obtained from a Japanese database. It remains unclear whether the results of the study can be generalized to other countries with different patient characteristics and healthcare systems.

5. Conclusions

This nationwide observational study suggested that early surgery within two days of hospital admission was not associated with a reduction in 30-day mortality in patients with geriatric distal femur fracture. However, early surgery was associated with decreased postoperative complications and lower total hospitalization costs.

Supplementary Materials: The following are available online at https://www.mdpi.com/article/10.3390/jcm10245800/s1, Figure S1: Distribution of propensity scores before matching, Figure S2: Distribution of propensity scores after matching; Figure S3: Kissing plot in propensity score matching, Table S1: International Classification of Diseases Tenth Revision (ICD-10) codes for complications, Table S2: International Classification of Diseases Tenth Revision (ICD-10) codes for comorbidities, Table S3: Postoperative complications in the original unmatched cohort and matched cohort.

Author Contributions: Conceptualization, N.Y., H.O., Y.T., M.N., Y.S. and T.N.; methodology, N.Y., H.O., Y.T. and T.Y.; software, H.O.; formal analysis, H.O., N.Y. and Y.T.; resources, H.O.; data curation, Y.M. and H.M.; writing—original draft, N.Y., H.O. and Y.T.; writing—review and editing, N.Y., H.O. and H.Y.; visualization, N.Y., H.O. and Y.T.; supervision, H.Y.; project administration, H.O.; funding acquisition, H.Y. All authors have read and agreed to the published version of the manuscript.

Funding: This work was supported by grants from the Ministry of Health, Labour and Welfare, Japan (21AA2007 and 20AA2005) and the Ministry of Education, Culture, Sports, Science and Technology, Japan (20H03907).

Institutional Review Board Statement: This study was performed in accordance with the amended Declaration of Helsinki and was approved by the Institutional Review Board of The University of Tokyo (approval number: 3501-(3); 25 December 2017).

Informed Consent Statement: The review board waived the requirement for informed consent because of the anonymous nature of the data. No information describing individual patients, hospitals, or treating physicians was obtained.

Data Availability Statement: The datasets analyzed during the current study are not publicly available owing to contracts with the hospitals providing data to the database.

Conflicts of Interest: The authors declare no conflict of interest.

References

1. Lundin, N.; Huttunen, T.T.; Enocson, A.; Marcano, A.I.; Felländer-Tsai, L.; Berg, H.E. Epidemiology and mortality of pelvic and femur fractures-a nationwide register study of 417,840 fractures in Sweden across 16 years: Diverging trends for potentially lethal fractures. *Acta Orthop.* **2021**, *92*, 323–328. [CrossRef]
2. Jennison, T.; Divekar, M. Geriatric distal femoral fractures: A retrospective study of 30 day mortality. *Injury* **2019**, *50*, 444–447. [CrossRef] [PubMed]
3. Wolf, O.; Mukka, S.; Ekelund, J.; Möller, M.; Hailer, N.P. How deadly is a fracture distal to the hip in the elderly? An observational cohort study of 11,799 femoral fractures in the Swedish Fracture Register. *Acta Orthop.* **2021**, *92*, 40–46. [CrossRef]
4. Carpintero, P.; Caeiro, J.R.; Carpintero, R.; Morales, A.; Silva, S.; Mesa, M. Complications of hip fractures: A review. *World J. Orthop.* **2014**, *5*, 402–411. [CrossRef]
5. Welford, P.; Jones, C.S.; Davies, G.; Kunutsor, S.K.; Costa, M.L.; Sayers, A.; Whitehouse, M.R. The association between surgical fixation of hip fractures within 24 hours and mortality: A systematic review and meta-analysis. *Bone Jt. J.* **2021**, *103*, 1176–1186. [CrossRef] [PubMed]
6. Klestil, T.; Röder, C.; Stotter, C.; Winkler, B.; Nehrer, S.; Lutz, M.; Klerings, I.; Wagner, G.; Gartlehner, G.; Nussbaumer-Streit, B. Impact of timing of surgery in elderly hip fracture patients: A systematic review and meta-analysis. *Sci. Rep.* **2018**, *8*, 13933. [CrossRef]
7. Myers, P.; Laboe, P.; Johnson, K.J.; Fredericks, P.D.; Crichlow, R.J.; Maar, D.C.; Weber, T.G. Patient Mortality in Geriatric Distal Femur Fractures. *J. Orthop. Trauma.* **2018**, *32*, 111–115. [CrossRef]
8. Moloney, G.B.; Pan, T.; Van Eck, C.F.; Patel, D.; Tarkin, I. Geriatric distal femur fracture: Are we underestimating the rate of local and systemic complications? *Injury* **2016**, *47*, 1732–1736. [CrossRef]
9. Streubel, P.N.; Ricci, W.M.; Wong, A.; Gardner, M.J. Mortality after distal femur fractures in elderly patients. *Clin. Orthop. Relat. Res.* **2011**, *469*, 1188–1196. [CrossRef] [PubMed]
10. Nyholm, A.M.; Palm, H.; Kallemose, T.; Troelsen, A.; Gromov, K.; DFDB Collaborators. No association between surgical delay and mortality following distal femoral fractures. A study from the danish fracture database collaborators. *Injury* **2017**, *48*, 2833–2837. [CrossRef]
11. Larsen, P.; Ceccotti, A.A.; Elsoe, R. High mortality following distal femur fractures: A cohort study including three hundred and two distal femur fractures. *Int. Orthop.* **2020**, *44*, 173–177. [CrossRef]
12. Brogan, K.; Akehurst, H.; Bond, E.; Gee, C.; Poole, W.; Shah, N.N.; McChesney, S.; Nicol, S. Delay to surgery does not affect survival following osteoporotic femoral fractures. *Injury* **2016**, *47*, 2294–2299. [CrossRef] [PubMed]
13. Smolle, M.A.; Hörlesberger, N.; Maurer-Ertl, W.; Puchwein, P.; Seibert, F.J.; Leithner, A. Periprosthetic fractures of hip and knee-A morbidity and mortality analysis. *Injury* **2021**, *52*, 3483–3488. [CrossRef] [PubMed]
14. Benchimol, E.I.; Smeeth, L.; Guttmann, A.; Harron, K.; Moher, D.; Petersen, I.; Sørensen, H.T.; von Elm, E.; Langan, S.M. The REporting of studies Conducted using Observational Routinely-collected health Data (RECORD) statement. *PLoS Med.* **2015**, *12*, e1001885. [CrossRef] [PubMed]
15. Yasunaga, H. Real World Data in Japan: Chapter II the Diagnosis Procedure Combination Database. *Ann. Clin. Epidemiol.* **2019**, *1*, 76–79. [CrossRef]
16. Yamana, H.; Moriwaki, M.; Horiguchi, H.; Kodan, M.; Fushimi, K.; Yasunaga, H. Validity of diagnoses, procedures, and laboratory data in Japanese administrative data. *J. Epidemiol.* **2017**, *27*, 476–482. [CrossRef]
17. The Ministry of Health, Labour and Welfare, Japan: Statistical Surveys 2015. Available online: https://www.mhlw.go.jp/stf/seisakunitsuite/bunya/open_data.html (accessed on 24 September 2021).
18. Sasabuchi, Y.; Matsui, H.; Lefor, A.K.; Fushimi, K.; Yasunaga, H. Timing of surgery for hip fractures in the elderly: A retrospective cohort study. *Injury* **2018**, *49*, 1848–1854. [CrossRef]
19. Pincus, D.; Ravi, B.; Wasserstein, D.; Huang, A.; Paterson, J.M.; Nathens, A.B.; Kreder, H.J.; Jenkinson, R.J.; Wodchis, W.P. Association Between Wait Time and 30-Day Mortality in Adults Undergoing Hip Fracture Surgery. *JAMA* **2017**, *318*, 1994–2003. [CrossRef]
20. Ogawa, T.; Yoshii, T.; Moriwaki, M.; Morishita, S.; Oh, Y.; Miyatake, K.; Nazarian, A.; Shiba, K.; Okawa, A.; Fushimi, K.; et al. Association between Hemiarthroplasty vs Total Hip Arthroplasty and Major Surgical Complications among Patients with Femoral Neck Fracture. *J. Clin. Med.* **2020**, *9*, 3203. [CrossRef]
21. Shigematsu, K.; Nakano, H.; Watanabe, Y. The eye response test alone is sufficient to predict stroke outcome—Reintroduction of Japan Coma Scale: A cohort study. *BMJ Open.* **2013**, *3*, e002736. [CrossRef]
22. Charlson, M.E.; Pompei, P.; Ales, K.L.; MacKenzie, C.R. A new method of classifying prognostic comorbidity in longitudinal studies: Development and validation. *J. Chronic. Dis.* **1987**, *40*, 373–383. [CrossRef]
23. Wada, T.; Yasunaga, H.; Yamana, H.; Matsui, H.; Matsubara, T.; Fushimi, K.; Nakajima, S. Development and validation of a new ICD-10-based trauma mortality prediction scoring system using a Japanese national inpatient database. *Inj. Prev.* **2017**, *23*, 263–267. [CrossRef] [PubMed]
24. Austin, P.C. Balance diagnostics for comparing the distribution of baseline covariates between treatment groups in propensity-score matched samples. *Stat. Med.* **2009**, *28*, 3083–3107. [CrossRef]
25. Edwin, L.; Barbara, S. *PSMATCH2: Stata Module to Perform Full Mahalanobis and Propensity Score Matching, Common Support Graphing, and Covariate Imbalance Testing*; Statistical Software Components: Boston, MA, USA, 2003.

26. Kammerlander, C.; Riedmüller, P.; Gosch, M.; Zegg, M.; Kammerlander-Knauer, U.; Schmid, R.; Roth, T. Functional outcome and mortality in geriatric distal femoral fractures. *Injury* **2012**, *43*, 1096–1101. [CrossRef] [PubMed]
27. Brox, W.T.; Roberts, K.C.; Taksali, S.; Wright, D.G.; Wixted, J.J.; Tubb, C.C.; Patt, J.C.; Templeton, K.J.; Dickman, E.; Adler, R.A.; et al. The American Academy of Orthopaedic Surgeons Evidence-Based Guideline on Management of Hip Fractures in the Elderly. *J. Bone Jt. Surg. Am.* **2015**, *97*, 1196–1199. [CrossRef]
28. Lévesque, L.E.; Hanley, J.A.; Kezouh, A.; Suissa, S. Problem of immortal time bias in cohort studies: Example using statins for preventing progression of diabetes. *BMJ* **2010**, *340*, 907–911. [CrossRef]

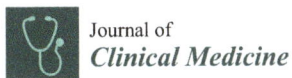

Article

Family Caregivers' Experiences with Tele-Rehabilitation for Older Adults with Hip Fracture

Patrocinio Ariza-Vega [1,2,3], Rafael Prieto-Moreno [2,3,*], Herminia Castillo-Pérez [4], Virginia Martínez-Ruiz [5,6,7], Dulce Romero-Ayuso [1] and Maureen C. Ashe [8]

1. Department of Physiotherapy, University of Granada, 18016 Granada, Spain; pariza@ugr.es (P.A.-V.); dulceromero@ugr.es (D.R.-A.)
2. Physical Medicine and Rehabilitation Service, Biohealth Research Institute, Virgen de las Nieves University Hospital, 18012 Granada, Spain
3. PA-HELP "Physical Activity for HEaLth Promotion" Research Group, Department of Physical and Sport Education, Faculty of Sports Sciences, University of Granada, 18071 Granada, Spain
4. Ciudad de Berja Nursing Home, Berja, 04760 Almería, Spain; hermicp11@gmail.com
5. Department of Preventive Medicine and Public Health, School of Medicine, University of Granada, 18016 Granada, Spain; virmruiz@ugr.es
6. Center for Biomedical Research in Network of Epidemiology and Public Health (CIBERESP), 28029, Madrid, Spain
7. Instituto de Investigación Biosanitaria de Granada (ibs.GRANADA), 18014 Granada, Spain
8. Centre for Hip Health and Mobility, Department of Family Practice, University of British Columbia, Vancouver, BC V5Z 1M9, Canada; maureen.ashe@ubc.ca
* Correspondence: rafapriemor@gmail.com

Abstract: Background: There is a knowledge gap for implementing tele-rehabilitation (telerehab) after hip fracture. We recently conducted a clinical trial (ClinicalTrials.gov Identifier: NCT02968589) to test a novel online family caregiver-supported rehabilitation program for older adults with hip fracture, called @ctivehip. In this qualitative substudy, our objective was to use semi-structured interviews to explore family caregivers experience with the telerehab program. Methods: Twenty-one family caregivers were interviewed between three and six months after the older adults completed @ctivehip. One occupational therapist with research and clinical experience, but not involved in the main trial, conducted and transcribed the interviews. We conducted a multi-step content analysis, and two authors completed one coding cycle and two recoding cycles. Results: Family caregivers who enrolled in @ctivehip were satisfied with the program, stated it was manageable to use, and perceived benefits for older adults' functional recovery after hip fracture. They also suggested improvements for the program content, such as more variety with exercises, and increased monitoring by health professionals. Conclusions: This work extends existing literature and generates research hypotheses for future studies to test telerehab content and program implementation.

Keywords: tele-rehabilitation; hip fracture; older people; family caregiver; information and communication technology

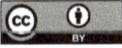

1. Introduction

Loss of functional independence [1], decreased social participation [1], and reduced quality of life [2] are some of the main consequences of hip fractures. Early hospital rehabilitation with follow-up post-discharge can support older adults' recovery of function [3]. Family caregivers play an essential role in helping older patients to complete activities of daily living (ADL) in the home setting [4,5]. The sudden and unexpected nature of hip fractures can impact both older adults and family caregivers, who as a result can experience increased stress and burden [6]. As a result, hip fracture is associated with worse overall health status in family caregivers [7]. These factors indicate a need for new post-discharge management strategies [8,9] to improve older adults' function post-hip fracture and reduce caregiver stress [10].

There are barriers to delivering rehabilitation after hip fracture, such as limited access to health professionals after discharge to home. Telerehabilitation (telerehab) is a promising management strategy to support recovery after discharge, and may be especially important in rural and remote areas with limited access to in-person rehabilitation [11]. Of note, there has been an increase in remote delivery of health care because of the SARS-CoV-2 (COVID-19) pandemic [12]. Based on previous studies, telerehab for musculoskeletal injuries or conditions were effective for improving physical function, quality of life, and psychological factors [13–16]. However, there is limited evidence for: (i) the effect of telerehab for older adults after hip fracture [17], and (ii) the inclusion of family caregivers in telerehab for hip fracture [18]. We focus on family caregivers to support older people using information and communication technologies (ICT), and to provide support for the telerehab program. Involving family caregivers in telerehab also addresses their request for more information on the recovery process [19]. Thus, we aimed to address these knowledge gaps [17] by designing and testing a telerehab program called @ctivehip for older adults with hip fracture and their family caregivers.

We previously published results from the main trial [20]—a choice-based multiple methods clinical trial comparing @ctivehip telerehab with home-based in-person rehabilitation for functional recovery of older adults with hip fracture [21]. The @ctivehip intervention consisted of: (i) web-based information to increase family caregivers' knowledge and skill development; (ii) a supported exercise and ADL program for older adults (delivered by the family caregiver); (iii) a specific section on family caregivers' health; and (iv) an option for family caregivers to video conference with health professionals.

The aim of the present exploratory study was to describe family caregivers experience with the @ctivehip telerehab program. We anticipated that family caregivers' feedback could be used to refine the intervention by identifying implementation opportunities and challenges from a person-centered approach.

2. Materials and Methods

2.1. Design

This was a substudy of a multiple methods clinical trial (Clinical Registration NCT0296 8589). We previously published the results of the main study (quantitative findings, primary outcome functional level) [20], and patients' and family caregivers' overall experience with hip fractures (qualitative findings) [22]. In this second qualitative study, we aimed to synthesize experiences of the family caregivers of older adults with hip fracture enrolled in the @ctivehip telerehab program. We were guided by the principles of interpretive description [23] when designing the interview guide, conducting interviews, and synthesizing findings.

2.2. Participants

A description of participant recruitment is provided elsewhere [21]; please see Figure 1. At the final assessment of the main trial (conducted at three months after hip fracture surgery), family caregivers were invited to participate in semi-structured interviews. For the present study, we summarize responses only from participants who requested @ctivehip (e.g., the intervention group). There were 23 family caregivers who agreed to participate and signed the study consent form. When we telephoned family caregivers three months later, two family caregivers did not answer the telephone after several attempts. Thus, 21 family caregivers representing 21 older adults with hip fracture were interviewed for the present study.

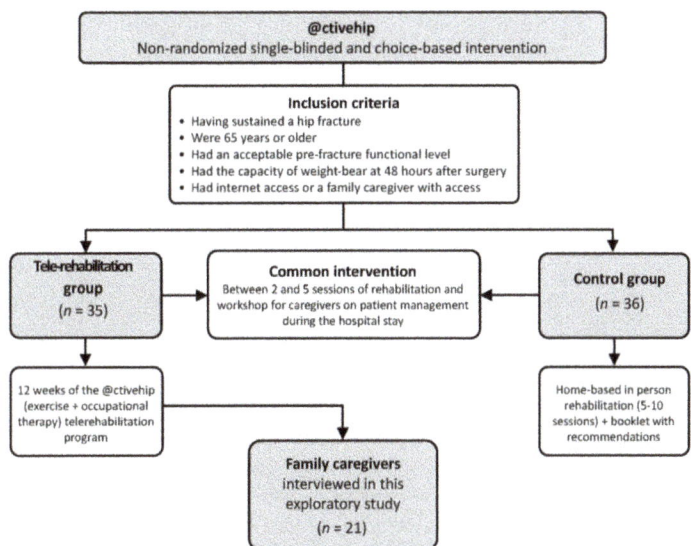

Figure 1. Flowchart for caregivers recruitment.

2.3. Semi-Structured Interviews

Between October 2017 and December 2018 an occupational therapist (OT), with related clinical experience but not involved in the main clinical trial, conducted the telephone interviews between three and six months after participants finished the main clinical trial. The virtual interviews were scheduled when family caregivers were at home, to minimize potential distractions. The OT recorded and transcribed the interviews within two days after each interview and kept field notes for reference during the analysis process. The interview guide is provided in Appendix A. During the interviews, the OT encouraged discussion using prompts such as "please explain how you did it", "tell me more about it", and follow-up questions to encourage participants to provide more details of their experience. To explore family caregivers' perceptions about the utility of, and satisfaction with, the telerehab program we asked participants to rate their experience using a scale of 0–10 points (0 = not useful and 10 = very useful; 0 = lowest level of satisfaction and 10 = highest level of satisfaction). On average, interviews lasted 18 (range 1–22) min.

2.4. Data Analysis

We followed the recommendations of Graneheim and Lundman [24] to conduct a multi-step content analysis. Two authors P.A.-V. and R.P.-M. first read the transcripts (in Spanish) several times. Following this they met three times to review data, create a coding framework, and synthesize findings. The process involved one coding cycle and two re-coding cycles [25] to increase confidence in the response classification. During this process, the authors identified meaning units, sorted them into subcategories, and then categories. Data (categories and quotes) were translated into English by the first and third authors (native Spanish speakers with proficiency in English) and reviewed by the last author (native English speaker). There was lengthy discussion between authors to ensure the cultural context was considered.

2.5. Trustworthiness of the Findings

We included several processes to increase trustworthiness of study findings [26]. First, the OT who conducted the interviews was experienced in the management of older adults with hip fracture, however they were not involved in the main clinical trial. Second, the interviews were recorded (with permission) and the interviewer took field notes. They also checked in with participants during the interview to clarify responses. Third, data were transcribed by the OT and one assistant within two days of the interview. Fourth, an audit trail was maintained throughout the process to summarize analysis steps and decisions. Fifth, a representative subgroup of participants checked a summary from emerging themes and quotes, and they were invited to add or change information. Finally, investigator triangulation was applied [27]. The first author (dual-trained physical therapist (PT) and OT with a doctoral degree) and third author (experienced OT with a research MSc) analyzed the data. Following this, the last author (PT and professor with a doctoral degree) reviewed the findings and discussed them multiple times with the first author.

We used NVivo 10 (QSR International, Doncaster, Australia) during data analysis to assist with data management (i.e., managing files, coding process, and analysis). We present participants age and scores for telerehab program utility and satisfaction using median (q25–q75) values.

3. Results

3.1. Demographics Characteristics

Twenty one family caregivers (16 women and five men; median (q25–q75) age 50 (43–54) years) participated in the present study. Most family caregivers were the offspring of the patients with a hip fracture (18/21; 86%) supported by other family caregivers (15/21; 71%), who lived with the patient (14/21; 67%), and more than half were also working (14/21; 67%) part-time or full-time. The median age of older adults with hip fracture was 78 (73–82) years; most were women (76%), and their functional level at the end of the telerehab program (12 weeks) was similar to their pre-fracture functional level assessed through the Functional Independence Measure (FIM) [28]. A detailed description of family caregivers' characteristics is provided in Table 1.

Table 1. Caregivers' characteristics.

Age	Gender	Relationship to Patient	Living with the Patient	Employment	Support of Other Caregivers (Number)
44	Woman	Daughter	No	Part-time	Yes (2)
53	Woman	Wife	Yes	Unemployed	Yes (1)
64	Woman	Daughter	Yes	Unemployed	Yes (2)
56	Woman	Daughter	Yes	Part-time	No (0)
42	Woman	Daughter	Yes	Part-time	Yes (3)
41	Woman	Daughter	Yes	Full-time	Yes (1)
38	Man	Son	No	Full-time	No (0)
40	Woman	Daughter	No	Full-time	Yes (1)
50	Woman	Daughter	Yes	Unemployed	No (0)
45	Woman	Daughter	Yes	Unemployed	Yes (2)
54	Woman	Niece	Yes	Full-time	No (0)
55	Woman	Niece	No	Part-time	No (0)
53	Woman	Daughter	No	Unemployed	Yes (2)
50	Man	Son	No	Unemployed	Yes (2)
54	Woman	Daughter	Yes	Part-time	Yes (1)
52	Woman	Daughter in law	Yes	Unemployed	No (0)
43	Man	Soon	Yes	Full-time	Yes (1)
44	Woman	Daughter	Yes	Full-time	Yes (1)
53	Man	Son	Yes	Part-time	Yes (2)
51	Man	Son	No	Full-time	Yes (3)
40	Woman	Daughter	Yes	Full-time	Yes (2)

3.2. Adherence to the Telerehab Program

Ten of twenty-one caregivers completed the program as intended (high fidelity at 12 weeks), and an additional six participants completed 8 weeks or more of the program

(76% in total). Half of the caregivers (10/21; 48%) stated their older family member completed the program, and then continued doing the exercises for a few more months. However, the remaining caregivers reported their family member stopped doing the exercises before the end of the 12 weeks. Most family caregivers (20/21; 95%) expressed 12 weeks was long enough to learn the program, or they believed their family member did not require rehabilitation beyond 12 weeks.

> " . . . We spent about one month doing the exercises with her. Afterwards she continued doing the exercises alone, but I think she did not do them for twelve weeks . . . She stopped when she felt she did not need to do [any] more . . . " (Caregiver 8)

The caregivers with lower adherence to the telerehab program (5/21) were all women, older than 50 years of age (range; 52–56 years) and had no support from other caregivers (4/5; 80%) or the support of one additional caregiver to help the patient with ADLs (1; 20%). From the five caregivers with lower program adherence, two were unemployed, two worked part-time, and one worked full-time.

3.3. Categories

There were two categories generated during data analysis: (1) the telerehab program was perceived to be useful for older adults' functional recovery without being onerous for family caregivers; and (2) there was room for improvement in the telerehab program. A visual summary of the main findings is provided in Figure 2.

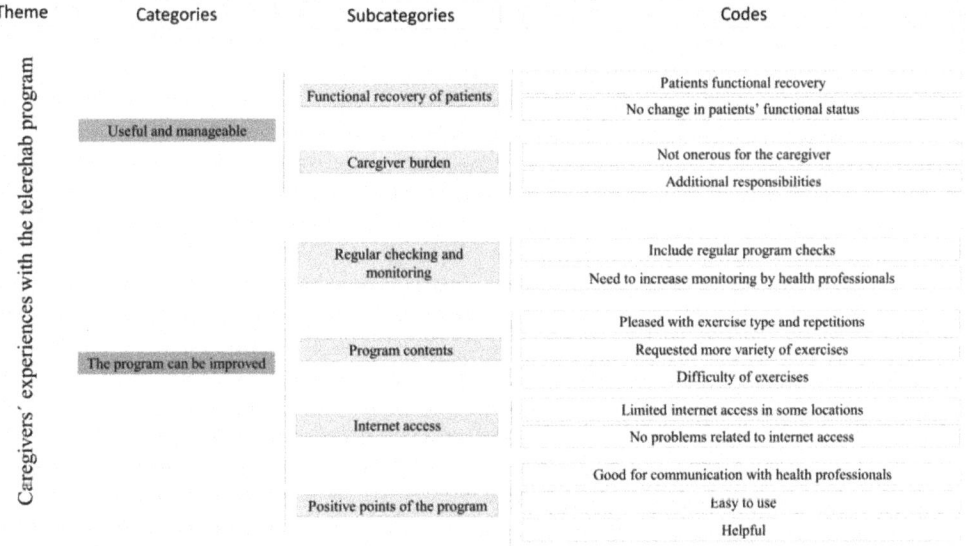

Figure 2. Caregivers experience with the telerehab program.

3.3.1. The telerehab clinical program: Useful and manageable

Caregiver support was essential for implementing @ctivehip. Overall, family caregivers were highly satisfied with the telerehab program and rated it useful (median (q25, q75): 8 (8-9)/10 points for utility and 9 (8–9.5)/10 points for satisfaction. Though the use of the program required more time and additional responsibilities for the caregivers, most participants stated there was no additional caregiving burden with using @ctivehip:

"... At first, it took a while but then we [created a] habit. I came home from work and connected the tablet. I helped her with the exercises that seemed more difficult." (Caregiver 12)

"... You need to [make time] to use the program ... my brother and I organized [it] between us and it was not too much burden ... " (Caregiver 15)

Although most caregivers noted improvement in patients' health after using @ctivehip, a few family caregivers reported no change in their family member's function with the program:

"... She could almost not walk and now she is completely independent ... " (Caregiver 15)

"... We started in the hospital, then he spent 3 months in my house doing the exercises and then he went home and continued doing them but without [the] internet ... He already memorized the exercises and keeps doing them because he says they are good for him and that the doctor told him he could continue doing them every day ... I would say that he is better than before the surgery ... " (Caregiver 4)

"... No, she won't be the same person anymore ... She is having a setback in general ... " (Caregiver 3)

3.3.2. Room for improvement

Based on the caregivers experience, there was an identified need to develop new approaches for health professionals to support them during the recovery process. Study participants provided valuable insights for how best to implement @ctivehip in the future. Although family caregivers were aware they could request a video-conference session with a health professional, they preferred a regular check-in within the telerehab program to verify everything was proceeding as planned. Some family caregivers further suggested regular health professional monitoring to support older adults' confidence with completing exercises:

"... I [missed] that the staff would call us from time to time to ask us how we were doing and to test if we were doing the exercises properly. ... I know we could have called to ask for a video conference, but we felt in some way alone ... " (Caregiver 13)

There were some differences among suggestions to improve the program content. Many family caregivers suggested the program should include more variety in the exercises to reduce the risk of boredom, and possibly increase older adults motivation. In contrast, some family caregivers were pleased with the repetition of the exercises, as it made them easier to remember:

"... All the exercises were very similar and became very monotonous and repetitive after the first week ... " (Caregiver 18)

"... I'm not an expert but I believe the exercises were [good] because my father memorized them every week and if he did not have internet one day, he would do it himself ... " (Caregiver 16)

Family caregivers rated the program's level of difficulty as either low or average. Nevertheless, eight family caregivers stated their family member avoided using weights to perform some exercises due to low confidence:

"... She did not do some exercises because she did not feel safe. For example, the exercises with the weights ... She did the exercises but without weights ... " (Caregiver 13)

Almost half of the caregivers stated they liked most components of the telerehab program, while seven family caregivers liked everything about the program. Constructive feedback on the program included difficulty accessing internet in some locations, and the exercises were repetitive (and possibly created boredom). Family caregivers also reported positive attributes of the program, such as usefulness for functional recovery (helpful and well-presented information, and ease of use).

4. Discussion

Telerehab is a rapidly growing mode of health care delivery, but there are known gaps for using ICTs for older adults with hip fracture [17]. Recognizing ICT barriers in the early discharge recovery period, we engaged family caregivers to facilitate the adoption of remote delivery of health care after hip fracture. Here we provide a detailed description of family caregivers experience using a telerehab program called @ctivehip. Overall, family caregivers reported a high level of satisfaction with the program, stated it was manageable to use, and reported it was useful for functional recovery. Importantly family caregivers provided valuable insights for future program content and implementation to strengthen delivery and uptake of the intervention.

Although participants chose to receive the telerehab program, our sample was similar to other studies where the caregiving was mainly provided by women [4,5] at middle-age [29,30] who were adult children, [6] and were supported by other family caregivers. [4,30] In our study most family caregivers worked full-time or part-time, in contrast to other studies where caregivers were mostly unemployed. [5,6] These characteristics can be influenced by social and cultural norms and by the organization of the social and healthcare systems. Our work provides a novel perspective on caregiving while employed showing similar adherence to the program between caregivers who were unemployed, and those with part-or full-time work. Further, caregivers with lower adherence to the program reported lower support from other caregivers. This finding generates hypotheses on support (amount and type) needed by caregivers to deliver and manage the program. Although telerehab in general may be cost-effective [31], future research is needed to determine the acceptability, costs, feasibility, and (cost) effectiveness of telerehab considering the caregivers perspective in a program like @ctivehip.

We observed a high level of satisfaction and perceived usefulness for family caregivers with the @ctivehip program. These factors may contribute to users' motivation to adopt and persist with the program, a key component of the technology acceptance model [32]. Our findings are similar to other ICT studies based on health communication and family caregivers' health literacy and caregiving skills [33,34]. Of note, in our study family caregivers did not perceive the program as onerous, even with the additional time commitment. Further, in our other qualitative study from @ctivehip, these same family caregivers in the intervention group reported lower levels of stress and anxiety and requested less social and health services compared with caregivers of patients who received only a few sessions of in-person rehabilitation [22]. An explanation for these findings may be related to the perceived benefits of the telerehab program: it was an opportunity for family members to receive education and skills training to prepare for the recovery process. Other studies reported family caregivers wanted role clarification and active participation in their family members recovery [10,18,22]. It is possible caregivers' observation of older adults' functional improvement with the program may have benefited both the caregiver (improved self-efficacy in caregiving) and the older adult with hip fracture (adoption and use of the program, mastery with exercises, improved self-efficacy, etc.) However, as we did not measure the effect of these factors in our study, we can only generate hypotheses on the "active ingredients" [35] or behavior change techniques associated with the telerehab program or its delivery.

Family caregivers requested regular communication with health professionals after hospital discharge (using a person-centered approach) to update and progress rehabilitation plans. At present we do not know if the family caregiver "regular check ins" need to be face-to-face or via ICTs. Technology may provide opportunities for more frequent communication with family caregivers and patients, especially during the transition back home [34]. An automatic system with personalized patient/caregiver feedback and monitoring to enhance motivation could be considered, similar to a system described in a pilot study of older adults with hip fracture [36]. We also recognize some patients and caregivers prefer face-to-face interactions [37]. Thus, health education should be individualized to each person, and consider internet resources available, motivation (habitual processes, emotional responses, and analytical decision-making), capability (knowledge and skills) and opportunities (context) of the patients, caregivers, and health professionals [37,38].

Family caregivers in our study requested more and varied exercise options within @ctivehip but, as some of the caregivers recognized, some patients did not use weights during the sessions for safety reasons. More frequent communication with health professionals could have addressed concerns, develop strategies, and explain why using weights (if possible) was recommended to increase strength and physical condition. It is difficult to know how the content of our telerehab program [21] compares with other published studies in this area [36,39,40] as previous work only provided a brief description of interventions.

We acknowledge that only half of participants completed the full program but overall, three-quarters completed eight weeks or more of the intervention. Reasons to explain the lack of fidelity to the program could be boredom related to the repetitive nature of the core exercises, participants higher level of function (pre-and post-intervention) reported in the main trial [20], or older adults (and family members) may have stopped the program when they felt independent in completing ADLs. The unified theory of acceptance and use of technology (UTAUT) describes factors which impact on technology adoption and use, such as social influence, effort expectancy, and performance expectancy [41]. Considering the UTAUT, possible elements to increase @ctivehip program adherence include reimagining work organization, with the inclusion of periodic health monitoring [42]; clear communication with patients and caregivers and a detailed explanation of the program [18,29]; discussing caregivers expectations [43]; and/or specific information on program progression (if/when appropriate). For example, progressing exercises with weights, if possible. Although we collected some implementation metrics, our future work needs to discern the optimal "dose" of the program, individualized for older adults following hip fracture.

Strengths and Limitations

We note some limitations within our study. First, due to the study's inclusion criteria, the older adults with hip fracture did not have cognitive impairment. Future studies should consider expanding the inclusion criteria to reflect a wider population of people who fracture their hip. Second, we conducted interviews three to six months after the telerehab program ended, and this delayed timing may have impacted family caregivers' responses. Third, we conducted short interviews although provided prompts and cues to explore caregivers' experience using the program. Fourth, group assignment was by choice, therefore participants who wanted to receive the telehealth program may have a different experience. Although many caregivers liked the program there were some perceived limitations such as the limited variety of exercises and monitoring. Fifth, we did not capture psychosocial factors such as caregivers' self-efficacy with delivering the telerehab program, but we recognize behavioral factors (for the older adult and family caregiver) are important to include in future research. Despite these limitations, our study provides valuable information to extend the limited evidence for ICTs for older community-dwelling adults with hip fracture [44,45] and their family caregivers [33].

5. Conclusions

To our knowledge, this is the first study to provide a detailed description of family caregivers' experience with a post-hip fracture telerehab program delivered before the SARS-CoV-2 (COVID-19) pandemic. Family caregivers who enrolled in the @ctivehip telerehab program were satisfied with the program, stated it was manageable, and reported perceived benefits for older adults' functional recovery after hip fractures. Family caregivers also provided helpful feedback to enhance program content and its delivery. Taken together, this work extends existing literature, and generates research hypotheses for future studies to test telerehab content and program implementation.

Author Contributions: Conceptualization, P.A.-V. and M.C.A.; methodology, P.A.-V., V.M.-R., D.R.-A. and M.C.A.; software, R.P.-M. and H.C.-P.; validation, P.A.-V., R.P.-M. and H.C.-P.; formal analysis P.A.-V. and M.C.A.; investigation, P.A.-V., R.P.-M., H.C.-P., V.M.-R., D.R.-A. and M.C.A.; resources,

R.P.-M. and H.C.-P.; data curation, P.A.-V., R.P.-M. and H.C.-P.; writing—original draft preparation, P.A.-V., and M.C.A.; writing—review and editing, P.A.-V., R.P.-M., H.C.-P., V.M.-R., D.R.-A. and M.C.A.; visualization, P.A.-V. and R.P.-M.; supervision, P.A.-V.; project administration, P.A.-V.; funding acquisition, P.A.-V. All authors have read and agreed to the published version of the manuscript.

Funding: This research was funded by EIT Health (210752).

Institutional Review Board Statement: The study was conducted according to the guidelines of the Declaration of Helsinki and Law 14/2007 on Biomedical Research and approved by the Ethics Committee of Research Center of Granada (CEI-GRANADA).

Informed Consent Statement: Informed consent was obtained from all subjects involved in the study.

Data Availability Statement: Not applicable.

Conflicts of Interest: The authors declare no conflict of interest.

Appendix A

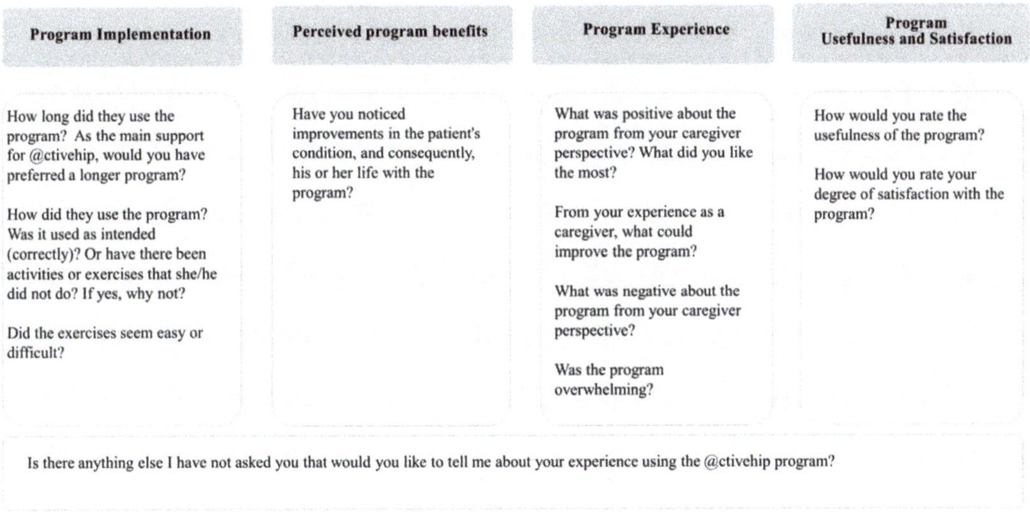

Program Implementation	Perceived program benefits	Program Experience	Program Usefulness and Satisfaction
How long did they use the program? As the main support for @ctivehip, would you have preferred a longer program? How did they use the program? Was it used as intended (correctly)? Or have there been activities or exercises that she/he did not do? If yes, why not? Did the exercises seem easy or difficult?	Have you noticed improvements in the patient's condition, and consequently, his or her life with the program?	What was positive about the program from your caregiver perspective? What did you like the most? From your experience as a caregiver, what could improve the program? What was negative about the program from your caregiver perspective? Was the program overwhelming?	How would you rate the usefulness of the program? How would you rate your degree of satisfaction with the program?

Is there anything else I have not asked you that would you like to tell me about your experience using the @ctivehip program?

Figure A1. Interview guide.

References

1. Dyer, S.M.; Crotty, M.; Fairhall, N.; Magaziner, J.; Beaupre, L.A.; Cameron, I.D.; Sherrington, C. A critical review of the long-term disability outcomes following hip fracture. *BMC Geriatr.* **2016**, *16*, 158. [CrossRef] [PubMed]
2. Orive, M.; Aguirre, U.; García-Gutiérrez, S.; Las Hayas, C.; Bilbao, A.; González, N.; Zabala, J.; Navarro, G.; Quintana, J.M. Changes in health-related quality of life and activities of daily living after hip fracture because of a fall in elderly patients: A prospective cohort study. *Int. J. Clin. Pract.* **2015**, *69*, 491–500. [CrossRef] [PubMed]
3. Perracini, M.R.; Kristensen, M.T.; Cunningham, C.; Sherrington, C. Physiotherapy following fragility fractures. *Injury* **2018**, *49*, 1413–1417. [CrossRef] [PubMed]
4. Rocha, S.A.; de Avila, M.A.G.; Bocchi, S.C.M. The influence of informal caregivers on the rehabilitation of the elderly in the postoperative period of proximal femoral fracture. *Rev. Gauch. Enferm.* **2016**, *37*, e51069.
5. Ariza-Vega, P.; Ortiz-Piña, M.; Kristensen, M.T.; Castellote-Caballero, Y.; Jiménez-Moleón, J.J. High perceived caregiver burden for relatives of patients following hip fracture surgery. *Disabil. Rehabil.* **2019**, *41*, 311–318. [CrossRef] [PubMed]

6. Martín-Martín, L.M.; Valenza-Demet, G.; Ariza-Vega, P.; Valenza, C.; Castellote-Caballero, Y.; Jiménez-Moleón, J.J. Effectiveness of an occupational therapy intervention in reducing emotional distress in informal caregivers of hip fracture patients: A randomized controlled trial. *Clin. Rehabil.* **2014**, *28*, 772–783. [CrossRef]
7. Siddiqui, M.Q.A.; Sim, L.; Koh, J.; Fook-Chong, S.; Tan, C.; Howe, T. Sen Stress levels amongst caregivers of patients with osteoporotic hip fractures - A prospective cohort study. *Ann. Acad. Med. Singapore* **2010**, *39*, 38–42.
8. Auais, M.; French, S.D.; Beaupre, L.; Giangregorio, L.; Magaziner, J. Identifying research priorities around psycho-cognitive and social factors for recovery from hip fractures: An international decision-making process. *Injury* **2018**, *49*, 1466–1472. [CrossRef]
9. McDonough, C.M.; Harris-Hayes, M.; Kristensen, M.T.; Overgaard, J.A.; Herring, T.B.; Kenny, A.M.; Mangione, K.K. Physical Therapy Management of Older Adults With Hip Fracture. *J. Orthop. Sport. Phys. Ther.* **2021**, *51*, CPG1–CPG81. [CrossRef] [PubMed]
10. Saletti-Cuesta, L.; Tutton, E.; Langstaff, D.; Willett, K. Understanding informal carers' experiences of caring for older people with a hip fracture: A systematic review of qualitative studies. *Disabil. Rehabil.* **2018**, *40*, 740–750. [CrossRef]
11. Peretti, A.; Amenta, F.; Tayebati, S.K.; Nittari, G.; Mahdi, S.S. Telerehabilitation: Review of the State-of-the-Art and Areas of Application. *JMIR Rehabil. Assist. Technol.* **2017**, *4*, e7. [CrossRef] [PubMed]
12. Wang, K.C.; Xiao, R.; Cheung, Z.B.; Barbera, J.P.; Forsh, D.A. Early mortality after hip fracture surgery in COVID-19 patients: A systematic review and meta-analysis. *J. Orthop.* **2020**, *22*, 584–591. [CrossRef]
13. Bodilsen, A.C.; Pedersen, M.M.; Petersen, J.; Beyer, N.; Andersen, O.; Smith, L.L.; Kehlet, H.; Bandholm, T. Acute hospitalization of the older patient: Changes in muscle strength and functional performance during hospitalization and 30 days after discharge. *Am. J. Phys. Med. Rehabil.* **2013**, *92*, 789–796. [CrossRef] [PubMed]
14. Petersen, W.; Karpinski, K.; Backhaus, L.; Bierke, S.; Häner, M. A systematic review about telemedicine in orthopedics. *Arch. Orthop. Trauma Surg.* **2021**, *141*, 1731–1739. [CrossRef] [PubMed]
15. Wang, Q.; Lee, R.L.T.; Hunter, S.; Chan, S.W.C. The effectiveness of internet-based telerehabilitation among patients after total joint arthroplasty: A systematic review and meta-analysis of randomised controlled trials. *J. Telemed. Telecare* **2021**, 1357633X2098029. [CrossRef]
16. Pastora-Bernal, J.M.; Martín-Valero, R.; Barón-López, F.J.; Estebanez-Pérez, M.J. Evidence of Benefit of Telerehabitation After Orthopedic Surgery: A Systematic Review. *J. Med. Internet Res.* **2017**, *19*, e142. [CrossRef] [PubMed]
17. Ashe, M.C.; Ekegren, C.L.; Chudyk, A.M.; Fleig, L.; Gill, T.K.; Langford, D.; Martin-Martin, L.; Ariza-Vega, P. Telerehabilitation for community-dwelling middle-aged and older adults after musculoskeletal trauma: A systematic review. *AIMS Med. Sci.* **2018**, *5*, 316–336. [CrossRef]
18. Asif, M.; Cadel, L.; Kuluski, K.; Everall, A.C.; Guilcher, S.J.T. Patient and caregiver experiences on care transitions for adults with a hip fracture: A scoping review. *Disabil. Rehabil.* **2020**, *42*, 3549–3558. [CrossRef] [PubMed]
19. Wolff, J.L.; Freedman, V.A.; Mulcahy, J.F.; Kasper, J.D. Family Caregivers' Experiences With Health Care Workers in the Care of Older Adults With Activity Limitations. *JAMA Netw. open* **2020**, *3*, e1919866. [CrossRef] [PubMed]
20. Ortiz-Piña, M.; Molina-Garcia, P.; Femia, P.; Ashe, M.C.; Martín-Martín, L.; Salazar-Graván, S.; Salas-Fariña, Z.; Prieto-Moreno, R.; Castellote-Caballero, Y.; Estevez-Lopez, F.; et al. Effects of Tele-Rehabilitation Compared with Home-Based in-Person Rehabilitation for Older Adult's Function after Hip Fracture. *Int. J. Environ. Res. Public Health* **2021**, *18*, 5493. [CrossRef]
21. Ortiz-Piña, M.; Salas-Fariña, Z.; Mora-Traverso, M.; Martín-Martín, L.; Galiano-Castillo, N.; García-Montes, I.; Cantarero-Villanueva, I.; Fernández-Lao, C.; Arroyo-Morales, M.; Mesa-Ruíz, A.; et al. A home-based tele-rehabilitation protocol for patients with hip fracture called @ctivehip. *Res. Nurs. Health* **2019**, *42*, 29–38. [CrossRef] [PubMed]
22. Ariza-Vega, P.; Castillo-Pérez, H.; Ortiz-Piña, M.; Ziden, L.; Palomino-Vidal, J.; Ashe, M.C. The Journey of Recovery: Caregivers' Perspectives From a Hip Fracture Telerehabilitation Clinical Trial. *Phys. Ther.* **2021**, *101*. [CrossRef] [PubMed]
23. Thorne, S.; Kirkham, S.R.; O'Flynn-Magee, K. The Analytic Challenge in Interpretive Description. *Int. J. Qual. Methods* **2004**, *3*, 1–11. [CrossRef]
24. Graneheim, U.H.; Lundman, B. Qualitative content analysis in nursing research: Concepts, procedures and measures to achieve trustworthiness. *Nurse Educ. Today* **2004**, *24*, 105–112. [CrossRef] [PubMed]
25. Saldaña, J. *The Coding Manual for Qualitative Researchers*, 3rd ed.; SAGE Publications Ltd.: London, UK, 2015; ISBN 9781446247365.
26. Shenton, A.K. Strategies for ensuring trustworthiness in qualitative research projects. *Educ. Inf.* **2004**, *22*, 63–75. [CrossRef]
27. Denzin, N. *Sociological Methods: A Sourcebook*; Aldine Transaction: Piscataway, NJ, USA, 2006; ISBN 9783540773405.
28. Takeda, H.; Kamogawa, J.; Sakayama, K.; Kamada, K.; Tanaka, S.; Yamamoto, H. Evaluation of clinical prognosis and activities of daily living using functional independence measure in patients with hip fractures. *J. Orthop. Sci. Off. J. Japanese Orthop. Assoc.* **2006**, *11*, 584–591. [CrossRef]
29. Giosa, J.L.; Stolee, P.; Dupuis, S.L.; Mock, S.E.; Santi, S.M. An examination of family caregiver experiences during care transitions of older adults. *Can. J. Aging* **2014**, *33*, 137–153. [CrossRef] [PubMed]
30. Liu, H.-Y.; Yang, C.-T.; Cheng, H.-S.; Wu, C.-C.; Chen, C.-Y.; Shyu, Y.-I.L. Family caregivers' mental health is associated with postoperative recovery of elderly patients with hip fracture: A sample in Taiwan. *J. Psychosom. Res.* **2015**, *78*, 452–458. [CrossRef]
31. Nelson, M.; Russell, T.; Crossley, K.; Bourke, M.; McPhail, S. Cost-effectiveness of telerehabilitation versus traditional care after total hip replacement: A trial-based economic evaluation. *J. Telemed. Telecare* **2021**, *27*, 359–366. [CrossRef] [PubMed]
32. Holden, R.J.; Karsh, B.T. The technology acceptance model: Its past and its future in health care. *J. Biomed. Inform.* **2010**, *43*, 159–172. [CrossRef] [PubMed]

33. Nahm, E.S.; Resnick, B.; Plummer, L.; Park, B.K. Use of discussion boards in an online hip fracture resource center for caregivers. *Orthop. Nurs.* **2013**, *32*, 89–95. [CrossRef] [PubMed]
34. Glenny, C.; Stolee, P.; Sheiban, L.; Jaglal, S. Communicating during care transitions for older hip fracture patients: Family caregiver and health care provider's perspectives. *Int. J. Integr. Care* **2013**, *13*. [CrossRef] [PubMed]
35. Michie, S.; Richardson, M.; Johnston, M.; Abraham, C.; Francis, J.; Hardeman, W.; Eccles, M.P.; Cane, J.; Wood, C.E. The behavior change technique taxonomy (v1) of 93 hierarchically clustered techniques: Building an international consensus for the reporting of behavior change interventions. *Ann. Behav. Med.* **2013**, *46*, 81–95. [CrossRef] [PubMed]
36. Bedra, M.; Finkelstein, J. Feasibility of post-acute hip fracture telerehabilitation in older adults. *Stud. Health Technol. Inform.* **2015**, *210*, 469–473. [CrossRef] [PubMed]
37. Yadav, L.; Gill, T.K.; Taylor, A.; De Young, J.; Chehade, M.J. Identifying Opportunities, and Motivation to Enhance Capabilities, Influencing the Development of a Personalized Digital Health Hub Model of Care for Hip Fractures: Mixed Methods Exploratory Study. *J. Med. Internet Res.* **2021**, *23*, e26886. [CrossRef] [PubMed]
38. Michie, S.; van Stralen, M.M.; West, R. The behaviour change wheel: A new method for characterising and designing behaviour change interventions. *Implement. Sci.* **2011**, *6*, 42. [CrossRef] [PubMed]
39. Kalron, A.; Tawil, H.; Peleg-Shani, S.; Vatine, J.J. Effect of telerehabilitation on mobility in people after hip surgery: A pilot feasibility study. *Int. J. Rehabil. Res.* **2018**, *41*, 244–250. [CrossRef] [PubMed]
40. Tappen, R.M.; Whitehead, D.; Folden, S.L.; Hall, R. Effect of a Video Intervention on Functional Recovery Following Hip Replacement and Hip Fracture Repair. *Rehabil. Nurs.* **2003**, *28*, 148–153. [CrossRef] [PubMed]
41. Ammenwerth, E. Technology Acceptance Models in Health Informatics: TAM and UTAUT. *Stud. Health Technol. Inform.* **2019**, *263*, 64–71. [CrossRef]
42. Mehta, S.J.; Hume, E.; Troxel, A.B.; Reitz, C.; Norton, L.; Lacko, H.; McDonald, C.; Freeman, J.; Marcus, N.; Volpp, K.G.; et al. Effect of Remote Monitoring on Discharge to Home, Return to Activity, and Rehospitalization After Hip and Knee Arthroplasty: A Randomized Clinical Trial. *JAMA Netw. open* **2020**, *3*, e2028328. [CrossRef] [PubMed]
43. Elliott, J.; Forbes, D.; Chesworth, B.M.; Ceci, C.; Stolee, P. Information sharing with rural family caregivers during care transitions of hip fracture patients. *Int. J. Integr. Care* **2014**, *14*. [CrossRef] [PubMed]
44. Ashe, M. Fracture Recovery for Seniors at Home: A Hip Fracture Recovery Guide for Patients & Families. 2015. Available online: http://www.hiphealth.ca/blog/FReSHStart (accessed on 8 December 2021).
45. Langford, D.P.; Fleig, L.; Brown, K.C.; Cho, N.J.; Frost, M.; Ledoyen, M.; Lehn, J.; Panagiotopoulos, K.; Sharpe, N.; Ashe, M.C. Back to the future – Feasibility of recruitment and retention to patient education and telephone follow-up after hip fracture: A pilot randomized controlled trial. *Patient Prefer. Adherence* **2015**, *9*, 1343–1351. [CrossRef] [PubMed]

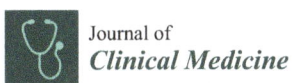

Article

Ethical Dilemmas with Regard to Elderly Patients with Hip Fracture: The Problem of Nonagenarians and Centenarians

Mario Herrera-Pérez [1,2], David González-Martín [1,*], Emilio J. Sanz [3] and José L. Pais-Brito [1,2]

1. Department of Orthopaedics, University Hospital of Canary Islands, 38320 Tenerife, Spain; herrera42@gmail.com (M.H.-P.); paisbrito@gmail.com (J.L.P.-B.)
2. Department of Surgery, School of Medicine, Universidad de La Laguna, 38320 Tenerife, Spain
3. Department of Pharmacology, School of Medicine, Universidad de La Laguna, 38320 Tenerife, Spain; esanz@ull.es
* Correspondence: davidglezmartin@gmail.com

Abstract: Hip fracture is the most feared complication of osteoporosis, producing up to 30% mortality at the first year. With the aging of society, it is increasingly common to deal with ethical dilemmas that involve decision making in the elderly patient with a hip fracture. The objectives of the present work are to describe the main bioethical dilemmas in this group of patients and their relationship with surgical delay. We conducted a retrospective descriptive study that studied an elderly population admitted to a University Hospital with a diagnosis of hip fracture. In total, 415 patients were analyzed. The majority received surgical treatment, a correct application of the principles of justice, non-maleficence and beneficence is verified, but a possible violation of the principle of autonomy is confirmed. Based on the results of this study, the elderly population may somehow lose their principle of autonomy when they enter a hospital due to a hip fracture. On the other hand, the so-called ageism due to ignorance can influence the surgical delay and therefore the mortality of these patients.

Keywords: autonomy; capacity; clinical ethics; informed consent; legal aspects

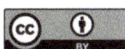

1. Introduction

Ageing populations are a global phenomenon with important biopsychosocial and economic impacts that will affect all areas of our lives. The global population over 60 years of age will increase from 900 million in 2015 to 2000 million in 2050, according to the World Health Organization (WHO) [1,2]. From a musculoskeletal perspective, old age means a higher level of osteoporosis, a silent, asymptomatic disease that produces bone fragility and when it manifests as fractures it can put the health of sufferers at risk. Of the various osteoporotic fractures, hip fractures are the most likely to cause mortality: the increased mortality in patients after a hip fracture compared with controls varies between 8% and 36% per year [1,3–6]. Hip fracture in the elderly represents approximately 40% of traumatology admissions in the developed world [1]. Therefore, because of its prevalence and clinical significance, especially in terms of mortality, it is an especially important area in biomedical traumatology research [2]. In the case of an elderly patient, over 85–90 years of age, with a hip fracture, the question arises as to whether it is ethically acceptable to subject the patient to surgery, assuming the risks (anesthesia, blood loss, convalescence) as opposed to the conservative attitude of no surgical intervention. It should be borne in mind that the patient is often vulnerable, not only because their advanced age may prevent them from being self-sufficient when it comes to daily living activities (walking, reading, seeing, hearing, etc.), but also because on many occasions there is an associated deterioration in mental function that hinders both the doctor–patient relationship and the decision-making process, which may be encompassed within the principle of autonomy [7]. All these circumstances described determine that, in many cases, the admitted elderly patient is considered ineligible to receive information, regardless of the assessment of their mental capacity to receive this, with the typical circumstance being arrived at where the family is informed before the patient, who should be the holder of the information. This is what many authors have called the tacit pact of silence or conspiracy of silence [8]. In this pact, the influence of ageism is crucial.

1.1. Ageism

This term was coined in 1968 by the gerontologist and psychiatrist Robert Butler, to refer to discrimination against older people, based on the terms sexism and racism [9,10]. Butler defined "ageism" as a combination of three connected elements. These include harmful attitudes towards older people, old age, and the ageing process; discriminatory practices against older people; and institutional practices and policies that perpetuate stereotypes about older people [11]. The fear of death and the fear of disability and dependency are the leading causes of ageism. In the social and health care system, ageism often manifests as ill-treatment, a lack of attention, and even the restriction of access to specific resources, as discussed later [9–11].

1.2. Legal Aspects

Elderly patients, regardless of their mental and physical capacities, have certain inviolable rights registered by multiple international treaties. Within this subsection, we consider three rights that should be considered. However, these are not the only ones (because there are also many others, such as confidentiality, as well as those contained in the Code of Medical Ethics): the right to non-discrimination (by age in this case), the right to accurate and truthful information, and the right not to receive treatment [12–14].

1.3. Bioethical Aspects of Caring for Elderly Patients

Clinical care and clinical ethics must be incorporated into geriatric care in order to develop high-quality care. Concerning the care of the elderly with hip fracture, the creation of orthogeriatric units has been a genuine revolution in the overall treatment of this, particularly vulnerable patients [15]. Incorporating values, together with objective facts, ensures that this care preserves the dignity of every elderly patient who receives health or social care. However, we are currently in a situation of moral pluralism in which it is not easy to reach agreements on what should and should not be carried out in the care of the elderly. Several methods have been developed in the field of bioethics that can help determine the ethical minimums required of any individual (professional, volunteer, politician, manager, and others.) about the care of the elderly [16]. Within the different methods that exist in the field of bioethics, and although the same problem can be approached from various perspectives, we consider principialism, based on the principles described in Beauchamp and Childress [16], and specifically that modified by Professor Diego Gracia Guillén, known as the "deliberative method", to be appropriate for the topic we are dealing with here: an elderly patient admitted to hospital which must be assessed for suitability for surgery [17,18].

1.4. Hip Fracture in the Elderly

In the developed world, it is also the most critical complication of osteoporosis in terms of mortality, morbidity, and cost [1,19]. Globally, there were around 1.3 million hip fractures in 1990, and according to estimates, there could be as many as 20 million cases in 2050 [20–22]. The mortality associated with hip fracture is 5–10% in the first month, 4% in-hospital mortality, and 30–33% in the first year after the fracture (although this is somewhat higher in men than women), figures that exceed those of the mortality due to colon, breast, or prostate cancer for the same age group. This mortality is related to respiratory complications, ischemic heart disease, and heart failure [23]. In total, 50% of patients do not recover the functional level they had before the fracture, close to 25% need care for long periods, and 20% have ongoing dependency: ultimately, only 5% return to their prior functional status [19,24].

It is expected that the global incidence of hip fractures will increase markedly in the coming decades [20,25,26]. Currently, according to the International Osteoporosis Foundation (IOF), around the world each year there are close to 9 million new osteoporotic fractures, of which 1.6 million are hip fractures; the forecasts for the year 2050 ranging from 4.5 to 6.3 million. This increase will be widespread, but especially dramatic in Asia. The current figure of hip fracture incidence in Europe comes from the report of Johnell and Kanis: they estimated that in Europe in the year 2030, around 1,000,000 hip fractures were suffered by men and women, making Europe the region with the highest number of hip fractures in the world, with 38% of the global total [27–29]. The expected increase in Europe is around 135% over the next 50 years, involving an estimated figure of close to a million new hip fractures a year. The morbidity and mortality rates are high, and this condition generates many disabilities, extended stays in chronic centers, and a considerable deterioration in the quality of life of the sufferer. If in 2000, 25,000 hospital beds were needed for treatment (0.88% of those available), in 2010 it was predicted that this number would be 30,000 (1.06% of those available), and by 2050 this figure would have almost doubled, meaning 2% of the available beds could be filled by hip fracture sufferers [24].

The main objectives of this work are:
(1) To describe the most frequent bioethical conflicts relating to elderly patients admitted to hospital with a hip fracture.
(2) To provide suggestions to help resolve the conflicts encountered.

2. Materials and Methods

Retrospective descriptive study of the main bioethical conflicts of patients admitted with a diagnosis of hip fracture in a university hospital from January 2017 to January 2019.

The inclusion criteria were:
- Hip fracture.
- Patients aged more than 65.

The exclusion criteria were:
- Inability to access medical history data (patient referred from another center).

For this study, we used the electronic medical record review from the orthopedic department from the past two years, on the medical practice carried out in the center regarding these patients. A search was made on the SAP system without providing any confidential patient data, collecting the following parameters:

- Age.
- The presence of dementia.
- Anesthetic risk according to the American Society of Anesthesiologists (ASA) score that distinguish between ASA I to ASA V, from lowest to highest risk) [30].
- Surgical delay and cause of that delay.
- Cause of non-surgical indication.

3. Results

Between January 2017 and February 2019, a total of 415 patients with a diagnosis of hip fracture were admitted to hospital (Table 1). Of these, 75% were women, with an average age of 88.2 (62–102 years), and 25% were men, with an average age of 84.3 (67–98 years). For the purposes of differentiated analysis, the series was split into three age groups: <90 years of age: 382 cases; 90–100 years of age: 25 cases; >100 years of age: 8 cases. The patients predominantly came in from their habitual residence (70%) but with nuances; in the age 90–100 group, all except one lived in a nursing home (24 cases), as did 6 of the centenarians. Dementia was present in 40% of the series, also differing according to age: 80% of patients older than 90 had mental deterioration. However, only 20% of our series (81 patients) were legally incapacitated.

Table 1. Demographics.

	Hip Fractures (n = 415)
Sex	Men 104 (25%) Women 311 (75%)
Age	Men 84.3 years (R 67–98) Women 88.2 years (R 62–102)
Age groups	<90 years→382 patients 90–100 years→25 patients >100 years→8 patients
Dementia	No 249 (60%) Yes 166 (40%)
Legal incapacity	No 334 (80%) Yes 81 (20%)
Comorbidities	≥3→100 (24%) Arterial hypertension→253 (61%) Diabetes→170 (41%) Dementia→166 (40%)

The delay to surgery was 3.6 days (1–17) and, in most cases, this was, firstly, due to the lack of availability of an operating room, and secondly, to optimize the medical care of the patients prior to surgery (Table 2). In 10% of the cases (42 patients), the surgical delay was longer than 48 h due to family members disagreeing about the suitability of surgical treatment for their relative (40 cases), and in 2 cases due to disagreements with anesthesiology. Of the entire series, only 18 patients did not undergo surgery (4.5% of the total), meaning 95.5% of the cases opted for an operation. The causes of non-surgical intervention were:

- Nine cases: worsening of the general state of health and death in the hospital environment.
- Five cases: joint decision made by the family and geriatrician due to the poor medical status at admission, tolerating conservative treatment and being discharged.
- Four cases: refusal of the family to assume the treatment risk (4 patients with advanced senile dementia aged 91, 89, 93, and 96), all of whom were discharged.

Regarding informed consent for surgery, for 55% of the patients in this series, the IC was signed by a relative or legal representative (100% of centenarian patients and 80% of nonagenarians), with the remaining 45% signed by the patients themselves.

Table 2. Results.

	Results
Surgical treatment	No 18 (4.5%) Yes 398 (95.5%)
Surgical delay	3.6 days (R 1–17)
Surgical delay causes	(1) Availability of operating theatres→116 (28%) (2) Medical optimisation→91 (22%) (3) Other (10%): Family discrepancy→40 (9%) Anesthesia discrepancy→2 (1%)
Informed consent Signatory	Patient 187 (45%) Relative or legal representative 228 (55%)

4. Discussion

Health-related ethical conflicts are a source of concern for many healthcare professionals involved in social and health care. An elderly patient with a hip fracture is an example of a vulnerable patient, not only because of the frequent associated comorbidity and sensory deficits, but also because of the aggravated situation caused by the fracture: pain and the need for hospital admission with the so-called loss of reference (loss of contact with family, caregivers, and the usual environment). These are, therefore, patients that we must protect in the broadest sense of the word. The four principles articulated in 1979, in the Belmont Report, were a milestone in medical practice. When making the most appropriate treatment decisions for an elderly patient with a hip fracture, the principles of non-maleficence, which ensure the life of individuals as a guarantee that they will not be harmed, either by the execution of a harmful action or by omission of an action due to avoiding harm, and the principle of justice, which ensures non-discrimination and equal access to social goods and resources (health in this case), come into play.

Regarding the results obtained in our study, it is noteworthy, in relation to the principle of autonomy, that in a high percentage of cases (55%) the patient was not correctly informed (or, at least, this is not recorded), and it was decided that the IC should be signed by relatives or representatives. If we subtract from this percentage those patients with dementia (40%), in at least 15% of the cases (60 patients) the decision to authorize surgery was not made by the patient. This is only legally admissible when the patient has impaired abilities. This is affirmed by Article 5.3 of the Law of Patient Autonomy [13] "where, in the opinion of the attending doctor, the patient lacks the capacity to understand the information because of their physical or mental condition, the information will be brought to the attention of persons that have family or de facto connections with them." However, this clarification is not found in the medical history of any of these 60 patients, which may be legally objectionable. This violation of the principle of autonomy in some cases also represents a paternalistic attitude on the part of the health professional, in contrast to the desirable participative decision-making model, since the patient must be correctly informed of their process, and this can only be explained by a flagrant lack of attention and respect for the dignity of the patient, since it was undoubtedly more comfortable for the treating physician to talk to the relatives (generally younger than the patient), and not make an effort to obtain authorization for surgery from the patient themselves, ignoring the fact that the vulnerability of a patient affected by illness does not deprive them of their personal autonomy and of their obligation to personally manage their own life and decisions. Regarding surgical delay, one of the main causes of mortality, even though the main reason for this was a lack of material resources (availability of the operating room), 10% of cases were due to ageism or age discrimination, since family members were not aware that surgery is indicated in almost 95% of cases. However, this may be better defined as ageism due to ignorance, as it is undoubtedly a lack of information on the suitability of surgical treatment despite age that made them doubt the pertinence of an operation.

A very interesting aspect to consider in elderly patients is the true concept of "old age"—should we consider a patient to be elderly when they are older than 80, 90, or 100 years of age? With the advances in multidisciplinary patient care after admission for hip fracture, their ability to withstand surgical aggression is increasing, with the geriatrician playing a key role in optimizing patients prior to surgery, leading to the momentum built in this field over recent years, and the creation of specialized orthogeriatric units [4,5,15,31,32]. Special mention should be made about the subgroup of nonagenarian patients, who are becoming increasingly frequent (25 cases in this series), as this subgroup is particularly critical due to the mental deterioration and the high medical comorbidity that is often present. Some authors state that the main criterion to follow in order to assess surgical treatment in patients over 90 years of age should be their mental state and their previous mobility. In 2005, Ooi et al. published an interesting study comparing patients over 90 years of age admitted for hip fracture, some treated surgically and others conservatively, including a 2-year follow-up period. They observed equally high mortality figures (49%) in both groups, whether they had been operated on or not; however, the same authors acknowledge that nonagenarian patients who had received surgery had a significantly increased walking capacity compared to those treated conservatively [33]. The first author to pose the dilemma of whether to operate, or not, on very elderly patients, i.e., nonagenarians, was Jennings in 1999, who, after studying a cohort of 50 hip fracture patients aged more than 90, concluded that although up to 50% of cases presented some type of postoperative complication, the majority of patients studied achieved the same mobility level they had prior to the fracture, and, therefore, considered that this type of surgery was equally beneficial in this age subgroup [34]. Along the same line, more recently an interesting article was published comparing the morbidity and mortality associated with hip fracture in nonagenarian and centenarian patients. No statistically significant differences were found between the two groups, so the authors do not consider advanced age as a factor of poor prognosis per se; however, they do place emphasis on the prior medical status of these patients [35].

The current problem is that the number of nonagenarian patients with hip fractures is still on the rise, and even more seriously, it is already relatively common to treat centenarian patients with hip fractures. In this sense, in 2004, authors from a public hospital in Edinburgh published the most complete study to date on the increased mortality in centenarian patients [36]. Comparing two groups of patients, 18 elderly patients aged over 100, with another 18 aged between 75–84 with similar levels of comorbidity, they reached the conclusion that the centenary group had a minimal increased mortality (51% versus 48%) although the percentage of post-surgery disability was higher in younger patients, perhaps because the centenarians already had more limited mobility. The presence of medical comorbidities in people with hip fractures is frequent. In a recent article, the main cause recorded for surgical delay was the presence of comorbidities that required the patient to be stabilized; the second was the presence of anticoagulation and antiaggregation [37–39]. In none of the articles we reviewed did we find that age is a negative factor when it comes to early surgery, as most authors recommend surgery in the first 48 h to avoid the appearance of possible complications [32,35,37].

Finally, the presence of some degree of senile dementia, present in 40% of our series, deserves separate consideration. Studies have shown that patients with dementia are at an increased risk of sustaining a hip fracture and tend to have worse functional outcomes than those who do not suffer this condition. Baker et al. recently presented an interesting article in which they analyzed the decision-making process in this particularly vulnerable group [15]. The authors conclude that the participation of geriatricians in this decision-making process is crucial when assessing the fragility of these patients, as part of the multidisciplinary team including orthopedic surgeons, anesthesiologists, nurses, and social agents, as occurs in our center [40–42].

There are limitations and strengths in our study that should be acknowledged. The main methodological limitation of this study is that it is a descriptive retrospective study. This is a single-center study, so the percentages described may not be representative of other centers. Its main strengths are the broad sample studied and the improvement actions proposed by the authors.

Based on the results of this study, the elderly population may somehow lose their principle of autonomy when they enter a hospital due to a hip fracture. On the other hand, the so-called ageism due to ignorance can influence the surgical delay and therefore the mortality of these patients. Finally, the authors consider that some proposals should be take into account when treating a frail and ancient population:

- Essential training in bioethics for postgraduates.
- Updating of the same staff, including knowledge of the basic legal framework that regulates patient rights.
- Dissemination of information to civil society on the reality of hip fractures to emphasize the seriousness of this genuine epidemic.

5. Conclusions

Based on the results of this study, the elderly population may somehow lose their principle of autonomy when they enter a hospital due to a hip fracture. On the other hand, the so-called ageism due to ignorance can influence the surgical delay and therefore the mortality of these patients.

Author Contributions: Conceptualization, M.H.-P.; methodology, M.H.-P.; formal analysis, M.H.-P.; investigation, M.H.-P.; data curation, D.G.-M. and M.H.-P.; writing—original draft preparation, M.H.-P. and D.G.-M.; writing—review and editing, J.L.P.-B. and D.G.-M.; supervision, E.J.S.; project administration, M.H.-P. All authors have read and agreed to the published version of the manuscript.

Funding: This research received no external funding.

Institutional Review Board Statement: We received an official statement from the medical/ethical board of the Hospital Universitario de Canarias that we were allowed to conduct the study (Code: 2018/57).

Informed Consent Statement: No informed consent is required for this type of publication.

Acknowledgments: The main author would like to thank to the medical residents in traumatology in University Hospital of Canary Islands and to his tutor and colleague Emilio Sanz, for introducing him to this new, limitless field.

Conflicts of Interest: The authors declare no conflict of interest.

References

1. Rapp, K.; Becker, C.; Lamb, S.E.; Icks, A.; Klenk, J. Hip fractures in institutionalized elderly people: Incidence rates and excess mortality. *J. Bone Miner. Res.* **2008**, *23*, 1825–1831. [CrossRef] [PubMed]
2. Herrera-Perez, M. Escalas de Valoración del Riesgo de Fractura en Pacientes Ingresados Por Fractura de Cadera. Ph.D. Thesis, Universidad de La Laguna, Tenerife, Spain, 2011.
3. Forsén, L.; Sogaard, A.; Meyer, H.E.; Edna, T.; Kopjar, B. Survival after hip fracture: Short- and long-term excess mortality according to age and gender. *Osteoporos. Int.* **1999**, *10*, 73–78. [CrossRef] [PubMed]
4. Lunney, J.R.; Lynn, J.; Foley, D.J.; Lipson, S.; Guralnik, J.M. Patterns of Functional Decline at the End of Life. *JAMA* **2003**, *289*, 2387–2392. [CrossRef] [PubMed]
5. Boyd, C.M.; Xue, Q.L.; Simpson, C.F.; Guralnik, J.M.; Fried, L.P. Frailty, hospitalization, and progression of disability in a cohort of disabled older women. *Am. J. Med.* **2005**, *118*, 1225–1231. [CrossRef]
6. Davison, J.; Bond, J.; Dawson, P.; Steen, I.N.; Kenny, R.A. Patients with recurrent falls attending Accident & Emergency benefit from multifactorial intervention—A randomised controlled trial. *Age Ageing* **2005**, *34*, 162–168. [PubMed]
7. Serra Rexach, J.A. Comunicación entre el paciente anciano y el médico. *Anales de Medicina Interna* **2003**, *20*, 57–58. [CrossRef]
8. Cejudo López, Á.; López López, B.; Duarte Rodríguez, M.; Crespo Serván, M.P.; Coronado Illescas, C.; de la Fuente Rodríguez, C. Silence pact from the perspective of caretakers of palliative care patients. *Enferm. Clin.* **2015**, *25*, 124–132. [CrossRef]
9. Wolinsky, F.D.; Miller, D.K.; Andresen, E.M.; Malmstrom, T.K.; Miller, J.P. Further evidence for the importance of subclinical functional limitation and subclinical disability assessment in gerontology and geriatrics. *J. Gerontol. B Psychol.Sci. Soc. Sci.* **2005**, *60*, S146–S151. [CrossRef]
10. Carlson, K.J.; Black, D.R.; Holley, L.M.; Coster, D.C. Stereotypes of Older Adults: Development and Evaluation of an Updated Stereotype Content and Strength Survey. *Gerontologist* **2020**, *60*, e347–e356. [CrossRef]
11. Donizzetti, A.R. Ageism in an Aging Society: The Role of Knowledge, Anxiety about Aging, and Stereotypes in Young People and Adults. *Int. J. Environ. Res. Public Health* **2019**, *16*, 1329. [CrossRef]
12. Consolidated Version of the Treaty of the European Union. Spanish State Official Newsletter, 30/3/2010. Available online: https://www.boe.es/doue/2010/083/Z00013-00046.pdf (accessed on 1 February 2017).
13. Ley 41/2002, 14 de noviembre, básica reguladora de la autonomía del paciente y de derechos y obligaciones en materia de información y documentación clínica. Boletín Oficial del Estado, 15 de noviembre de 2002, núm. 274. pp. 40126–40132. Available online: https://www.boe.es/eli/es/l/2002/11/14/41/con (accessed on 1 March 2017).
14. Ley 14/1986, 25 de abril, General de Sanidad. Boletín Oficial del Estado, 29 de abril de 1986, núm. 102. pp. 15207–15224. Available online: https://www.boe.es/eli/es/l/1986/04/25/14 (accessed on 1 March 2017).
15. Baker, A.C.; Ambrose, C.G.; Knudson, P.L.; Saraykar, S.S.; Piller, L.B.; McCurdy, S.A.; Rianon, N.J. Factors Considered by Interprofessional Team for Treatment Decision in Hip Fracture with Dementia. *J. Am. Geriatr. Soc.* **2019**, *67*, 1132–1137. [CrossRef] [PubMed]
16. Beauchamp, T.L.; Childress, J.F. *Principles of Biomedical Ethics*; Oxford University Press: New York, NY, USA, 1979.
17. Gracia, D. *Fundamentos de Bioética*, 3rd ed.; Editorial Triacastela: Madrid, Spain, 2008.
18. Gracia, D. Spanish bioethics comes into maturity: Personal reflections. *Camb. Q. Heal. Ethics* **2009**, *18*, 219–227. [CrossRef] [PubMed]
19. Gill, T.M.; Allore, H.G.; Holford, T.R.; Guo, Z. Hospitalization, restricted activity, and the development of disability among older persons. *JAMA* **2004**, *292*, 2115–2124. [CrossRef] [PubMed]

20. Gullberg, B.; Johnell, O.; Kanis, J.A. World-wide projections for hip fracture. *Osteoporos. Int.* **1997**, *7*, 407–413. [CrossRef] [PubMed]
21. Sosa, M.; Arbelo, A.; Lainez, P.; Navarro, M.C. Datos actualizados sobre la epidemiología de la fractura osteoporótica en España. *Rev. Esp. Enf. Metab. Óseas.* **1998**, *7*, 174–179.
22. Serra, J.A.; Garrido, G.; Vidán, M.; Marañón, E.; Brañas, F.; Ortiz, J. Epidemiología de la fractura de cadera en ancianos en España. Epidemiology of hip fractures in the elderly in Spain. *An. Med. Interna.* **2002**, *19*, 389–395.
23. Chatterton, B.D.; Moores, T.S.; Ahmad, S.; Cattell, A.; Roberts, P.J. Cause of death and factors associated with early in-hospital mortality after hip fracture. *Bone Joint J.* **2015**, *97*, 246–251. [CrossRef]
24. Dyer, S.M.; Crotty, M.; Fairhall, N.; Magaziner, J.; Beaupre, L.A.; Cameron, I.D.; Sherrington, C. Fragility Fracture Network (FFN) Rehabilitation Research Special Interest Group. A critical review of the long-term disability outcomes following hip fracture. *BMC Geriatr.* **2016**, *16*, 158. [CrossRef]
25. Sanz-Reig, J.; Salvador Marín, J.; Fernández Martínez, J.; Orozco Beltrán, D.; Martínez López, J.F. Factores de riesgo para la demora quirúrgica en la fractura de cadera. *Rev. Esp. Cir. Ortop. Traumatol.* **2017**, *61*, 162–169. [CrossRef]
26. Cordero, J.; Maldonado, A.; Iborra, S. Surgical delay as a risk for wound infection after hip fracture. *Injury* **2016**, *47* (Suppl. 3), S56–S60. [CrossRef]
27. Johnell, O.; Kanis, J.A. Epidemiology of osteoporotic fractures. *Osteoporos. Int.* **2005**, *16* (Suppl. 2), S3–S7. [CrossRef] [PubMed]
28. Cooper, C.; O'Neill, T.; Silman, A. The epidemiology of vertebral fractures. European Vertebral Osteoporosis Study Group. *Bone* **1993**, *14* (Suppl. 1), S89–S97. [CrossRef]
29. Sosa, M.; Segarra, M.C.; Hernández, D.; Gonzalez, A.; Limiñana, J.M.; Betancor, P. Epidemiology of proximal femoral fracture in Gran Canaria (Canary Islands). *Age Ageing* **1993**, *22*, 285–288. [CrossRef] [PubMed]
30. Sidi, A.; Lobato, E.B.; Cohen, J.A. The American Society of Anesthesiologists´physical status: Category V revisited. *J. Clin. Abesth.* **2000**, *12*, 328–334. [CrossRef]
31. Mercado, C. Dilemas bioéticos en geriatría: Toma de decisiones médicas. *Acta Bioeth.* **2001**, *7*, 129–141. [CrossRef]
32. Vidán, M.T.; Sánchez, E.; Gracia, Y.; Marañón, E.; Vaquero, J.; Serra, J.A. Causes and effects of surgical delay in patients with hip fracture: A cohort study. *Ann. Intern. Med.* **2011**, *155*, 226–233. [CrossRef]
33. Ooi, L.H.; Wong, T.H.; Toh, C.L.; Wong, H.P. Hip fractures in nonagenarians–a study on operative and non-operative management. *Injury* **2005**, *36*, 142–147. [CrossRef]
34. Jennings, A.G.; de Boer, P. Should we operate on nonagenarians with hip fractures? *Injury* **1999**, *30*, 169–172. [CrossRef]
35. Barceló, M.; Francia, E.; Romero, C.; Ruiz, D.; Casademont, J.; Torres, O.H. Hip fractures in the oldest old. Comparative study of centenarians and nonagenarians and mortality risk factors. *Injury* **2018**, *49*, 2198–2202. [CrossRef]
36. Oliver, C.W.; Burke, C. Hip fractures in centenarians. *Injury* **2004**, *35*, 1025–1030. [CrossRef]
37. Correoso-Castellanos, S.; Lajara-Marco, F.; Díez-Galán, M.M.; Blay-Dominguez, E.; Bernáldez-Silvetti, P.F.; Palazón-Banegas, M.A.; Lozano Requena, J.A. Analysis of surgical delay and its influence on morbimortality in patients with hip fracture. *Rev. Esp. Cir. Ortop. Traumatol.* **2019**, *63*, 246–251. [CrossRef]
38. Serbest, S.; Tiftikci, U.; Tosun, H.B.; Gumustas, S.A.; Uludag, A. Is there a relationship between fracture healing and mean platelet volume? *Ther. Clin. Risk Manag.* **2016**, *12*, 1095–1099. [CrossRef] [PubMed]
39. Serbest, S.; Tiftikçi, U.; Tosun, H.B.; Kısa, Ü. The Irisin Hormone Profile and Expression in Human Bone Tissue in the Bone Healing Process in Patients. *Med. Sci. Monit.* **2017**, *23*, 4278–4283. [CrossRef] [PubMed]
40. González-Martín, D.; González-Casamayor, S.; Herrera-Pérez, M.; Guerra-Ferraz, A.; Ojeda-Jiménez, J.; Pais-Brito, J.L. Is Stem Revision Necessary for Vancouver B2 Periprosthetic Hip Fractures? Analysis of Osteosynthesis Results from 39 Cases. *J. Clin. Med.* **2021**, *10*, 5288. [CrossRef]
41. González-Martín, D.; Pais-Brito, J.L.; González-Casamayor, S.; Guerra-Ferraz, A.; Martín-Vélez, P.; Herrera-Pérez, M. Periprosthetic Hip Fractures with a Loose Stem: Open Reduction and Internal Fixation Versus Stem Revision. *J. Arthroplast.* **2021**, *36*, 3318–3325. [CrossRef]
42. González-Martín, D.; Pais-Brito, J.L.; González-Casamayor, S.; Guerra-Ferraz, A.; Ojeda-Jiménez, J.; Herrera-Pérez, M. New Sub-Classification of Vancouver B2 Periprosthetic Hip Fractures According to Fracture Pattern. *Injury* **2022**, *53*, 1218–1224. [CrossRef]

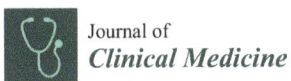

Article

Peri-Implant Distal Radius Fracture: Proposal of a New Classification

Leonardo Stramazzo [1,†], Giuseppe Rovere [2,†], Alessio Cioffi [1], Giulio Edoardo Vigni [1], Nicolò Galvano [1], Antonio D'Arienzo [3], Giulia Letizia Mauro [4], Lawrence Camarda [1,*] and Michele D'Arienzo [1]

[1] Department of Orthopaedic Surgery (DICHIRONS), University of Palermo, 90133 Palermo, Italy; stramazzoleonardo@gmail.com (L.S.); ale.cioffi90@gmail.com (A.C.); giulio.vigni@gmail.com (G.E.V.); nicologalvano@libero.it (N.G.); michele.darienzo@unipa.it (M.D.)
[2] Department of Orthopaedics and Traumatology, Fondazione Policlinico Universitario A. Gemelli IRCCS, Università Cattolica del Sacro Cuore, 00168 Rome, Italy; rovere292@hotmail.com
[3] Department of Orthopaedic Surgery, University of Pisa, 56126 Pisa, Italy; antu84@gmail.com
[4] Department of Physical Medicine and Rehabilitation, University of Palermo, 90133 Palermo, Italy; giulia.letiziamauro@unipa.it
* Correspondence: lawrence.camarda@unipa.it
† These authors contributed equally to this work.

Abstract: A peri-implant fracture near the volar plate of the distal radius represents a rarity and can be associated with a mechanical failure of the devices. A literature review was conducted including all fractures that occurred around a volar wrist plate, which could be associated with an ulna fracture. All articles published until December 2021 were considered according to the guidelines presented in the PRISMA Statement. The search was conducted with the PubMed electronic database, Cochrane Database of Systematic Reviews, Medline, Embase, and Google Scholar. Only nine cases of these fractures were reported in the literature. The causes could be due to delayed union/non-union of the old fracture after low energy traumas, high energy trauma in patients with poor bone quality, or hardware mechanical failure. Furthermore, the literature review of peri-implant radius fracture shows different level of radius fracture and types of implant failure. In accordance with these different cases, a new classification of peri-implant fracture of the distal radius is proposed.

Keywords: wrist fracture; plate breakage; plate bending; peri-implant fracture

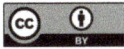

1. Introduction

Distal radius fractures (DRF) are frequent fractures in the adult population and represent one third of all fractures in the elderly, with an incidence of 190/100,000 per year [1,2]. The surgical management of DRF has undergone extensive changes over the last four decades, from casting to K-wire fixation followed by locked plate fixation. Volar locking plates are being increasingly used for the stabilization of distal radius fractures [3]. Complication rates after volar locking plate fixation of DRF range from 3 to 36% and are widely reported in the literature: sensibility change, tendon irritation or rupture, hardware malfunction, infection, complex regional pain syndrome, and arthritis [4,5]. Mechanical failure of the volar locking plate device is considered to be a rare complication, with failure being defined as plate breakage/bending, screw breakage/loosening, or collapse of articular fragments resulting in intra-articular screw extrusion. Non-prosthetic peri-implant fracture (NPPIF) as a distinct clinical entity is very rare, and only a few articles are reported in the literature [6–14]. With the term NPPIF, we referred to an acute bone fracture during a trauma that occurs around implants [15], and it did not include failures of primary fracture fixation such as an implant breakage due to non-union.

In this article, we review all cases of peri-implant radius fracture reported in the literature, and a new classification is proposed according to the different levels of the fracture and the type of plate failure.

2. Material and Methods

A review of the literature was performed to investigate all cases of peri-implant radius fracture according to the guidelines presented in the PRISMA Statement (Preferred Reporting Items for Systematic Reviews and Meta-Analyses) [16]. All cases included were of peri-implant radius fractures that occurred around a previous fixation of a wrist fracture with a volar plate in patients over 18 years of age. Cases with an ulna fracture associated with the radius fracture were also considered, including only the detailed cases described regarding the fracture and its treatment. The search was conducted with the PubMed electronic database, Cochrane Database of Systematic Reviews, Medline, Embase, and Google Scholar. The search was conducted including all studies published until December 2021. The following MeSH entries were used for research articles: peri-implant wrist fracture, breakage plate, bending plate, fracture plate wrist, radius hardware failure, radius refracture. All journals were included, and all relevant studies were considered for this study. No filters were applied to the search strategies, and only papers published in English were considered for inclusion. Three reviewers (L.S., A.C., and L.C.) independently conducted the research. Papers were initially identified based on the title and abstract. Investigators separately reviewed the abstract of each publication and then performed an accurate reading of all extended papers to minimize bias. The researchers (L.S., A.C.) checked all the references from the identified articles in order to not miss any relevant study.

3. Results

Nine manuscripts fulfilled the inclusion criteria and were included in the review [6–14] (Table 1 and Figure 1). The articles included in this review were all case report studies (nine patients). In four patients, hardware failure occurred after small efforts or low energy traumas [6–8,12]; in four cases, the new fracture occurred a few months after the fixation and along the old line of fracture [6–8,14]. Loss of reduction with implant failure was presented in two cases without trauma or particular efforts [13,14]. In one case, the fixation failure occurred after seven days [13]. The causes of these fractures were due to delayed union/non-union (promoted by patient's comorbidity or by smoking habit) or to implant design failure (high rigidity of the hardware, number and direction of proximal and distal locking screws). In four patients, the fractures occurred years later from the primary surgery when the old fracture was already healed [9–12]. In this case, fractures occurred following a high energy trauma (three patients) and in a patient affected by osteoporosis and poor bone quality.

Regardless of the type of trauma, the condition of the plate or site of the fracture can vary. In fact, in three cases, the plate was bent, and in all these cases the fracture occurred under the plate. One patient was treated with close reduction and plate alignment [8], while two other patients were treated with plate removal and a new plate placement [9,10]. One of these cases was associated with a compound ulna fracture that did not require surgical fixation [10]. In four cases, the new fracture occurred along the old line of fracture with the loosening of the previous reduction [6,7,13,14]. In all these cases, the plate was broken and different treatments were reported. In three cases, the broken plate was removed and a new reduction with a new plate was performed [6,13,14]. In the other case, a closed reduction and splint immobilization was performed due to comorbidities of the patient [7]. In the last two cases reported in the literature, the plate was whole and the fracture occurred proximally to the plate and was associated with an ulna fracture; in both cases, the authors opted for a substitution of the old implant with a longer volar plate and synthesis of the ulna fracture with a plate [11,12].

Table 1. Literature review of perisynthesic fractures of the distal radius with their main features.

Authors Year of Publication	Years Old	Sex	Time from Primary Implant	Type of Trauma	Site of the Fracture	Plate Condition	Ulnar Fracture	Neuro-Vascular Compromise	Treatment
De Baere et al., 2007	58	F	3.5 months	Effort	Loss of previous reduction	Broken	No	No	Substitution of old implant with new plate
Yukata et al., 2009	82	F	3 months	Effort	Loss of previous reduction	Broken	No	No	Splint
Imade et al., 2009	56	M	7 days	Unknown	Loss of previous reduction	Broken	No	No	Substitution of old implant with new plate
Geurts et al., 2012	78	F	6 months	Accidental fall	Under the plate	Bent	No	Yes	Close reduction and alignment of the plate
Khan et al., 2012	30	M	2 months	Unknown	Loss of previous reduction	Broken	No	No	Substitution of old implant with new plate
Lucke-Wold et al., 2016	73	F	3 years	Traffic accident	Under the plate	Bent	Yes	No	Substitution of old implant with new plate
Kanji et al., 2017	50	M	11 years	Traffic accident	Under the plate	Bent	No	Yes	Substitution of old implant with new plate
Barrera-Ochoa et al., 2017	34	M	9 years	Traffic accident	Proximally to the plate	Whole	Yes	No	Substitution of old implant with a longer volar plate and a plate for the ulna
Stramazzo et al., 2020	61	F	4 years	Accidental fall	Proximally to the plate	Whole	Yes	No	Substitution of old implant with a longer volar plate and a plate for the ulna

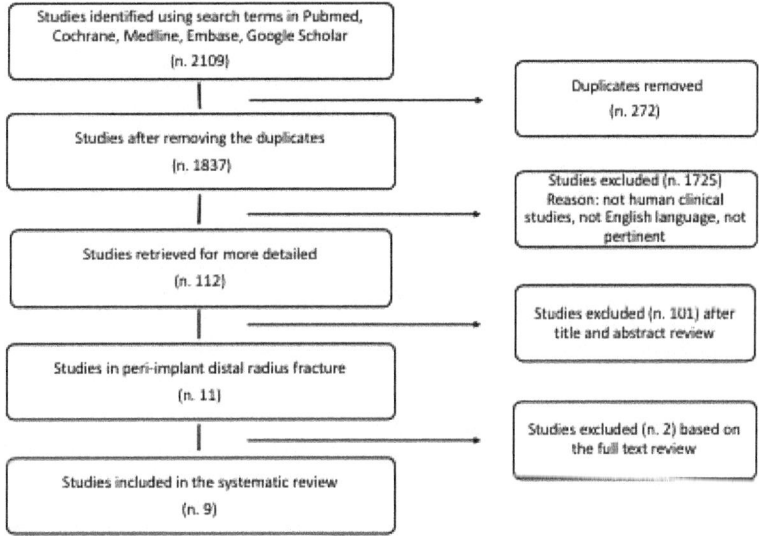

Figure 1. Flow diagram that describes the number of studies identified, included, and excluded as well as the reasons for exclusion.

4. Discussion

Peri-implant distal radius fractures are rare, but their number will go up due to the increased use of volar plates for wrist fractures fixation [17]. The causes of these different fractures include patient factors (comorbidity such as osteoporosis, smoking), biological factors (complex fractures), and mechanical factors (no bone graft, unfilled screw holes, and insufficient immobilization). In a recent systematic review of 52 articles, Yamamoto et al. analyzed the hardware removal and complication rate of using a volar locking plate for a distal radius fracture; they did not specifically talk of peri-implant fractures or damaged plates, but they generally reported a hardware problem in 14% of cases and refracture in 1% [18]. A recent study on early postoperative complications that occurred in 594 patients with a distal radius fracture treated with a volar locking plate and a minimum 1-month evaluation reported only two cases of peri-plate fracture. They occurred proximally to the plate, and any cases of plate breakage or bending were reported [19].

Based on the type of fracture, it will be necessary to investigate the precise position of the fracture in relation to the plate and its condition. Further, is mandatory to evaluate the location of the previous wrist fracture in order to plan the surgical treatment. In 2017, Chan and coll. proposed a classification of non-prosthetic peri-implant fractures (NPPIF), which considers the type of implant (nail or plate), the type of fracture (close or far to the implant) in any part of the body, and the healing of the old fracture. However, the authors did not consider the failure of the old plate such as breakage or mobilization [15].

According to the literature review, a classification for the peri-implant wrist fractures was proposed by the senior author (Michele D'Arienzo), and it can be comparable to Duncan's classification for periprosthetic hip fractures [20–22]. This new classification, which we prefer to define "perisynthesic" by analogy with periprosthetic, contemplates three types: A, B, and C, based on the location of the fracture and the type of plate failure (bending or breakage) (Figure 2). We call A1 fractures those of radial styloid and A2 those of the medial part of distal epiphysis of the radius. The type B fractures are radius ones that occur under the plate, and we distinguish them as type B1 if there is a bending of the plate and B2 if the plate is broken. In type C, radius fracture occurs proximally to the plate and we call them C1 or C2, depending on whether they occur within 3.5 cm from the plate or beyond 3.5 cm. If there is an association with a fracture of the ulna, we associate the letter U with these abbreviations (e.g., A1U or B2U).

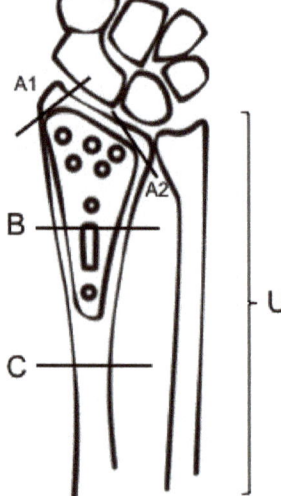

Figure 2. Michele D'Arienzo Classification of perisynthesic fractures of the distal radius with different levels.

According to this new classification, we propose the following therapeutic algorithm: for A1 and A2 fractures, we suggest non-invasive treatment in the case of compound fractures or surgical treatment in relation to the type of displacement (K-wires, screws). For type B1 and B2 fractures, it is necessary to replace the old plate with a new implant, though in the literature it is also reported that two cases were successfully treated with closed reduction and immobilization [7,8]. In the case of C1 fractures, it is necessary to replace the old plate with a longer plate, while in C2 the fracture is located at a distance such from the old implant that there is enough space to insert a new plate proximally. These must eventually be associated with a reduction and synthesis of the ulna according to level and eventual displacement of the fracture.

5. Conclusions

A peri-implant fracture near the volar plate of the distal radius represents a very rare injury, but, considering the growing use of plates, its frequency will probably increase. A trauma of high energy associated with poor bone quality (osteoporosis) can determine a re-fracture around the plate, even if the previous implant was stable, as a low energy trauma in delayed union/non-union fracture can do it too. In addition, the new trauma can cause the bending or the breakage of the plate. In the literature, there is not an exhaustive classification for these types of lesions, and our classification describes a specific point of perisynthesic fracture and the treatment algorithm.

Author Contributions: Conceptualization, M.D., L.C., L.S. and G.R.; methodology, M.D., L.S. and G.R.; software, G.R.; validation, M.D., G.L.M., G.E.V. and L.S.; formal analysis, G.R.; investigation, A.D., G.R., L.S., N.G. and A.C.; resources, L.S and G.R; data curation, L.S.; writing—original draft preparation, L.S. and G.R.; writing—review and editing, L.S., G.R., M.D. and L.C.; visualization, L.S.; supervision, L.C. and M.D. All authors have read and agreed to the published version of the manuscript.

Funding: This research received no external funding.

Institutional Review Board Statement: Not applicable.

Informed Consent Statement: Not applicable.

Data Availability Statement: Not applicable.

Conflicts of Interest: The authors declare that they have no conflict of interest.

References

1. Wilcke, M.K.; Hammarberg, H.; Adolphson, P.Y. Epidemiology and changed surgical treatment methods for fractures of the distal radius: A registry analysis of 42,583 patients in Stockholm County, Sweden, 2004–2010. *Acta Orthop.* **2013**, *84*, 292–296. [CrossRef] [PubMed]
2. Jupiter, J.B.; Marent-Huber, M.; L.C.P Study Group. Operative management of distal radial fractures with 2.4- millimeter locking plates: A multicenter prospective case series. *J. Bone Jt. Surg. Am.* **2010**, *92*, 96–106. [CrossRef] [PubMed]
3. Arora, R.; Gabl, M.; Erhart, S.; Schmidle, G.; Dallapozza, C.; Lutz, M. Aspects of current management of distal radius fractures in the elderly individuals. *Geriatr. Orthop. Surg. Rehabil.* **2011**, *2*, 187–194. [CrossRef]
4. Foo, T.L.; Gan, A.W.; Soh, T.; Chew, W.Y. Mechanical failure of the distal radius volar locking plate. *J. Orthop. Surg.* **2013**, *21*, 332–336. [CrossRef]
5. Wilson, J.; Viner, J.J.; Johal, K.S.; Woodruff, M.J. Volar Locking Plate Fixations for Displaced Distal Radius Fractures: An Evaluation of Complications and Radiographic Outcomes. *Hand* **2018**, *13*, 466–472. [CrossRef]
6. De Baere, T.; Lecouvet, F.; Barbier, O. Breakage of a volar locking plate after delayed union of a distal radius fracture. *Acta Orthop. Belg.* **2007**, *73*, 785–790.
7. Yukata, K.; Doi, K.; Hattori, Y.; Sakamoto, S. Early breakage of a titanium volar locking plate for fixation of a distal radius fracture: Case report. *J. Hand Surg. Am.* **2009**, *34*, 907–909. [CrossRef]
8. Geurts, G.F.; Van Riet, R.P.; Verstreken, F. Successful closed reduction of refractured wrist with a bent volar distal radius plate. *Acta Orthop. Belg.* **2012**, *78*, 126–128.
9. Kanji, R.; Nutt, J.; Stavropoulos, S.; Elmorsy, A.; Schneider, H. Distal radius re-fracture with bending of implant and neurovascular compromise. *J. Clin. Orthop. Trauma* **2017**, *8*, S40–S42. [CrossRef]

10. Lucke-Wold, B.P.; Bonasso, P.C.; Jacob, G. Re-fracture of Distal Radius and Hardware Repair in the Setting of Trauma. *Med. Stud. Res. J.* **2017**, *5*, 2–7. [CrossRef]
11. Barrera-Ochoa, S.; Nuñez, J.H.; Mir, X. Peri-implant radial and ulnar shaft fractures after volar locking plate fixation of the distal radius. *J. Hand Surg. Eur. Vol.* **2018**, *43*, 209–210. [CrossRef] [PubMed]
12. Stramazzo, L.; Cioffi, A.; Rovere, G.; Vigni, G.E.; Galvano, N.; Sallì, M.; D'Arienzo, A.; Camarda, L.; D'Arienzo, M. A rare case of peri-implant distal radius fracture. *Trauma Case Rep.* **2020**, *9*, 100387. [CrossRef] [PubMed]
13. Imade, S.; Matsuura, Y.; Miyamoto, W.; Nishi, H.; Uchio, Y. Breakage of a volar locking compression plate in distal radial fracture. *Inj. Extra* **2009**, *40*, 77–80. [CrossRef]
14. Khan, S.K.; Gozzard, C. Union of an intra-articular distal radius fracture after successive failures of three locking plates: A case report. *Strateg. Trauma Limb. Reconstr.* **2012**, *7*, 45–50. [CrossRef]
15. Chan, L.W.M.; Gardner, A.W.; Wong, M.K.; Chua, K.; Kwek, E.B.K. Non-prosthetic peri-implant fractures: Classification, management and outcomes. *Arch. Orthop. Trauma Surg.* **2018**, *138*, 791–802. [CrossRef]
16. Moher, D.; Liberati, A.; Tetzlaff, J.; Altman, D.G. Preferred reporting items for systematic reviews and meta-analyses: The PRISMA statement. *Ann. Intern. Med.* **2009**, *18*, 264–269. [CrossRef]
17. Snoddy, M.C.; An, T.J.; Hooe, B.S.; Kay, H.F.; Lee, D.H.; Pappas, N.D. Incidence and reasons for hardware removal following operative fixation of distal radius fractures. *J. Hand Surg. Am.* **2015**, *40*, 505–507. [CrossRef]
18. Yamamoto, M.; Fujihara, Y.; Fujihara, N.; Hirata, H. A systematic review of volar locking plate removal after distal radius fracture. *Injury* **2017**, *48*, 2650–2656. [CrossRef]
19. Soong, M.; Van Leerdam, R.; Guitton, T.G.; Got, C.; Katarincic, J.; Ring, D. Fracture of the distal radius: Risk factors for complications after locked volar plate fixation. *J. Hand Surg. Am.* **2011**, *36*, 3–9. [CrossRef]
20. Duncan, C.P.; Masri, B.A. Fractures of the femur after hip replacement. *Instr. Course Lect.* **1995**, *44*, 293–304.
21. Camarda, L.; Martorana, U.; D'Arienzo, M. A case of bilateral luxatio erecta. *J. Orthop. Traumatol.* **2009**, *10*, 97–99. [CrossRef] [PubMed]
22. Bonetti, M.A.; Rovere, G.; Fulchignoni, C.; De Santis, V.; Ziranu, A.; Maccauro, G.; Pataia, E. Autologous fat transplantation for the treatment of trapeziometacarpal joint osteoarthritis. *Orthop. Rev.* **2020**, *12*, 8666.

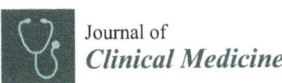

Review

Biological Approach in the Treatment of External Popliteal Sciatic Nerve (Epsn) Neurological Injury: Review

Alejandro León-Andrino [1], David C. Noriega [1,2,*], Juan P. Lapuente [3], Daniel Pérez-Valdecantos [4], Alberto Caballero-García [5], Azael J. Herrero [6] and Alfredo Córdova [4]

1. Department of Orthopedic Surgery, Clinic University Hospital of Valladolid, 47005 Valladolid, Spain; aaleon@saludcastillayleon.es
2. Department of Surgery, Ophthalmology, Otorhinolaryngology and Physiotherapy, Faculty of Medicine, University of Valladolid, 47005 Valladolid, Spain
3. SCO (Scientific Chief Officer) Laboratorio de Biología Molecular y Celular R4T, University Hospital of Fuenlabrada, 28942 Fuenlabrada, Spain; jplapuente@yahoo.es
4. Biochemistry, Molecular Biology and Physiology, Faculty of Health Sciences, GIR Physical Exercise and Aging, University of Valladolid, Campus Duques de Soria, 42004 Soria, Spain; danielperezvaldecantos@gmail.com (D.P.-V.); a.cordova@uva.es (A.C.)
5. Department of Anatomy and Radiology, Faculty of Health Sciences, GIR Physical Exercise and Aging, University of Valladolid, Campus Duques de Soria, 42004 Soria, Spain; alberto.caballero@uva.es
6. Department of Health Sciences, Miguel de Cervantes European University, 47012 Valladolid, Spain; jaherrero@uemc.es
* Correspondence: drdcnoriegagonz@gmail.com or davidcesar.noriega@uva.esm

Abstract: The external popliteal sciatic nerve (EPSN) is the nerve of the lower extremity most frequently affected by compressive etiology. Its superficial and sinuous anatomical course is closely related to other rigid anatomical structures and has an important dynamic neural component. Therefore, this circumstance means that this nerve is exposed to multiple causes of compressive etiology. Despite this fact, there are few publications with extensive case studies dealing with treatment. In this review, we propose to carry out a narrative review of the neuropathy of the EPSN, including an anatomical reminder, its clinical presentation and diagnosis, as well as its surgical and biological approach. The most novel aspect we propose is the review of the possible role of biological factors in the reversal of this situation.

Keywords: external popliteal sciatic nerve (EPSN); common peroneal nerve; compression; neurolysis; foot drop; growth factors

1. Introduction

Traumatic peripheral nerve injury is a difficult and controversial issue for the orthopaedic surgeon and a challenge for rehabilitation. Despite the introduction of microsurgical techniques by Kurze [1], nerve repair and functional recovery is mostly incomplete and always difficult to predict. Moreover, nerve injuries remain the main causes of reduced functional capacity and generate high socio-economic costs due to the long rehabilitation times required, as well as the disability sequelae that may eventually result [2,3].

Fibular or peroneal neuropathy is the most common lower limb neuropathy and the third most common focal neuropathy found in general, after median and ulnar neuropathies [4]. Following high tibial and fibular osteotomies, an incidence of peroneal neuropathy has been observed in 2–27% of patients [4]. Following knee dislocations, common peroneal nerve injury has been observed in 16–40% of patients. In children, peroneal neuropathy of the common peroneal nerve was also observed to be affected most frequently (59%), followed by the deep (12%) and superficial (5%) peroneal nerves [5].

To the best of our current knowledge about nerve trauma and neuronal regeneration, the solution to improve the outcome of peripheral nerve repair is biological rather than surgical or rehabilitative [3,6,7]. Progress can only come from understanding and being able to modulate the different biological phases involved in the repair of peripheral nerve injuries, as there are phenomena of nerve regeneration fatigue, fascicle mismatches, and effector degeneration [8].

The mechanisms of injury are mainly contusions, compression, traction, focal ischaemia, and total or partial section. In practice, all degrees of involvement are observed, from conduction blocks to neurapraxia, axonotmesis, and neurotmesis. The most frequent causes of nerve involvement in the lower extremity are: penetrating trauma; fractures; dislocations; and iatrogenesis during injection or surgery, especially total knee arthroplasty [2,9–11]. The pathogenesis of these lesions progress in complexity from neurapraxia (a punctual conduction block due to myelin damage, as in compressive neuropathies) to axonotmesis (an axonal injury, due to crushing or traction, with irreversible damage associated with denervation time of the target muscle, but with a favourable prognosis of the nerve) and to neurotmesis (a complete section of the nerve with destruction of the endoneurial tubes that requires surgical treatment for resolution, and appears in penetrating wounds or ischemic processes) [11].

Microscopic techniques have shown that nerve morphology is normal and neuromuscular junctions are maintained in chronic compression lesions. However, the myelin sheath is thinner and degraded, and there is decreased internodal length (the distance between adjacent nodes of Ranvier) [12].

The main mechanical characteristic of the peripheral nerve is the tensile strength with a non-linear behaviour between weight and deformation. Under constant elongation, the nerve tension is reduced to 30% in the first 10 min and very little more in the next 20 min. This relaxation phenomenon (creep) is useful in sutures and nerve grafts, as the remaining tension will be lower after a short time [13].

Regarding the mechanisms thought to lead to compression injuries, from an anatomical point of view, the narrowing of the openings causes an increase in pressure at that site, compresses the blood vessels, and leads to nerve ischaemia. Another proposed mechanism is that, as a result of lower pressure, which decreases venous return, it can lead to venous stasis. Over time, this situation can lead to extraneural oedema, with a consequent increase in fibrous tissue around the nerve [14].

Not all cases resolve favourably because up to 33% of cases in peripheral nerve injuries have incomplete recovery with poor functional outcomes. Partial recovery has been observed, sometimes with a complete loss of motor and sensory function, and with chronic pain and muscle atrophy [1,15,16]. Compression of the EPSN is associated with peripheral neuropathy [17].

Nowadays, more and more importance is being given to the role that biological therapy can play after surgery for peripheral nerve disorders. This paper reviews the general aspects of surgery in traumatic compression of the EPSN. Special emphasis is placed on the possibilities of biological treatment for nerve regeneration after surgery.

To conduct the narrative review, a comprehensive literature search was performed using PubMed, Ovid MEDLINE, and EMBASE databases and the following search terms: ("nerve" OR "nerve trauma" OR "neurological surgery" OR "peripheral nerve injuries" OR "nerve repair" OR "nerve regeneration" OR "paralysis of the external popliteal" OR "compression and entrapment neuropathy" OR "fibular nerve compression" OR "peroneal nerve" OR "repair Schwann cell" OR "neurotrophic factors" OR "nerve regeneration" OR "mesenchymal stem cells" OR "fibroblast growth factors" OR "adipose stem cells" OR "platelet-derived growth factors" OR "myelination". We first selected the articles based on what we found in the abstracts, which led to a more exhaustive selection by reading the selected articles. We must take into account that many of them are very similar and do not contribute more than other articles.

2. Anatomy of the EPSN

The EPSN is the external division branch of the sciatic nerve. As it passes through the thigh, it is responsible for the innervation of the short head of the biceps femoris. From its origin, it descends outwards, following the biceps cruris tendon, and then it branches off and becomes independent of the sciatic nerve at the level of the popliteal fossa (Figure 1). The global function of the EPSN is dorsiflexion of the ankle at the moment of foot stance, directing the toe outward [18,19].

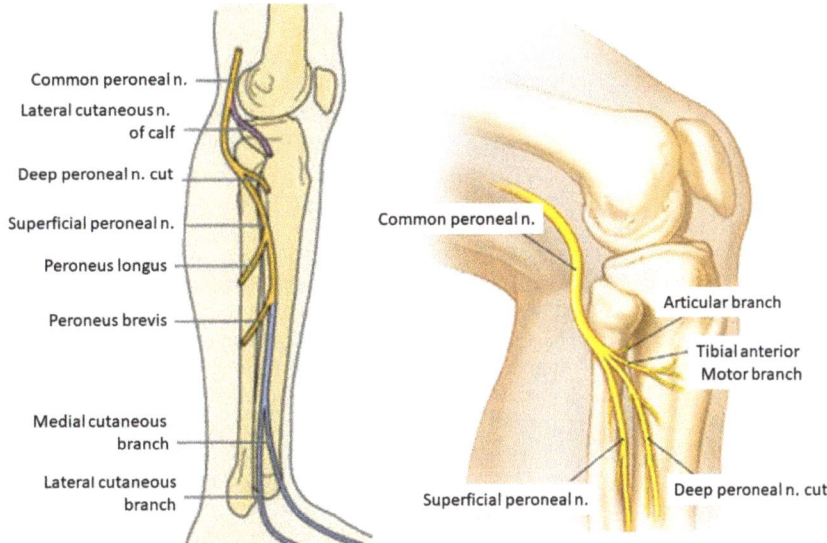

Figure 1. Anatomical presentation of the bifurcations of the sciatic nerve in the popliteal fossa.

3. Compression of the EPSN

There are several causes of nerve injury, the most frequent being the compressive cause; however, in this review, we do not wish to expand on this aspect. Schematically, the etiology may be due to: sustained nerve compression; trauma; peripheral neuropathies; very strenuous exercise; viral infection; and idiopathy [20–24]. From a pathophysiological point of view, nerve compression causes alterations in the intraneural blood microcirculation and axonal lesions, and alterations in the supporting connective tissue, among others [16,21]. These alterations, maintained over time, lead to demyelination, conduction disorders, and degeneration of nerve fibres [8,19,25–27].

Endoneural oedema increases hydrostatic pressure leading to endothelial hypoxia and consequent axonal damage [28,29]. Segmental axonal ischaemia is produced by a decrease in blood flow involving a loss of energy for transport and dysfunction of the sodium pump system. The cell membrane is also affected by the energy failure and has a consequent loss of conduction and transmission through the axon [30].

The part of the axon that has lost contact with the neuronal body is destroyed, and its myelin is phagocytosed by Schwann cells and macrophages. The whole process is known as Wallerian degeneration [26]. As a result of the process, the muscle fibres atrophy very rapidly in the absence of nerve stimuli, and are irreversibly damaged by 18 months. They are then replaced by fatty and fibrous tissue [31,32].

4. Clinical

When it comes to sciatic neuropathy, the clinical picture is usually more frequently seen with a lesion at the level of the common division of the fibula than at the tibial division. The common division of the fibula, compared to the tibial division, has fewer and larger fascicles and has less supporting tissue, and is therefore thought to be more vulnerable to compression. In addition, the common division of the fibula is tighter and more secure at the sciatic notch and the neck of the fibula. This makes it potentially more prone to stretch injury [33–35].

Clinically, EPSN neuropathy is manifested by weakness in dorsiflexion and eversion of the foot, often causing the person to stub their toe when walking. Inversion of the foot and plantar flexion must be preserved. The toes cannot be extended, with the flexors predominating and causing claw foot [21,36–38].

The onset of symptoms varies depending on the cause and extent of the injuries. It may appear abruptly or progressively and start with one symptom or another without the onset of other symptoms [39]. If the lesion is irritative rather than destructive, there may be neuropathic pain, which increases at night, with activity and stretching. Possible symptoms include the Valleix phenomenon, wherein the nerve is sensitive to palpation. Also positivity to the Tinel test, wherein a sensation of electrical discharge is felt along the nerve pathway due to direct percussion on it. In addition, vegetative changes may appear in the autonomic territory of the injured nerve [40].

5. Diagnosis

Patient history and clinical examination are key in the diagnosis of nerve entrapment. The examination should include a provocative sign using Tinel's sign and/or nerve blocks. Peripheral nerve injuries are initially assessed according to the crush dynamics of the nerve injury. During the clinical examination, motor power, sensation, and autonomic nerve functions are also explored [35,40].

When approaching the diagnosis, we should start with electromyography (EMG) [4,41–43]. Nerve conduction studies and EMG can identify axonal injury but cannot precisely localise the site of nerve injury. EMG is not valid until 3 weeks have passed and Wallerian degeneration has occurred [35].

Magnetic resonance neurography (MRN) is a new technique to detect peripheral nerve lesions [44,45], and can visualise nerve lesions even at the fascicular microstructural level [46].

The echography offers a less expensive and non-invasive option to guide treatment. Unlike electrodiagnostic studies alone, ultrasound can detect anatomical causes such as scarring, lesions, infiltration of bony fragments, and motion-tethered nerves. Contralateral comparison is often helpful for determining the type of lesion [39,47].

6. Treatment

In medicine, there is often a tendency to think that nerve injuries cannot be repaired, but fortunately, this is not the case. This may be due to confusion between the central nervous system (CNS) and the peripheral nervous system (PNS) injuries. Currently, CNS lesions cannot regenerate with surgical intervention; however, PNS lesions can regenerate after intervention. Moreover, it is currently not only limited to nerve regeneration by surgery. In addition, experimental molecular and bioengineering strategies are currently being developed to overcome nerve regeneration and recovery in patients [21,34].

6.1. Surgical Treatment

First, when the intrinsic compressive etiology is demonstrated by a space-occupying lesion, for example, by MRN, the lesion will be removed and analysed histologically, as shown in Figure 2A,B.

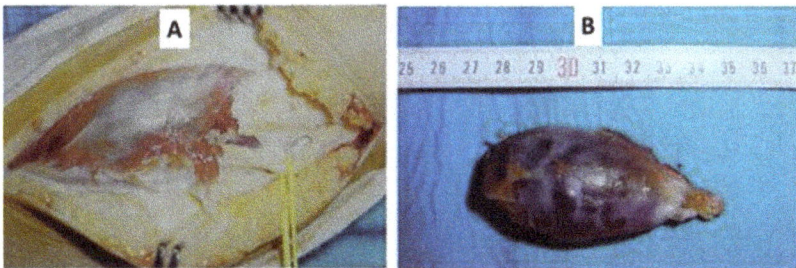

Figure 2. (**A**) Intraoperative image of upper tibio-peroneal cyst compressing the EPSN. (**B**) Sample of the superior tibio-peroneal cyst compressing the EPSN.

Another procedure is neurolysis, but its problem is that there is a risk of damaging undamaged nerve bundles. External neurolysis consists of freeing the nerve from its scar environment and involves fibrosis of the epineurium and the elements surrounding the nerve. Internal neurolysis requires the release of compressed fascicular groups, but the risk of injury to the inter-fascicular communications is significant. Both of these are shown in Figure 3A,B.

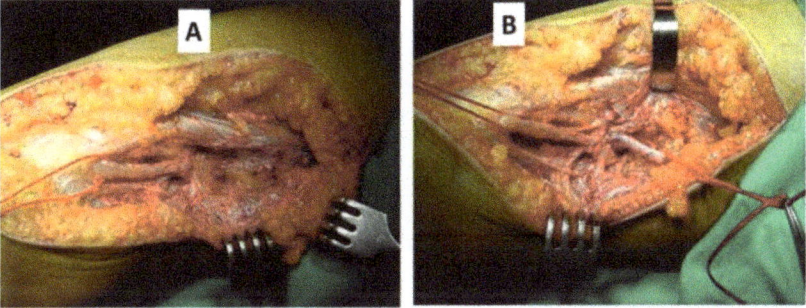

Figure 3. (**A**) Intraoperative image of fibrosis encompassing the EPSN. (**B**) Intraoperative image of the NPCE after neurolysis; note the macroscopic appearance of the nerve in its compressed section.

Grafts are indicated in cases where a suture would be under too much tension or where there is loss of substance between the two ends of the nerve [48,49]. It is always an autograft that must be revascularized from the tissue in which it is placed. This is why only small-diameter nerves can be used, as if the nerve is too thick, it will necrose in the central part.

Another surgical technique is neurotisation, which consists of driving a healthy nerve into a denervated nerve or territory when suturing or grafting is impossible. It is mainly used in brachial plexus injuries, as the absence of healthy donor nerves forces the use of nerves from adjacent regions. In the case of peroneal nerve involvement, transpositions of posterior tibial branches and functional branches of the superficial peroneal nerve, to the deep branch of the peroneal nerve, are performed, as well as innervation of the tibialis anterior muscle, with favourable results in motor recovery [50–52].

6.2. Biological Treatment

There is now a growing body of research into various cellular, molecular, and bio-engineering strategies to promote the repair and recovery of nerve damage. A number of technologies are now available that may help to improve the treatment of peripheral nerve injuries. Their use as an adjunct to surgical nerve repair may help to address the biological limitations of nerve regeneration. Many of the analgesic therapy clinical trials do not discriminate about the type of pain they treat. Cell therapies have emerged as promising potential therapeutics in both spinal cord regeneration and central neuropathic pain mitigation, but most clinical trials are animal-based.

In our opinion, biological techniques could be a paradigm shift in treatment and prognosis after peripheral nerve injury. In principle, we have to consider that nerve fibres regenerate spontaneously, depending on the size of the condition, the neuroma, and the formation of scar tissue [53].

Mesenchymal stem cells (MSCs) used for injuries of the musculoskeletal system can be obtained from the patient's fat, bone marrow, or even the umbilical cord. Although the mechanism of action is not yet fully elucidated, the use of MSCs is based on their anti-inflammatory property, which can lead to a decrease in the inflammatory response [54].

We must consider that it is possible that peripheral nerves could also be regenerated by the ability of peripheral neurons and Schwann cells (SC) to stimulate appropriate growth [39,55,56]. Early in development, neural crest cells produce SC precursors and other cells (neuronal and non-neuronal) [57–59].

In the repair process, Schwann cells provide the signals necessary for the survival and adaptation of injured neurons, axonal regeneration, and reinnervation. Conversion into reparative Schwann cells involves cell dedifferentiation and activation [55]. In this regard, it has already been described that SCs play a key role in the regeneration of axons in peripheral nerve grafts. With myelination, Schwann cells organize themselves. Many axons are introduced deeply into the cellular grafts, but not the acellular peripheral nerve grafts [59–61].

Nowadays, the use of biological techniques to deliver growth factors after nerve injury, which also promotes the reprogramming of Schwann cells, can accelerate this regeneration rate [55,62]. Likewise, in our group and in reference to vertebral disc regeneration, we used autologous and allogeneic mesenchymal stromal cells (MSC), which demonstrated their viability, safety, and strong indications of clinical efficacy one year after cell transplantation in the treatment of vertebral discs. They appear to be a valid alternative for the treatment of degenerative disc disease, as they can provide effective and long-lasting pain relief [63,64].

Following nerve injury, Schwann cells are reprogrammed, which involves the activation of repair-supporting elements, including macrophage recruitment, increased cytokines, increased trophic factors, and the removal of destroyed myelin through the autophagic capacity of the SCs themselves [65].

Studies on the importance and utility of stem cells have reported that bone marrow stem cells (BMSCs) have the capacity to differentiate into neuronal lines. These include SC-like cells, astrocytes, and oligodendrocytes [66,67]. It has been reported [68] that BMSCs can restore peripheral nerves through neutrophilic elements, and indirectly by altering SCs [68,69].

Neurotrophins (nerve growth factors) are released from the nerve ending during the process of nerve regeneration. They are released especially after nerve injury and promote nerve differentiation and growth [70].

After nerve injury, the production of nerve growth factor (NGF) is stimulated and plays a key role in the survival of sensory neurons [52]. Other growth factors, such as glial growth factor (GGF), glial cell-derived neurotrophic factor (GDNF), fibroblast growth factor (FGF), neurotrophin-3 (NT-3), ciliary neurotrophic factor, and leupeptin, are also produced in nerve regeneration [53,62,71–73].

In addition, other neurotrophic factors and surface proteins that promote axonal elongation include artemin, brain-derived neurotrophic factor (BDNF), neurotrophin-3 (NT-3), vascular endothelial growth factor (VEGF), erythropoietin, pleiotrophin, p75NTR, and N-cadherin [32,63,70,74,75].

In a study from Nath et al. [50], NGF, GGF, GDNF, and NT-3 were applied to small animal models of nerve gap injuries. These authors observed clear histological and electro-physiological improvements [51]. A study comparing NGF-seeded conduits with nerve autografts demonstrated high functional results in the autograft group. This confirms that the application of growth factors in this type of pathology could further enhance axonal regeneration [76].

Moreover, adipose-derived stem cells (ASCs) have been reported to be able to differentiate into cell types contained in different germ layers [75,77] and can effectively support nerve repair [6,78–80].

ASCs increased the regeneration and proliferation of proliferating Schwann cells. Indeed, Kingham et al. [81] observed that treatment of ASCs with a combination of mitogenic and distinct elements led to the expression of the glial cell markers S100B, glial fibrillary acidic protein, and the neurotrophic receptor p75 [82–87].

The compounds used in Kingham's induction protocol have different biological functions. For example, forskolin activates adenylyl cyclase, which causes an increase in the level of intracellular cyclic adenosine monophosphate (cAMP), which promotes and enhances the mitogenic responses of SCs [72], in response to that of the growth factors of PDGF and bFGF/FGF2 [78]. Neuregulin-1 (NRG1) is also involved in SC development and progression. It determines the differentiation of Schwann cells into myelinating or non-myelinating cells. This NRG1 generates a cascade of events that promotes SC differentiation and expansion. NRG1 levels will determine axon size, allowing myelinating Schwann cells to optimise myelin sheath thickness [79,80].

Furthermore, ASCs have yielded positive results in studies on a large number of peripheral nerve lesions [81,83], despite uncertainty about their precise dynamics. It is likely that ASCs produce an excess of growth factors, which are critical in the functioning of the peripheral nervous system [87,88].

As indicated by Mathot et al. [6] in a recent review, these adipose tissue-derived mesenchymal stem cells (MSCs) produced by ASCs can successfully differentiate into Schwann-like cells, with the potential to enhance peripheral nerve repair/reconstruction.

7. Conclusions

Compression injuries of the EPSN are the most frequent in the lower limb. In this review we highlighted the importance and relevance that biological treatment can have as a complement to traditional surgical treatments. The application of biological growth factors will undoubtedly help to achieve stable nerve recovery. Future research should examine the specific pain response.

Author Contributions: Conceptualization: A.L.-A. and D.C.N.; validation: J.P.L., D.P.-V. and A.C.-G.; resources: A.C.-G and D.P.-V.: writing—original draft preparation: A.L.-A., A.J.H., J.P.L. and A.C.: writing—review and editing: D.C.N. and A.C.; supervision: A.L.-A., A.J.H., D.C.N. and A.C.-G.; project administration: D.C.N., A.L.-A. and A.C.-G.; funding acquisition: A.C.-G. All authors have read and agreed to the published version of the manuscript.

Funding: This study was supported by Caja Rural de Soria (Soria, Spain).

Institutional Review Board Statement: Not applicable.

Informed Consent Statement: Not applicable.

Data Availability Statement: Not applicable.

Conflicts of Interest: The authors declare no conflict of interest.

References

1. Kurze, T. Microtechniques in neurological surgery. *Neurosurgery* **1964**, *11*, 128–137. [CrossRef] [PubMed]
2. Huckhagel, T.; Nüchtern, J.; Regelsberger, J.; Gelderblom, M.; Lefering, R.; TraumaRegister DGU®. Nerve trauma of the lower extremity: Evaluation of 60,422 leg injured patients from the TraumaRegister DGU® between 2002 and 2015. *Scand. J. Trauma Resusc. Emerg. Med.* **2018**, *26*, 40. [CrossRef] [PubMed]
3. Grinsell, D.; Keating, C.P. Peripheral nerve reconstruction after injury: A review of clinical and experimental therapies. *BioMed Res. Int.* **2014**, *2014*, 698256. [CrossRef] [PubMed]
4. Marciniak, C. Fibular (peroneal) neuropathy: Electrodiagnostic features and clinical correlates. *Phys. Med. Rehabil. Clin. N. Am.* **2013**, *24*, 121–137. [CrossRef] [PubMed]

5. Moatshe, G.; Dornan, G.J.; Løken, S.; Ludvigsen, T.C.; Laprade, R.F.; Engebretsen, L. Demographics and injuries associated with knee dislocation: A prospective review of 303 patients. *Orthop. J. Sports Med.* **2017**, *5*, 2325967117706521. [CrossRef]
6. Wang, M.L.; Rivlin, M.; Graham, J.G.; Beredjiklian, P.K. Peripheral nerve injury, scarring, and recovery. *Connect. Tissue Res.* **2019**, *60*, 3–9. [CrossRef]
7. Mathot, F.; Shin, A.Y.; Van Wijnen, A.J. Targeted stimulation of MSCs in peripheral nerve repair. *Gene* **2019**, *710*, 17–23. [CrossRef]
8. Sumner, A.J. Aberrant reinnervation. *Muscle Nerve* **1990**, *13*, 801–803. [CrossRef]
9. Piton, C.; Fabre, T.; Lasseur, E.; André, D.; Geneste, M.; Durandeau, A. Les lésions du nerf fibulaire commun: Approche étiologique et thérapeutique. A propos de 146 cas traités chirurgicalement [Common fibular nerve lesions. Etiology and treatment. Apropos of 146 cases with surgical treatment]. *Rev. Chir. Orthop. Reparatrice Appar. Mot.* **1997**, *83*, 515–521.
10. Beccari, S.; Turki, M.; Zinelabidine, M.; Ennouri, K.H.; Tarhouni, L.; Bahri, H. Une étiologie rare de paralysie du nerf sciatique poplité externe: L'entorse de la cheville. À propos de 6 cas. *J. Traumatol Sport* **2000**, *17*, 208–212.
11. Sunderland, S. *Nerves and Nerves Injuries*, 2nd ed.; Churchill Livinstone: Edinburg, UK, 1978.
12. Menorca, R.M.; Fussell, T.S.; Elfar, J.C. Nerve physiology: Mechanisms of injury and recovery. *Hand Clin.* **2013**, *29*, 317–330. [CrossRef] [PubMed]
13. Kendall, J.P.; Stokes, I.A.; O'Hara, J.P.; Dickson, R.A. Tension and creep phenomena in peripheral nerve. *Acta Orthop. Scand.* **1979**, *50*, 721–725. [CrossRef] [PubMed]
14. Pham, K.; Gupta, R. Understanding the mechanisms of entrapment neuropathies. Review article. *Neurosurg. Focus* **2009**, *26*, E7. [CrossRef] [PubMed]
15. Noble, J.; Munro, C.A.; Prasad, V.S.S.V.; Midha, R. Analysis of upper and lower extremity peripheral nerve injuries in a population of patients with multiple injuries. *J. Trauma Inj. Infect. Crit. Care* **1998**, *45*, 116–122. [CrossRef]
16. Atkins, S.; Smith, K.G.; Loescher, A.R.; Boissonade, F.M.; O'Kane, S.; Ferguson, M.W.; Robinson, P.P. Scarring impedes regeneration at sites of peripheral nerve repair. *NeuroReport* **2006**, *17*, 1245–1249. [CrossRef]
17. Piñeiro, L.; Rey, R.R.; Sabina, A.G.; Secades, R.M.; Pais, M.J.G. Paralysis of the external popliteal sciatic nerve associated with daptomycin administration. *J. Clin. Pharm. Ther.* **2018**, *43*, 578–580. [CrossRef]
18. Pérez, L.M.; Vived, Á.M.; Gil, D.R. *Manual y Atlas Fotográfico de Anatomía del Aparato Locomotor*; Panamericana: Madrid, Spain, 2010.
19. Sánchez-Martín, M.M. *Traumatología y Ortopedia*; Universidad de Valladolid: Valladolid, Spain, 2002.
20. Cortet, B.; Bourgeois, P. Causes et mécanismes des souffrances sciatiques [Causes and mechanisms of sciatic pains]. *Rev. Prat.* **1992**, *42*, 539–543.
21. Poage, C.; Roth, C.; Scott, B. Peroneal Nerve Palsy: Evaluation and Management. *J. Am. Acad. Orthop. Surg.* **2016**, *24*, 1–10. [CrossRef]
22. Chow, A.L.; Levidy, M.F.; Luthringer, M.; Vasoya, D.; Ignatiuk, A. Clinical Outcomes After Neurolysis for the Treatment of Peroneal Nerve Palsy: A Systematic Review and Meta-Analysis. *Ann. Plast. Surg.* **2021**, *87*, 316–323. [CrossRef]
23. Waldman, S.D. *Waldman's Comprehensive Atlas of Diagnostic Ultrasound of Painful Conditions*, 1st ed.; Wolters Kluwer: Philadelphia, PA, USA, 2016.
24. Martyn, C.N.; Hughes, R.A. Epidemiology of peripheral neuropathy. *J. Neurol. Neurosurg. Psychiatry* **1997**, *62*, 310–318. [CrossRef]
25. Kitamura, T.; Kim, K.; Morimoto, D.; Kokubo, R.; Iwamoto, N.; Isu, T.; Morita, A. Dynamic factors involved in common peroneal nerve entrapment neuropathy. *Acta Neurochir.* **2017**, *159*, 1777–1781. [CrossRef] [PubMed]
26. Dahlin, L.B.; Lundborg, G. The neurone and its response to peripheral nerve compression. *J. Hand Surg. Br. Eur. Vol.* **1990**, *15*, 5–10. [CrossRef]
27. Gutiérrez-Mendoza, I. Generalidades y fisiopatología de la compresión nerviosa. *Orthotips AMOT* **2014**, *10*, 9–14.
28. Eversmann, W.W., Jr. Compression and entrapment neuropathies of the upper extremity. *J. Hand Surg. Am.* **1983**, *8 Pt 2*, 759–766. [CrossRef]
29. Rydevik, B.L. The effects of compression on the physiology of nerve roots. *J. Manip. Physiol. Ther.* **1992**, *15*, 62–66.
30. Artico, M.; Pastore, F.S.; Nucci, F.; Giuffre, R. 290 surgical procedures for ulnar nerve entrapment at the elbow: Physiopathology, clinical experience and results. *Acta Neurochir.* **2000**, *142*, 303–308. [CrossRef]
31. Radosevich, J. (Ed.) *Apoptosis and Beyond: The Many Ways Cells Die*; Wiley Blackwell: Hoboken, NJ, USA, 2018.
32. Dy, C.J.; Brogan, D.M.; Wagner, E.R. *Peripheral Nerve Issues after Orthopedic Surgery: A Multidisciplinary Approach to Prevention, Evaluation and Treatment*, 1st ed; Springer: Berlin/Heidelberg, Germany, 2021.
33. Seddon, H.J. Three Types of Nerve Injury. *Brain* **1943**, *66*, 237–288. [CrossRef]
34. Tubbs, R.S.; Rizk, E.; Shoja, M.M.; Loukas, M.; Barbaro, N.; Spinner, R.J. *Nerves and Nerve Injuries*; Academic Press (Elsevier): Waltham, MA, USA, 2015.
35. Distad, B.J.; Weiss, M.D. Clinical and Electrodiagnostic Features of Sciatic Neuropathies. *Phys. Med. Rehabil. Clin. N. Am.* **2013**, *24*, 107–120. [CrossRef]
36. Anderson, J.C. Common Fibular Nerve Compression: Anatomy, Symptoms, Clinical Evaluation, and Surgical Decompression. *Clin. Podiatr. Med. Surg.* **2016**, *33*, 283–291. [CrossRef]
37. Garg, B.; Poage, C. Peroneal Nerve Palsy: Evaluation and Management. *J. Am. Acad. Orthop. Surg.* **2016**, *24*, e49. [CrossRef]
38. Tzika, M.; Paraskevas, G.; Natsis, K. Entrapment of the superficial peroneal nerve: An anatomical insight. *J. Am. Podiatr. Med. Assoc.* **2015**, *105*, 150–159. [CrossRef] [PubMed]

39. Fortier, L.M.; Markel, M.; Thomas, B.G.; Sherman, W.F.; Thomas, B.H.; Kaye, A.D. An Update on Peroneal Nerve Entrapment and Neuropathy. *Orthop. Rev.* **2021**, *13*, 24937. [CrossRef] [PubMed]
40. Riccio, M.; Marchesini, A.; Pugliese, P.; De Francesco, F. Nerve repair and regeneration: Biological tubulization limits and future perspectives. *J. Cell. Physiol.* **2019**, *234*, 3362–3375. [CrossRef] [PubMed]
41. Hobson-Webb, L.D.; Juel, V.C. Common Entrapment Neuropathies. *Contin. Lifelong Learn. Neurol.* **2017**, *23*, 487–511. [CrossRef]
42. Karakis, I.; Khoshnoodi, M.; Liew, W.; Nguyen, E.S.; Jones, H.R.; Darras, B.T.; Kang, P.B. Electrophysiologic features of fibular neuropathy in childhood and adolescence. *Muscle Nerve* **2017**, *55*, 693–697. [CrossRef]
43. Roy, P.C. Electrodiagnostic evaluation of lower extremity neurogenic problems. *Foot Ankle Clin.* **2011**, *16*, 225–242. [CrossRef]
44. Bendszus, M.; Stoll, G. Technology insight: Visualizing peripheral nerve injury using MRI. *Nat. Clin. Pract. Neurol.* **2005**, *1*, 45–53. [CrossRef]
45. Grant, G.A.; Britz, G.W.; Goodkin, R.; Jarvik, J.G.; Maravilla, K.; Kliot, M. The utility of magnetic resonance imaging in evaluating peripheral nerve disorders. *Muscle Nerve* **2002**, *25*, 314–331. [CrossRef]
46. Stoll, G.; Bendszus, M.; Perez, J.; Pham, M. Magnetic resonance imaging of the peripheral nervous system. *J. Neurol.* **2009**, *256*, 1043–1051. [CrossRef]
47. Tsukamoto, H.; Granata, G.; Coraci, D.; Paolasso, I.; Padua, L. Ultrasound and neurophysiological correlation in common fibular nerve conduction block at fibular head. *Clin. Neurophysiol.* **2014**, *125*, 1491–1495. [CrossRef]
48. Pabari, A.; Yang, S.Y.; Seifalian, A.M.; Mosahebi, A. Modern surgical management of peripheral nerve gap. *J. Plast. Reconstr. Aesthetic Surg.* **2010**, *63*, 1941–1948. [CrossRef] [PubMed]
49. Bamba, R.; Loewenstein, S.N.; Adkinson, J.M. Donor site morbidity after sural nerve grafting: A systematic review. *J. Plast. Reconstr. Aesthetic Surg.* **2021**, *74*, 3055–3060. [CrossRef] [PubMed]
50. Chen, H.; Meng, D.; Yin, G.; Hou, C.; Lin, H. Translocation of the soleus muscular branch of the tibial nerve to repair high common peroneal nerve injury. *Acta Neurochir.* **2019**, *161*, 271–277. [CrossRef] [PubMed]
51. Nath, R.K.; Lyons, A.B.; Paizi, M. Successful management of foot drop by nerve transfers to the deep peroneal nerve. *J. Reconstr. Microsurg.* **2008**, *24*, 419–427. [CrossRef] [PubMed]
52. El-Taher, M.; Sallam, A.; Saleh, M.; Metwally, A. Foot Reanimation Using Double Nerve Transfer to Deep Peroneal Nerve: A Novel Technique for Treatment of Neurologic Foot Drop. *Foot Ankle Int.* **2021**, *42*, 1011–1021. [CrossRef]
53. Siemionow, M.; Brzezicki, G. Chapter 8: Current techniques and concepts in peripheral nerve repair. *Int. Rev. Neurobiol.* **2009**, *87*, 141–172. [CrossRef]
54. Lapuente, J.P.; Dos-Anjos, S.; Blázquez-Martínez, A. Intra-articular infiltration of adipose-derived stromal vascular fraction cells slows the clinical progression of moderate-severe knee osteoarthritis: Hypothesis on the regulatory role of intra-articular adipose tissue. *J. Orthop. Surg. Res.* **2020**, *15*, 137. [CrossRef]
55. Jessen, K.R.; Mirsky, R. The repair Schwann cell and its function in regenerating nerves. *J. Physiol.* **2016**, *594*, 3521–3531. [CrossRef]
56. Mirsky, R.; Jessen, K.R.; Brennan, A.; Parkinson, D.; Dong, Z.; Meier, C.; Parmantier, E.; Lawson, D. Schwann cells as regulators of nerve development. *J. Physiol.* **2002**, *96*, 17–24. [CrossRef]
57. Woodhoo, A.; Alonso, M.B.; Droggiti, A.; Turmaine, M.; D'Antonio, M.; Parkinson, D.B.; Wilton, D.K.; Al-Shawi, R.; Simons, P.; Shen, J.; et al. Notch controls embryonic Schwann cell differentiation, postnatal myelination and adult plasticity. *Nat. Neurosci.* **2009**, *12*, 839–847. [CrossRef]
58. Monk, K.R.; Feltri, M.L.; Taveggia, C. New insights on Schwann cell development. *Glia* **2015**, *63*, 1376–1393. [CrossRef] [PubMed]
59. Salzer, J.L. Schwann cell myelination. *Cold Spring Harb. Perspect. Biol.* **2015**, *7*, a020529. [CrossRef] [PubMed]
60. Berry, M.; Hall, S.; Follows, R.; Rees, L.; Gregson, N.; Sievers, J. Response of axons and glia at the site of anastomosis between the optic nerve and cellular or acellular sciatic nerve grafts. *J. Neurocytol.* **1988**, *17*, 727–744. [CrossRef] [PubMed]
61. Fu, H.; Hu, D.; Chen, J.; Wang, Q.; Zhang, Y.; Qi, C.; Yu, T. Repair of the Injured Spinal Cord by Schwann Cell Transplantation. *Front. Neurosci.* **2022**, *16*, 800513. [CrossRef]
62. Lee, S.K.; Wolfe, S.W. Peripheral nerve injury and repair. *J. Am. Acad. Orthop. Surg.* **2000**, *8*, 243–252. [CrossRef]
63. Noriega, D.C.; Ardura, F.; Hernández-Ramajo, R.; Martín-Ferrero, M.Á.; Sánchez-Lite, I.; Toribio, B.; Alberca, M.; García, V.; Moraleda, J.M.; González-Vallinas, M.; et al. Treatment of Degenerative Disc Disease with Allogeneic Mesenchymal Stem Cells: Long-term Follow-up Results. *Transplantation* **2021**, *105*, e25–e27. [CrossRef]
64. Noriega, D.C.; Ardura, F.; Hernández-Ramajo, R.; Martín-Ferrero, M.Á.; Sánchez-Lite, I.; Toribio, B.; Alberca, M.; García, V.; Moraleda, J.M.; Sánchez, A.; et al. Intervertebral Disc Repair by Allogeneic Mesenchymal Bone Marrow Cells: A Randomized Controlled Trial. *Transplantation* **2017**, *101*, 1945–1951. [CrossRef]
65. Chen, Z.L.; Yu, W.M.; Strickland, S. Peripheral regeneration. *Annu. Rev. Neurosci.* **2007**, *30*, 209–233. [CrossRef]
66. Kitada, M. Mesenchymal cell populations: Development of the induction systems for Schwann cells and neuronal cells and finding the unique stem cell population. *Anat. Sci. Int.* **2012**, *87*, 24–44. [CrossRef]
67. Scuteri, A.; Miloso, M.; Foudah, D.; Orciani, M.; Cavaletti, G.; Tredici, G. Mesenchymal stem cells neuronal differentiation ability: A real perspective for nervous system repair? *Curr. Stem Cell Res. Ther.* **2011**, *6*, 82–92. [CrossRef]
68. Cai, S.; Shea, G.K.; Tsui, A.Y.; Chan, Y.S.; Shum, D.K. Derivation of clinically applicable schwann cells from bone marrow stromal cells for neural repair and regeneration. *CNS Neurol. Disord.-Drug Targets* **2011**, *10*, 500–508. [CrossRef] [PubMed]
69. Wakao, S.; Matsuse, D.; Dezawa, M. Mesenchymal stem cells as a source of Schwann cells: Their anticipated use in peripheral nerve regeneration. *Cells Tissues Organs* **2014**, *200*, 31–41. [CrossRef] [PubMed]

70. Konofaos, P.; Ver Halen, J.P. Nerve repair by means of tubulization: Past, present, future. *J. Reconstr. Microsurg.* **2013**, *29*, 149–164. [CrossRef]
71. Klimaschewski, L.; Claus, P. Fibroblast Growth Factor Signalling in the Diseased Nervous System. *Mol. Neurobiol.* **2021**, *58*, 3884–3902. [CrossRef] [PubMed]
72. Grothe, C.; Nikkhah, G. The role of basic fibroblast growth factor in peripheral nerve regeneration. *Anat. Embryol.* **2001**, *204*, 171–177. [CrossRef]
73. Boyd, J.G.; Gordon, T. Neurotrophic factors and their receptors in axonal regeneration and functional recovery after peripheral nerve injury. *Mol. Neurobiol.* **2003**, *27*, 277–324. [CrossRef]
74. Scheib, J.; Höke, A. Advances in peripheral nerve regeneration. *Nat. Rev. Neurol.* **2013**, *9*, 668–676. [CrossRef]
75. Wood, M.D.; Mackinnon, S.E. Pathways regulating modality-specific axonal regeneration in peripheral nerve. *Exp. Neurol.* **2015**, *265*, 171–175. [CrossRef]
76. Spector, J.G.; Derby, A.; Lee, P.; Roufa, D.G. Comparison of Rabbit Facial Nerve Regeneration in Nerve Growth Factor-Containing Silicone Tubes to that in Autologous Neural Grafts. *Ann. Otol. Rhinol. Laryngol.* **1995**, *104*, 875–885. [CrossRef]
77. De Francesco, F.; Ricci, G.; D'Andrea, F.; Nicoletti, G.F.; Ferraro, G.A. Human Adipose Stem Cells: From Bench to Bedside. *Tissue Eng. Part B Rev.* **2015**, *21*, 572–584. [CrossRef]
78. Nicoletti, G.F.; De Francesco, F.; D'Andrea, F.; Ferraro, G.A. Methods and procedures in adipose stem cells: State of the art and perspective for translation medicine. *J. Cell. Physiol.* **2015**, *230*, 489–495. [CrossRef] [PubMed]
79. Allbright, K.O.; Bliley, J.M.; Havis, E.; Kim, D.Y.; Dibernardo, G.A.; Grybowski, D.; Waldner, M.; James, I.B.; Sivak, N.; Rubin, J.P.; et al. Delivery of adipose-derived stem cells in poloxamer hydrogel improves peripheral nerve regeneration. *Muscle Nerve* **2018**, *58*, 251–260. [CrossRef] [PubMed]
80. Fernandes, M.; Valente, S.G.; Sabongi, R.G.; Gomes Dos Santos, J.B.G.; Leite, V.M.; Ulrich, H.; Nery, A.A.; da Silva Fernandes, M.J. Bone marrow-derived mesenchymal stem cells versus adipose-derived mesenchymal stem cells for peripheral nerve regeneration. *Neural Regen. Res.* **2018**, *13*, 100–104. [CrossRef] [PubMed]
81. Kingham, P.J.; Kalbermatten, D.F.; Mahay, D.; Armstrong, S.J.; Wiberg, M.; Terenghi, G. Adipose-derived stem cells differentiate into a Schwann cell phenotype and promote neurite outgrowth In Vitro. *Exp. Neurol.* **2007**, *207*, 267–274. [CrossRef] [PubMed]
82. Alsmadi, N.Z.; Bendale, G.S.; Kanneganti, A.; Shihabeddin, T.; Nguyen, A.H.; Hor, E.; Dash, S.; Johnston, B.; Granja-Vazquez, R.; Romero-Ortega, M.I. Glial-derived growth factor and pleiotrophin synergistically promote axonal regeneration in critical nerve injuries. *Acta Biomater.* **2018**, *78*, 165–177. [CrossRef] [PubMed]
83. Kim, H.A.; Ratner, N.; Roberts, T.M.; Stiles, C.D. Schwann cell proliferative responses to cAMP and Nf1 are mediated by cyclin D1. *J. Neurosci.* **2001**, *21*, 1110–1116. [CrossRef]
84. Davis, J.B.; Stroobant, P. Platelet-derived growth factors and fibroblast growth factors are mitogens for rat Schwann cells. *J. Cell Biol.* **1990**, *110*, 1353–1360. [CrossRef]
85. Nave, K.A.; Salzer, J.L. Axonal regulation of myelination by neuregulin 1. *Curr. Opin. Neurobiol.* **2006**, *16*, 492–500. [CrossRef]
86. Garratt, A.N.; Britsch, S.; Birchmeier, C. Neuregulin, a factor with many functions in the life of a schwann cell. *BioEssays* **2000**, *22*, 987–996. [CrossRef]
87. Faroni, A.; Terenghi, G.; Reid, A.J. Adipose-derived stem cells and nerve regeneration: Promises and pitfalls. *Int. Rev. Neurobiol.* **2013**, *108*, 121–136. [CrossRef]
88. Walocko, F.M.; Khouri, R.K., Jr.; Urbanchek, M.G.; Levi, B.; Cederna, P.S. The potential roles for adipose tissue in peripheral nerve regeneration. *Microsurgery* **2016**, *36*, 81–88. [CrossRef] [PubMed]

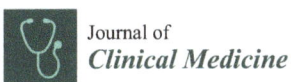

Article

Association of Thiazide Use in Patients with Hypertension with Overall Fracture Risk: A Population-Based Cohort Study

Cheng-Hsun Chuang [1,2,3], Shun-Fa Yang [1,4], Pei-Lun Liao [4], Jing-Yang Huang [1,4], Man-Yee Chan [5,*] and Chao-Bin Yeh [1,2,3,*]

[1] Institute of Medicine, Chung Shan Medical University, Taichung 402, Taiwan; skdef37372@hotmail.com.tw (C.-H.C.); ysf@csmu.edu.tw (S.-F.Y.); wchinyang@gmail.com (J.-Y.H.)
[2] Department of Emergency Medicine, School of Medicine, Chung Shan Medical University, Taichung 402, Taiwan
[3] Department of Emergency Medicine, Chung Shan Medical University Hospital, Taichung 402, Taiwan
[4] Department of Medical Research, Chung Shan Medical University Hospital, Taichung 402, Taiwan; liaopeilun0410@gmail.com
[5] Department of Dentistry, Taichung Tzu Chi Hospital, Buddhist Tzu Chi Medical Foundation, Taichung 427, Taiwan
* Correspondence: hychung@tzuchi.com.tw (M.-Y.C.); sky5ff@gmail.com (C.-B.Y.)

Abstract: Thiazide diuretics have long been widely used as antihypertensive agents. In addition to reducing blood pressure, thiazides also control calcium homeostasis and increase bone density. We hypothesized that the use of thiazides in patients with hypertension would reduce overall fracture risk. We used the Taiwan National Health Insurance Research Database to find patients with a hypertension diagnosis who accepted antihypertensive treatment from 2000 to 2017. The patients were further classified into thiazide users and nonthiazide users. Multivariable Cox regression analysis and Kaplan–Meier survival analysis were performed to estimate the adjusted hazard ratios (aHRs) and cumulative probability of fractures. After 1:1 propensity score matching by sex, age, urbanization level of place of residence, income, comorbidities, and medications, there were 18,483 paired thiazide users and non-users, respectively. The incidence densities of fractures (per 1000 person-months) were 1.82 (95% CI: 1.76–1.89) and 1.99 (95% CI: 1.92–2.06) in the thiazide and nonthiazide groups, respectively. The results indicated a lower hazard ratio for fractures in thiazide users (aHR = 0.93, 95% CI: 0.88–0.98). Kaplan–Meier survival analysis revealed a significantly lower cumulative incidence of fractures in the thiazide group (log-rank test; $p = 0.0012$). In conclusion, our results reveal that thiazide use can reduce fracture risk. When antihypertensive agents are being considered, thiazide may be a better choice if the patient is at heightened risk of fracture.

Keywords: thiazide; hypertension; risk of fracture

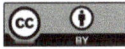

1. Introduction

With an aging worldwide population, the importance of effectively treating muscle loss and osteoporosis is increasing. The characteristic of osteoporosis is bone mass loss and microarchitectural deterioration of bone tissue. Osteoporotic bone can easily fracture even in a minor collision [1], and osteoporotic fractures are one of the most common injuries encountered in the emergency department [2]. The most osteoporotic fracture locations were distal radius, proximal femur, and vertebral compression fractures. Calcium is the most abundant mineral in the body, 99% of which is found in the teeth and bones. Apart from bone, the two main organ systems responsible for calcium homeostasis are the intestines and kidneys [3–5]. Vitamin D improves the ability of the intestines to absorb calcium [6], and a calcium plus vitamin D supplement has been used to prevent osteoporotic fractures. A meta-analysis revealed a significant 15% reduction in the risk of total fractures and a 30% reduction in the risk of hip fractures when patients use calcium plus vitamin D supplementation for fracture prevention [7]. The kidneys play a key role in both calcium reabsorption and excretion. Approximately 200 mg of calcium per day is typically excreted by adults through the kidneys via urine [8], but this value varies by diet and serum parameters. Reducing the excretion of calcium from urine is one strategy to maintain adequate calcium in the human body [9].

In older people, hypertension is a common disease, and initial control through non-drug therapies, such as lifestyle modifications, body weight management, and increased exercise, is recommended [10,11]. Antihypertensive medications are used if non-drug therapy cannot achieve adequate blood pressure control. Many types of antihypertensive drugs have been developed. The four main classes of medications used in combination therapies for the treatment of hypertension are thiazide diuretics, calcium channel blockers (CCBs), angiotensin-converting enzyme inhibitors (ACEIs), and angiotensin receptor blockers (ARBs). The combination use of antihypertensive medications can achieve synergistic effects in blood pressure reduction with fewer doses [12–14]. Physicians select an antihypertensive treatment for a patient according to their underlying diseases or contraindications [15,16]. Patients with a reduced ejection fraction should initially be treated with a beta-blocker and an ACEI or ARB [16]. Patients with chronic kidney disease and proteinuria should be treated with an ACEI or ARB plus a thiazide diuretic or CCB [17]. If patients with diabetes mellitus have proteinuria, combination therapy should include an ACEI or ARB [18].

Thiazide diuretics have long been widely used as antihypertensive agents. Thiazides are defined as a third-line antihypertensive because they are less effective at reducing blood pressure than are ACEIs or ARBs. Thiazides inhibit the Na+/Cl cotransporter (NCC) in the convoluted renal distal tubule. The NCC facilitates the reabsorption of sodium from the distal tubules to the interstitium. A decrease in sodium reabsorption results in an increase in urine output, leading to a decrease in plasma volume and decreased blood pressure.

In addition to reducing blood pressure, thiazides control calcium homeostasis and increase bone density. Thiazides reduce urinary calcium excretion and stimulate osteoblast differentiation and bone mineral formation [7]. The mechanism by which thiazides reduce calcium excretion remains unclear. In some studies, thiazide has been used in idiopathic hypercalciuria [19]. Li et al. reported that the long-term use of thiazide diuretics reduces the incidence of recurrent renal calculi and the 24-h urinary calcium level [20]. By reducing calcium loss, the bone density and calcium within bones increase. Aung et al. reported that thiazide could reduce the incidence of hip fractures [21].

In perimenopausal or postmenopausal women, osteoporotic fractures are one of the common complications [22]. Several therapies have been proposed to prevent them. Calcium plus vitamin D, hormone therapy, or combination therapy are the current primary treatments to protect against osteoporotic fractures [23].

Our primary outcome of the study was the fracture rate of the hypertensive participant and the adjusted hazard ratio between the thiazide user and the non-user for hypertension using data from the Taiwan National Health Research Database of Taiwan (NHIRD). Our second objective was to determine whether thiazide can prevent fractures in perimenopausal or postmenopausal women.

2. Materials and Methods

2.1. Study Design and Population

As stated, we used data from Taiwan's NHIRD; Taiwan implemented National Health Insurance (NHI) in 1995, and the database contains NHI claims data for more than 99% of Taiwan's population and provides a means to explore the risk factors or effects of disease interventions. This study used a retrospective cohort design with NHIRD data from 2000 to 2017. Diseases were diagnosed using the International Classification of Diseases, Ninth [Tenth] Edition, Clinical Modification (ICD-9(10)–CM). This study was approved by the

Institutional Review Board of Chung Shan Medical University Hospital (approval number CS2-20036).

2.2. Study Population

Records from 2000 to 2017 were collected from the NHIRD, and the study population included patients with hypertension (ICD-9-CM codes 401-405 and ICD-10-CM codes I10-I15). Patients must have used a hypertension medication within 1 year of diagnosis, including beta-blockers (anatomic therapeutic chemical [ATC] code: C07), CCBs (ATC code: C08), alpha-blockers (ATC code: C02CA), and ACEIs or ARBs (ATC code: C09).

We identified a total of 498,738 patients with hypertension. After accounting for the excluded conditions, we finally included 216,867 patients for data analysis. We divided patients into two groups: hypertension with thiazide use (HT-with-thiazide) and hypertension without thiazide use (HT-without-thiazide). A total of 18,620 patients were placed in the HT-without-thiazide group and 198,247 patients were placed in the HT-without-thiazide group. The index date was defined as the first day 365 days after the diagnosis of hypertension. This setting is because we defined patients who continuously used thiazide for 1 year as stable users and assumed that these stable users would continue to use thiazide during follow-up.

2.3. Characteristics, Comorbidities, and Outcomes

We identified baseline demographic characteristics (as reported within 365 days before the index date), such as age and sex, and the comorbidities and medications of each participant to evaluate their health status. Baseline comorbidities included diabetes mellitus, hyperlipidemia, ischemic heart disease, cerebrovascular accident, abnormal renal function, chronic obstructive pulmonary disease (COPD), cancer, and depressive disorders. Baseline medications included beta-blockers, CCBs, ACEIs, ARBs, corticosteroids, non-steroidal anti-inflammatory drugs (NSAIDs), proton-pump inhibitors, and hormonal medications.

The study outcome was defined as the diagnosis of a fracture, differentiated into skull, spine and trunk, upper limb, lower limb, and pathological fractures. All study individuals were followed up from the index date to either the study outcome, the occurrence of fracture due to car accident, death, or the end of the study (31 December 2017).

2.4. Statistical Analysis

Statistical analysis was performed using SAS version 9.4 (SAS Institute, Cary, NC, USA), and a p-value of <0.05 was considered statistically significant. HT-with-thiazide patients were matched with HT-without-thiazide patients by age (± 1 year) and sex at a 1:4 ratio. To reduce potential confounding bias due to measured factors, 1:1 propensity score matching (PSM) was performed by using the greedy nearest neighbor algorithm and noreplacement matching with a caliper width of 0.01; matched variables included birth year, sex, age (± 1 year) at the index date, index year, comorbidities, and medication. The absolute standardized difference (ASD) was used to evaluate the differences in covariates between the two study groups; an ASD value of <0.1 indicated that the item was balanced between the groups.

Categorical data were presented as numbers and percentages, and the differences in categorical variables were compared using the chi-square test. Incidence rates with corresponding confidence intervals (CI) and crude hazard ratios (HRs) were calculated using Poisson regression. After the proportional hazards assumption was tested, a Cox proportional hazards model analysis was performed to estimate the HRs for mortality and 95% CIs. Cumulative fracture probabilities were assessed using Kaplan–Meier analysis, in which statistical significance was determined using the results of a log-rank test.

3. Results

3.1. Characteristics of the Participants

The selection flow chart for this study is presented in Figure 1. A total of 18,593 patients were included in the HT-with-thiazide group, and an additional 74,372 patients were sex and age (±1 years) matched at a 1:4 ratio to form the HT-without-thiazide control group (Supplementary Table S1). After 1:1 PSM matching by sex, age, urbanization level of place of residence, income, comorbidities, and medications, 18,483 HT with-thiazide and HT without-thiazide participants were obtained; 58% of the patients were male, and 41% were female. Over 57% were aged 46 to 60 years. The baseline characteristics are presented in Table 1.

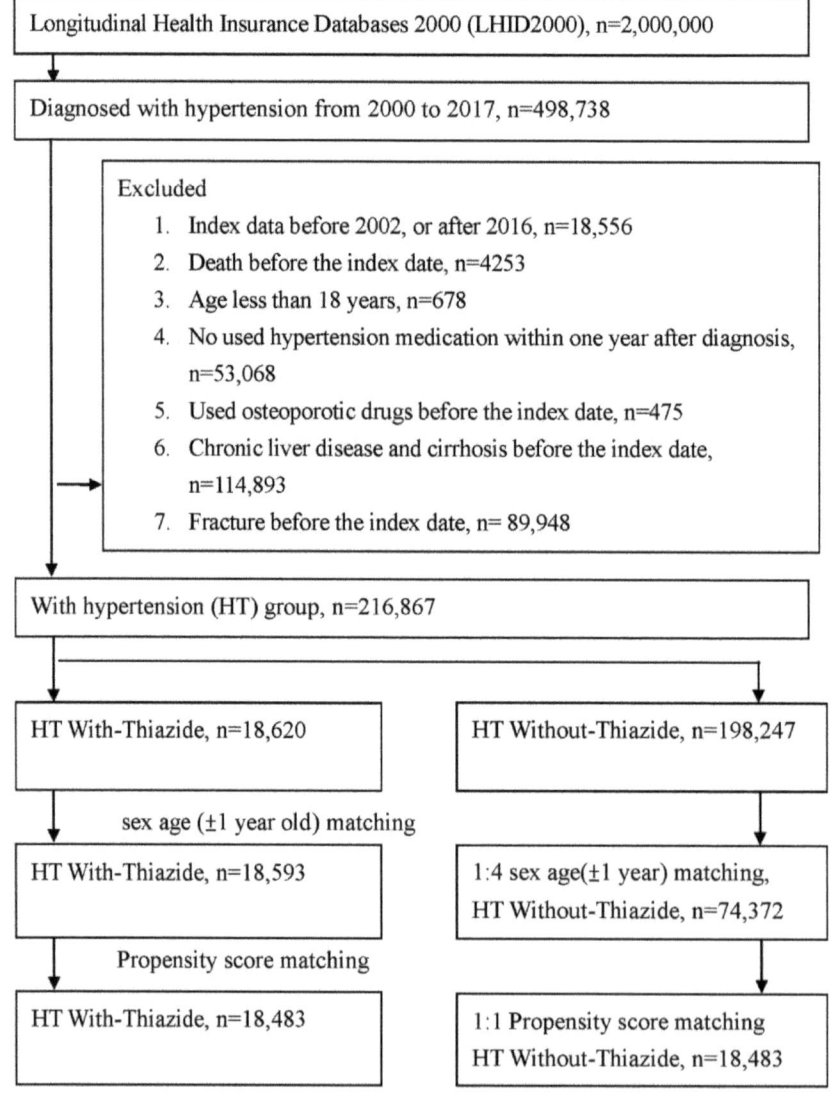

Figure 1. Study flowchart of patient selection.

Table 1. Baseline characteristics among study groups.

Variables	After PSM		ASD
	Without-Thiazide n = 18,483	With-Thiazide n = 18,483	
Index year			0.0244
2002–2006	5573 (30.15%)	5660 (30.62%)	
2007–2011	5831 (31.55%)	5842 (31.61%)	
2012–2016	7079 (38.3%)	6981 (37.77%)	
Sex			0.0020
Female	7689 (41.6%)	7707 (41.7%)	
Male	10,794 (58.4%)	10,776 (58.3%)	
Age at index			0.0000
19–45	3463 (18.74%)	3543 (19.17%)	
46–60	10,616 (57.44%)	10,544 (57.05%)	
≥61	4404 (23.83%)	4396 (23.78%)	
Urbanization			0.0412
Urban	11,580 (62.65%)	11,534 (62.4%)	
Sub-urban	5731 (31.01%)	5753 (31.13%)	
Rural	1172 (6.34%)	1196 (6.47%)	
Income			0.0061
1–22,000	6218 (33.64%)	6271 (33.93%)	
>22,000	12,265 (66.36%)	12,212 (66.07%)	
Comorbidities			
Diabetes mellitus	5530 (29.92%)	5493 (29.72%)	0.0044
Hyperlipidemia	7209 (39%)	7124 (38.54%)	0.0094
Ischemic heart disease	3281 (17.75%)	3302 (17.87%)	0.0030
Cerebrovascular accident	2198 (11.89%)	2297 (12.43%)	0.0164
Abnormal renal function	1140 (6.17%)	1199 (6.49%)	0.0131
COPD	1132 (6.12%)	1210 (6.55%)	0.0173
Cancer	482 (2.61%)	575 (3.11%)	0.0302
Depressive disorders	459 (2.48%)	508 (2.75%)	0.0166
Medication			
Beta- blockers	8035 (43.47%)	7934 (42.93%)	0.0110
CCBs	10,960 (59.3%)	10,928 (59.12%)	0.0035
Alpha-blockers	880 (4.76%)	979 (5.3%)	0.0245
ACEI/ARB	17,326 (93.74%)	17,326 (93.74%)	0.0000
corticosteroids	9427 (51%)	9460 (51.18%)	0.0036
NSAIDs	12,540 (67.85%)	12,402 (67.1%)	0.0159
PPIs	989 (5.35%)	1087 (5.88%)	0.0230
Hormonal medications	818 (4.43%)	859 (4.65%)	0.0107

ASD: Absolute Standardized Difference; COPD: Chronic Obstructive Pulmonary Disease; CCBs: Calcium Channel Blockers; ACEIs: Angiotensin-Converting Enzyme Inhibitors; ARB: Angiotensin Receptor Blockers; NSAIDs: Non-Steroidal Anti-Inflammatory Drugs; PPIs: Proton Pump Inhibitors.

3.2. Risk of Fracture between HT with Thiazide and HT-without Thiazide Group

As Table 2 indicates, the incidence densities of fractures (per 1000 person-months) were 1.83 (95% CI: 1.76–1.90) and 1.97 (95% CI: 1.94–2.01) in the sex- and age-matched HT-with-thiazide and HT-without-thiazide cohorts, respectively (Supplementary Table S2). After PSM, the values were 1.82 (95% CI: 1.76–1.89) and 1.99 (95% CI: 1.92–2.06) in the HT-with-thiazide and HT-without thiazide cohorts, respectively, and the aHR for the HR-with-thiazide group was 0.93 (95% CI: 0.88–0.98). Kaplan Meier survival analysis revealed a significantly lower cumulative incidence of fractures in the HT-with-thiazide group (log-rank test; p = 0.0012; Figure 2).

Table 2. Incidence density of fracture.

Variables	After PSM	
	Without-Thiazide	With-Thiazide
Number	18,483	18,483
Follow up person months	1,428,347	1,457,827
New fracture case *	2848	2666
Incidence rate * (95% C.I.)	1.99 (1.92–2.06)	1.82 (1.76–1.89)
Crude Relative risk (95% C.I.)	Reference	0.92 (0.87–0.97)
Adjusted hazard ratio [†] (95% C.I.)	Reference	0.93 (0.88–0.98)
Competing Risk (95% C.I.)	Reference	0.93 (0.88–0.98)

* per 1000 person-months. [†] Adjusted variables including age, sex, comorbidities and medication.

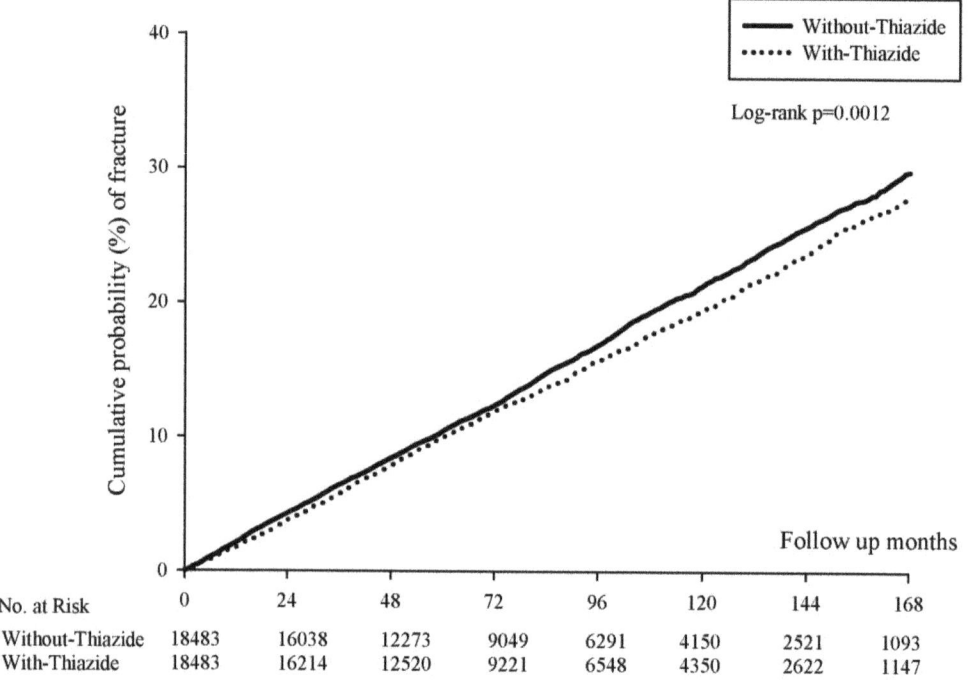

Figure 2. Kaplan–Meier curves of the cumulative proportions of fracture in the use of thiazide and without the use of thiazide.

Multiple cox regression revealed that the aHR of fractures for the HT-with-thiazide group was significantly lower than that of the HT-without-thiazide group. Other significant risk factors for fractures were sex; age; urbanization level; income; the comorbidities of diabetes mellitus, hyperlipidemia, cerebrovascular accident, abnormal renal function, and COPD; and the medications of corticosteroids and NSAIDs (Supplementary Table S3).

In Figure 3, subgroup analysis revealed that the aHR for women and men was 0.98 (95% CI: 0.91–1.05) and 0.86 (95% CI: 0.80–0.93), respectively, and the HR-with-thiazide group exhibited a significantly reduced risk compared to the HR-without-thiazide group. For the age 41 to 50 years group, the aHR was 0.87 (95% CI: 0.76–0.99). For the with-CCBs group, the aHR was 0.92 (95% CI: 0.86–0.90). For the with-ACEI or ARBs group, the aHR was 0.91 (95% CI: 0.86–0.96).

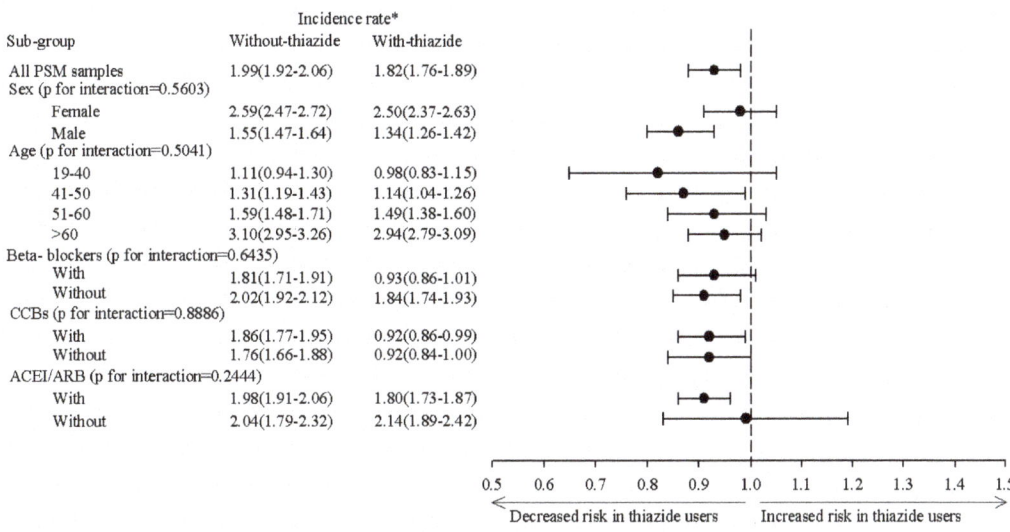

Figure 3. Subgroup analysis of adjusted hazard ratio for fractures in patients with thiazide compared with patients without thiazide. * per 1000 person-months; aHR (adjusted Hazard Ratio) adjusted variables including age, sex, comorbidities and medication; CCBs: Calcium Channel Blockers; ACEIs: Angiotensin-Converting Enzyme Inhibitors; ARB: Angiotensin Receptor Blockers.

4. Discussion

Hypertension is a common chronic disease among older adults. Several hypotheses accounting for the pathophysiology have been proposed. One of the hypotheses concerns maladaptation to a high-salt diet. Hypertension may be a physiological response intended to excrete excess salt. Natriuresis is a key treatment for hypertension [24]. Diuretics could remove excessive salt to achieve hypertension control. A review concluded that the use of a low-dose thiazide reduced all mortality and morbidity in adult patients with moderate-to-severe primary hypertension [25].

Older people are also more susceptible to osteoporotic fractures and even low-energy injuries due to low bone density and being prone to falls. Hip fracture is also one of the risks associated with higher mortality and morbidity among older adults. The cumulative mortality rate for 12 months was 33%, and the 1-year mortality rate increased significantly by 2% per year [26] Several cost-effective pharmacologic treatments may be used to prevent fractures, such as vitamin D and calcium supplements and bisphosphonates [27]. Denosumab is an effective option for preventing fracture, which reduces bone resorption to achieve bone mass preservation [28].

Our study aimed to determine whether thiazide could be used to reduce fracture risk in patients with hypertension. This has remained controversial in prior research. A meta-analysis determined that the use of thiazide was associated with reduced risk in case-control studies but not in cohort studies. That study concluded that the use of thiazide might not protect against fractures [29]. However, some studies have different conclusions. A recent study using a Swedish database concluded that the use of bendroflumethiazide or hydrochlorothiazide could reduce the risk of hip fractures [30]. That study also noted that the choice of antihypertensive can influence fracture risk. A recent meta-analysis including 22 observational studies concluded the use of thiazide was associated with a lower fracture rate of the hip [31]. A meta-analysis that compared patients with diuresis with and without thiazide determined that thiazide reduced overall fracture risk by 14% and hip fracture risk by 18% [32].

In the present population-based retrospective cohort study, we determined that patients with hypertension and thiazide had a lower overall fracture risk. The adjusted risk ratio for the HT-with-thiazide group was 0.926, indicating thiazide has a protective effect against fracture for patient hypertension.

A meta-analysis found the protective effect on fracture risk is associated with the long duration and continuity of thiazide use [33]. Similar to our study, the protective effect seems more significant after 72 months from Kaplan–Meier curves (Figure 2). Another meta-analysis concluded that the association between the use of thiazide and risk of osteoporotic fracture is not significant. However, this study also concluded that the different general status of a patient might have different levels of benefit [34]. This study gave us an important implication that we should find the specific population that could benefit from thiazide diuretics for preventing fracture. In our study, subgroup analysis was used to determine whether thiazide could protect against fractures in perimenopausal and postmenopausal women.

A retrospective cohort study using the MJ Health Database in Taiwan indicated that the mean age at menopause for women in Taiwan is 50.2 [35]. The adjusted fracture risk ratio was 0.88 in a subgroup of females aged 41–50. (95% C.I. 0.73–1.06) The possible explanation is sample size was not large enough to meet statistical significance. The adjusted fracture risk ratio was 0.87 in a group aged 41–50. (95% C.I. 0.76–0.99) A possible explanation for this is as follows: As people reach their forties and start to lose protection from hormones, thiazide can compensate to improve calcium reabsorption and increase bone density. However, during their fifth decade or older, people completely lose the protection of hormones. Bone mineral loss accelerates and worsens, and thiazide does not provide sufficient protection.

Bone mineral density (BMD) measurements provide a snapshot of bone health, including the presence of osteoporosis and the risk of fractures. Two randomized controlled trials revealed that thiazide achieved significant benefits in BMD in postmenopausal women [36,37]. To sum up, thiazide could produce a positive effect on BMD, but increased BMD does not necessarily indicate reduced fracture risk.

A meta-analysis revealed that the risk of osteoporotic fractures among individuals with hypertension was higher than individuals without hypertension, with an odds ratio of 1.33 [38]. A longitudinal study indicated that hypertension is an independent risk factor for fractures in women but not men [39]. Although our study observed that thiazide had a protective effect on fracture in patients with hypertension, we were unable to determine whether the protective effect originates from the control of blood pressure or thiazide facilitating calcium reabsorption.

The most common indication for thiazide is hypertension; others include edema or ascites secondary to cirrhosis or heart failure. In several studies, the research participants were not specifically individuals with hypertension [21,29,40]. Different from those studies, the participants in our study used thiazide specific for hypertension.

Our study has several limitations. First, the claims records in the NHIRD are mainly used to calculate medical unit services and service costs. Several key indicators recorded in clinical practice are not included in the database, such as the severity, type, and mechanism of patient fractures. We used PSM to eliminate possible confounding factors that were recorded in the database. Second, the retrospective cohort design of this study excluded causal inference and limited the precision of our study. Therefore, we matched the study group with the control group by propensity score to reduce this bias. Third, BMD is a useful indicator of bone health. A previous study concluded that thiazide could improve BMD [41]. However, BMD values are not recorded in the NHIRD. Further cohort studies or studies using hospital electronic medical records systems might help to clarify the relationships between BMD and the use of thiazide.

5. Conclusions

In conclusion, our study revealed that thiazide use for hypertension can reduce overall fracture risk. When deciding between antihypertensive agents, thiazide may be a favorable choice if the patient is at elevated risk of fragility fractures. Through subgroup analysis, we also determined that women over 40 years of age who used thiazide were at a reduced risk of fractures. This could be an indication for the use of antihypertensive medications in perimenopausal women.

Supplementary Materials: The following supporting information can be downloaded at: https://www.mdpi.com/article/10.3390/jcm11123304/s1, Table S1: Baseline characteristics among study groups. Table S2: Incidence density of fracture. Table S3: Multiple Cox proportional hazard regression results for fracture.

Author Contributions: Conceptualization, C.-H.C., M.-Y.C. and C.-B.Y.; formal analysis, S.-F.Y., P.-L.L. and J.-Y.H.; writing—original draft preparation, C.-H.C., M.-Y.C. and C.-B.Y.; writing—review and editing, C.-H.C., M.-Y.C. and C.-B.Y. All authors have read and agreed to the published version of the manuscript.

Funding: This research received no external funding.

Institutional Review Board Statement: The study was conducted according to the guidelines of the Declaration of Helsinki and approved by the Ethical Review Board of the Chung Shan Medical University Hospital (CS2-20036) approved our study.

Informed Consent Statement: Patient consent was waived by both the National Health Insurance Administration and the Institutional Review Board of Chung Shan Medical University Hospital due to the database-processing nature of the current study.

Data Availability Statement: Restrictions apply to the availability of these data. Data were obtained from the National Health Insurance database and are available from the authors with the permission of the National Health Insurance Administration of Taiwan.

Acknowledgments: This study was partly based on data from the NHIRD provided by the NHI Administration, Ministry of Health and Welfare, and managed by the Health and Welfare Data Science Center (HWDC) in Taiwan. The interpretation and conclusions contained herein do not represent those of the NHI Administration, Ministry of Health and Welfare, or National Health Research Institutes.

Conflicts of Interest: The authors declare no conflict of interest.

References

1. Lupsa, B.C.; Insogna, K. Bone Health and Osteoporosis. *Endocrinol. Metab. Clin. N. Am.* **2015**, *44*, 517–530. [CrossRef] [PubMed]
2. Ensrud, K.E. Epidemiology of fracture risk with advancing age. *J. Gerontol. Ser. A Biol. Sci. Med. Sci.* **2013**, *68*, 1236–1242. [CrossRef] [PubMed]
3. Song, L. Calcium and Bone Metabolism Indices. *Adv. Clin. Chem.* **2017**, *82*, 1–46. [CrossRef] [PubMed]
4. Moe, S.M. Calcium Homeostasis in Health and in Kidney Disease. *Compr. Physiol.* **2016**, *6*, 1781–1800. [CrossRef]
5. Arfat, Y.; Rani, A.; Jingping, W.; Hocart, C.H. Calcium homeostasis during hibernation and in mechanical environments disrupting calcium homeostasis. *J. Comp. Physiol. B Biochem. Syst. Environ. Physiol.* **2020**, *190*, 1–16. [CrossRef]
6. Binkley, N. Vitamin D and osteoporosis-related fracture. *Arch. Biochem. Biophys.* **2012**, *523*, 115–122. [CrossRef]
7. Weaver, C.M.; Alexander, D.D.; Boushey, C.J.; Dawson-Hughes, B.; Lappe, J.M.; LeBoff, M.S.; Liu, S.; Looker, A.C.; Wallace, T.C.; Wang, D.D. Calcium plus vitamin D supplementation and risk of fractures: An updated meta-analysis from the National Osteoporosis Foundation. *Osteoporos. Int.* **2016**, *27*, 367–376. [CrossRef]
8. Blaine, J.; Chonchol, M.; Levi, M. Renal control of calcium, phosphate, and magnesium homeostasis. *Clin. J. Am. Soc. Nephrol. CJASN* **2015**, *10*, 1257–1272. [CrossRef]
9. Beto, J.A. The role of calcium in human aging. *Clin. Nutr. Res.* **2015**, *4*, 1–8. [CrossRef]
10. Sainani, G.S. Non-drug therapy in prevention and control of hypertension. *J. Assoc. Physicians India* **2003**, *51*, 1001–1006.
11. Vertes, V. Weight reduction for control of systemic hypertension. *Am. J. Cardiol.* **1987**, *60*, 48–54. [CrossRef]
12. Tsioufis, C.; Thomopoulos, C. Combination drug treatment in hypertension. *Pharmacol. Res.* **2017**, *125*, 266–271. [CrossRef] [PubMed]
13. Düsing, R.; Waeber, B.; Destro, M.; Santos Maia, C.; Brunel, P. Triple-combination therapy in the treatment of hypertension: A review of the evidence. *J. Hum. Hypertens.* **2017**, *31*, 501–510. [CrossRef] [PubMed]

14. Gorostidi, M.; de la Sierra, A. Combination therapy in hypertension. *Adv. Ther.* **2013**, *30*, 320–336. [CrossRef] [PubMed]
15. Taylor, A.A.; Pool, J.L. Clinical pharmacology of antihypertensive therapy. *Semin. Nephrol.* **2005**, *25*, 215–226. [CrossRef] [PubMed]
16. Frank, J. Managing hypertension using combination therapy. *Am. Fam. Physician* **2008**, *77*, 1279–1286.
17. Wenzel, R.R. Renal protection in hypertensive patients: Selection of antihypertensive therapy. *Drugs* **2005**, *65* (Suppl. S2), 29–39. [CrossRef]
18. Smith, D.K.; Lennon, R.P.; Carlsgaard, P.B. Managing Hypertension Using Combination Therapy. *Am. Fam. Physician* **2020**, *101*, 341–349.
19. Escribano, J.; Balaguer, A.; Pagone, F.; Feliu, A.; Roqué, I.F.M. Pharmacological interventions for preventing complications in idiopathic hypercalciuria. *Cochrane Database Syst. Rev.* **2009**, *2009*, Cd004754. [CrossRef]
20. Li, D.F.; Gao, Y.L.; Liu, H.C.; Huang, X.C.; Zhu, R.F.; Zhu, C.T. Use of thiazide diuretics for the prevention of recurrent kidney calculi: A systematic review and meta-analysis. *J. Transl. Med.* **2020**, *18*, 106. [CrossRef]
21. Aung, K.; Htay, T. Thiazide diuretics and the risk of hip fracture. *Cochrane Database Syst. Rev.* **2011**, *10*, Cd005185. [CrossRef] [PubMed]
22. Langdahl, B.L. Osteoporosis in premenopausal women. *Curr. Opin. Rheumatol.* **2017**, *29*, 410–415. [CrossRef] [PubMed]
23. Sullivan, S.D.; Lehman, A.; Nathan, N.K.; Thomson, C.A.; Howard, B.V. Age of menopause and fracture risk in postmenopausal women randomized to calcium + vitamin D, hormone therapy, or the combination: Results from the Women's Health Initiative Clinical Trials. *Menopause* **2017**, *24*, 371–378. [CrossRef] [PubMed]
24. Ferdinand, K.C.; Nasser, S.A. Management of Essential Hypertension. *Cardiol. Clin.* **2017**, *35*, 231–246. [CrossRef]
25. Wright, J.M.; Musini, V.M.; Gill, R. First-line drugs for hypertension. *Cochrane Database Syst. Rev.* **2018**, *4*, Cd001841. [CrossRef]
26. Guzon-Illescas, O.; Perez Fernandez, E.; Crespí Villarias, N.; Quirós Donate, F.J.; Peña, M.; Alonso-Blas, C.; García-Vadillo, A.; Mazzucchelli, R. Mortality after osteoporotic hip fracture: Incidence, trends, and associated factors. *J. Orthop. Surg. Res.* **2019**, *14*, 1–9. [CrossRef]
27. Li, N.; Cornelissen, D.; Silverman, S.; Pinto, D.; Si, L.; Kremer, I.; Bours, S.; de Bot, R.; Boonen, A.; Evers, S.; et al. An Updated Systematic Review of Cost-Effectiveness Analyses of Drugs for Osteoporosis. *PharmacoEconomics* **2021**, *39*, 181–209. [CrossRef]
28. Pang, K.L.; Low, N.Y.; Chin, K.Y. A Review on the Role of Denosumab in Fracture Prevention. *Drug Des. Dev. Ther.* **2020**, *14*, 4029–4051. [CrossRef]
29. Charkos, T.G.; Liu, Y.; Jin, L.; Yang, S. Thiazide Use and Fracture Risk: An updated Bayesian Meta-Analysis. *Sci. Rep.* **2019**, *9*, 19754. [CrossRef]
30. Bokrantz, T.; Schiöler, L.; Boström, K.B.; Kahan, T.; Mellström, D.; Ljungman, C.; Hjerpe, P.; Hasselström, J.; Manhem, K. Antihypertensive drug classes and the risk of hip fracture: Results from the Swedish primary care cardiovascular database. *J. Hypertens.* **2020**, *38*, 167–175. [CrossRef]
31. Langerhuizen, D.W.G.; Verweij, L.P.E.; van der Wouden, J.C.; Kerkhoffs, G.; Janssen, S.J. Antihypertensive drugs demonstrate varying levels of hip fracture risk: A systematic review and meta-analysis. *Injury* **2022**, *53*, 1098–1107. [CrossRef] [PubMed]
32. Xiao, X.; Xu, Y.; Wu, Q. Thiazide diuretic usage and risk of fracture: A meta-analysis of cohort studies. *Osteoporos. Int.* **2018**, *29*, 1515–1524. [CrossRef] [PubMed]
33. Kruse, C.; Eiken, P.; Vestergaard, P. Continuous and long-term treatment is more important than dosage for the protective effect of thiazide use on bone metabolism and fracture risk. *J. Intern. Med.* **2016**, *279*, 110–122. [CrossRef] [PubMed]
34. Wang, J.; Su, K.; Sang, W.; Li, L.; Ma, S. Thiazide Diuretics and the Incidence of Osteoporotic Fracture: A Systematic Review and Meta-Analysis of Cohort Studies. *Front. Pharmacol.* **2019**, *10*, 1364. [CrossRef] [PubMed]
35. Shen, T.Y.; Strong, C.; Yu, T. Age at menopause and mortality in Taiwan: A cohort analysis. *Maturitas* **2020**, *136*, 42–48. [CrossRef]
36. Reid, I.R.; Ames, R.W.; Orr-Walker, B.J.; Clearwater, J.M.; Horne, A.M.; Evans, M.C.; Murray, M.A.; McNeil, A.R.; Gamble, G.D. Hydrochlorothiazide reduces loss of cortical bone in normal postmenopausal women: A randomized controlled trial. *Am. J. Med.* **2000**, *109*, 362–370. [CrossRef]
37. Bolland, M.J.; Ames, R.W.; Horne, A.M.; Orr-Walker, B.J.; Gamble, G.D.; Reid, I.R. The effect of treatment with a thiazide diuretic for 4 years on bone density in normal postmenopausal women. *Osteoporos. Int.* **2007**, *18*, 479–486. [CrossRef]
38. Li, C.; Zeng, Y.; Tao, L.; Liu, S.; Ni, Z.; Huang, Q.; Wang, Q. Meta-analysis of hypertension and osteoporotic fracture risk in women and men. *Osteoporos. Int.* **2017**, *28*, 2309–2318. [CrossRef]
39. Yang, S.; Nguyen, N.D.; Center, J.R.; Eisman, J.A.; Nguyen, T.V. Association between hypertension and fragility fracture: A longitudinal study. *Osteoporos. Int.* **2014**, *25*, 97–103. [CrossRef]
40. Lin, S.M.; Yang, S.H.; Cheng, H.Y.; Liang, C.C.; Huang, H.K. Thiazide diuretics and the risk of hip fracture after stroke: A population-based propensity-matched cohort study using Taiwan's National Health Insurance Research Database. *BMJ Open* **2017**, *7*, e016992. [CrossRef]
41. Dalbeth, N.; Gamble, G.D.; Horne, A.; Reid, I.R. Relationship between Changes in Serum Urate and Bone Mineral Density during Treatment with Thiazide Diuretics: Secondary Analysis from a Randomized Controlled Trial. *Calcif. Tissue Int.* **2016**, *98*, 474–478. [CrossRef] [PubMed]

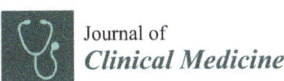

Systematic Review

Comparison between Vascular and Non-Vascular Bone Grafting in Scaphoid Nonunion: A Systematic Review

Gianluca Testa *, Ludovico Lucenti, Salvatore D'Amato, Marco Sorrentino, Pierluigi Cosentino, Andrea Vescio and Vito Pavone

Department of General Surgery and Medical-Surgical Specialties, Section of Orthopaedics and Traumatology, A.O.U. Policlinico Rodolico—San Marco, University of Catania, 95123 Catania, Italy; ludovico.lucenti@gmail.com (L.L.); salvatoredamato2419@gmail.com (S.D.); marcosor95@icloud.com (M.S.); pierluigi-cosentino@hotmail.it (P.C.); andreavescio88@gmail.com (A.V.); vitopavone@hotmail.com (V.P.)
* Correspondence: gianpavel@hotmail.com

Abstract: Background: Scaphoid fractures correspond to 60% of all carpal fractures, with a risk of 10% to progress towards non-union. Furthermore, ~3% present avascular necrosis (AVN) of the proximal pole, which is one of the main complications related to the peculiar vascularization of the bone. Scaphoid non-union can be treated with vascularized and non-vascularized bone grafting. The aim of the study is to evaluate the rates of consolidation of scaphoid non-union treated using two types of grafts. Methods: A systematic review of two electronic medical databases was carried out by two independent authors, using the following inclusion criteria: non-union of the proximal pole of the scaphoid bone, treated with vascular bone grafting (VBG) or non-vascular bone grafting (NVBG), with or without the use of internal fixation, patients aged $\geq$ 10 years old, and a minimum of 12 months follow-up. Research of any level of evidence that reports clinical results and regarding non-union scaphoid, either using vascularized or non-vascularized bone grafting, has been included. Results: A total of 271 articles were identified. At the end of the first screening, 104 eligible articles were selected for the whole reading of the text. Finally, after reading the text and the control of the reference list, we selected 26 articles following the criteria described above. Conclusions: The choice of the VBG depends mainly on the defect of the scaphoid and on the surgeon's knowledge of the different techniques. Free vascular graft with medial femoral condyle (MFC) seems to be a promising alternative to local vascularized bone grafts in difficult cases.

Keywords: scaphoid; non-union; vascular bone grafting; non-vascular bone grafting

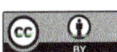

1. Introduction

Scaphoid fractures are the most common wrist fractures, accounting for 60% of all carpal fractures. Although consolidation can occur without needing surgical treatment, the non-union rate is ~10% [1]. The main risk factor for non-union is fragment dislocation, associated with non-union rates of up to 55% [2]. Additionally, the displacement and time of surgery may play an important role: Davis suggests that all fractures with >3 mm displacement should be operated on early to prevent the development of non-union [3].

Avascular necrosis (AVN) is one of the most feared complications. It has an estimated occurrence of 3% of all cases of scaphoid fractures; it occurs mainly in the proximal pole, probably due to the particular vascularization of this bone [4,5]. Magnetic resonance imaging (MRI) is recommended to diagnose AVN. However, the gold standard is an intraoperative evaluation of the absence of bleeding in the proximal fragment [6]. Plain radiographs of the hand and wrist are partially valuable for diagnosing and evaluating displacement. However, scaphoid views are the most useful. Therefore, MRI or CT scans are indicated in most scaphoid fractures [7,8].

When a scaphoid non-union occurs because of late diagnosis or failed treatment, it can cause a scaphoid non-union advance collapse (SNAC), a condition characterized by progressive deformity and degenerative changes ranging between radial styloid arthritis and pancarpal arthritis. The resultant wrist architecture is known as dorsal intercalated segment instability (DISI) deformity, which affects the patient in terms of a limited range of movement, grip strength, and daily living activities [9,10].

The risk of developing wrist osteoarthritis increases in proportion to the time elapsed between injury and surgery [11,12]. Surgical treatment involves reducing and fixation of the scaphoid, either with a non-vascularized bone graft (NVBG) or vascularized bone graft (VBG).

There is little evidence about the best type of graft in the current literature. In a systematic review, Munk et al. found a slightly higher union rate in pedicled vascularized grafts (90%) compared to non-vascularized bone grafts with internal fixation (84%) [13]. Many authors agree that a vascularized bone graft is preferred in avascular necrosis and proximal pole non-union, especially when vascularity is compromised and augmentation of the local biology is needed [14]. More recently, a vascularized graft from the medial femoral condyle has been described for scaphoid waist non-union, with the advantage of lower donor site morbidity [15]. Although free vascularized bone grafts are increasingly used and may have a better union rate than pedicled bone grafts [16], this major surgery should be reserved for the failure of conservative treatment or when a small proximal pole needs to be reconstructed. The aim of the treatment of scaphoid non-union is pain relief, better hand function, and the prevention of late-onset painful post-traumatic osteoarthritis [17]. Following the non-union, progressively degenerative changes may occur with the formation of cysts, bony resorption with loss of bone stock, and the development of apex dorsal angulation or the humpback deformity [9]. The importance of vascularity has been enforced by finding that conventional NVBGs could only achieve a 47% union rate in the presence of AVN. However, in the absence of AVN, NVBGs could achieve union rates of 94% [18]. It was widely believed that providing adequate blood flow would help treat cases of non-union. Several in vivo studies have aimed to demonstrate that VBGs accelerated bone healing by preserving osteocytes and preventing the slower creeping substitution; canine models demonstrated increased blood flow and superior mechanical properties in VBGs compared to NVBGs [14,19].

This systematic review aims to evaluate the available literature on the rates of consolidation of scaphoid non-union treated using two types of grafts (VBG and NVBG) to help decision making in the management of these injuries and to establish the outcomes of bone grafting surgery.

2. Materials and Methods

2.1. Research Selection

According to the Preferred Reporting Items for Systematic Reviews and Meta-Analyses (PRISMA) guidelines [20], two databases (PubMed and Google Scholar) were revised by two authors (DAS and SM). The keywords used in the research were "scaphoid" AND (non-union OR ill-union OR pseudoarthrosis OR delayed healing OR avascular necrosis), AND (surgical OR operating OR surgery OR grafting OR non-conservative OR not bloodless) AND (vascularized OR non-vascularized). For every original article included in the research, a standard form of input data was used to extrapolate the number of patients, gender, the average age at the time of treatment, type of grafting, donor site, complications, and mean follow-up, post-surgery immobilization, and research year. The quality assessment of the research was carried out double-blind by two independent reviewers (AV and GT). Any disagreement on data was resolved by consulting a senior surgeon (VP).

2.2. Inclusion and Exclusion Criteria

All articles identified in our systematic review included the treatment of scaphoid non-union using vascular bone grafting (VBG) or non-vascular bone grafting (NVBG). The initial screening of the titles and the abstracts was carried out using the following criteria of inclusion: non-union of the proximal pole of the scaphoid bone, treatment with VBG or

NVBG with or without the use of internal fixation, patients ≥ 10 years old, and a minimum of 6 months follow-up.

The exclusion criteria were all the articles that did not mention the use of bone grafting to treat the scaphoid non-union and those that did not refer to the avascular necrosis of the proximal pole. Studies focused on other topics or without a clear reference on post-surgical grafting results and those with a limited science-based methodology or no available abstracts or full text have been excluded.

2.3. Assessment of Bias Risk

In this systematic review, the bias risk evaluation was carried out using the ROBINS-I tool for non-randomized studies: it consists of a three-step assessment. The first step concerns the initial planning of the systematic review. The second step is evaluating the common biases that can be found in these studies. The third step concerns the overall bias risk. Two authors (AV and GT) carried out the evaluation independently. Any discrepancies were discussed with the senior researcher (VP) for the final decision. All evaluators agreed on the final decision of each assessment step (Table 1).

Table 1. The main results of the non-scaphoid unions included metanalysis, systematic reviews, case studies, cohort studies, and prospective and retrospective series.

Ref	Author	Level of Evidence/Type of Paper	N of Patients	Surgery	FU	Results	Limit of the Study
[21]	Korompilias et al.	IV Therapeutic	23	VBG	24 m	Fixation of the bone graft with 1 or 2 K-wires + external fixator has clear advantages: to provide better wrist support than a brace or cast, and secondarily to be able to perform a post-operative MRI to assess the vascularity of the proximal pole once the K-wires are removed upon obtaining the union.	Absence of a comparison group Lack of a postoperative CT scan in all patients
[22]	Mouilhade et al.		15	VBG		Zaidemberg graft allows better vision of the proximal pole of the scaphoid and does not destabilize the extrinsic volar ligaments of the carpus. The Kuhlmann graft allows for easier height restoration and better graft adaptation to the scaphoid surface.	Anatomical/cadaveric comparative study
[23]	Barrera-Ochoa et al.	IV Therapeutic	32	VBG	12 m	Vascularized periosteal flaps (VPFs) represent an additional method to conventional VBGs; it improves difficult non-union in the presence of poor prognostic factors in children, adolescents, and adults.	The technique combines 2 procedures, each of which could be considered individual. Absence of comparisons with other techniques. Small sample size and short follow-up
[24]	Severo et al.	Review		VBG vs. NVBG		There is a preference in the literature for vascularized bone grafts over conventional NVBG. The 1,2-intercompartmental supraretinacular artery pedicled (ICSRA-VBG) technique provides easy visualization and dissection of the pedicle, which makes this technique critical for treating scaphoid non-union with AVN of the proximal pole.	
[13]	Munk et al.	Review	5246	VBG vs. NVBG	12 m	The addition of internal fixation of an NVBG does not significantly increase the union rate of a scaphoid non-union. With a VBG, there is an increase in union rate and a reduction in immobilization time.	

Table 1. Cont.

Ref	Author	Level of Evidence/Type of Paper	N of Patients	Surgery	FU	Results	Limit of the Study
[25]	Hovius et al.	Review	5745	VBG vs. NVBG	12 m	The study shows that NVBG is used as the standard treatment for simple, non-displaced non-unions. When AVN, proximal pole non-union, and/or pseudoarthrosis is present, a vascularized graft is preferred.	
[26]	Capo et al.	Case report	1	NVBG	12 m	Despite a chronic non-union of the scaphoid (28 years), surgical treatment has allowed healing and good clinical-functional outcomes. The natural history of chronic scaphoid non-union does not always result in the progressive degeneration of the radioscaphoid joint.	
[27]	Rahimnia et al.	Retrospective study	41	VBG	12 m	Patients who achieve full scaphoid union report significantly better outcomes in radio-ulnar deviation and handgrip strength ($p < 0.03$; $p < 0.04$). Smoking represents the main negative prognostic factor affecting non-union.	Small sample size and many patients lost to follow-up. Not able to determine the time of union. Not evaluated the revascularization of scaphoid bone
[28]	Tsumura et al.	IV Therapeutic	19	VBG	12 m	1,2-ICSRA VGB with a dorsomedial approach was useful for treating scaphoid non-union with a humped deformity. The study shows that taking up to about 15 mm in length and width and about 10 mm in thickness from the graft should be sufficient to correct most back deformities.	There is not a statistical analysis of outcomes. Small sample size and short follow-up No control group
[29]	Moon et al.	Review	1	NVBG	12 m	The findings suggest that NVBG can result in high union rates when the scaphoid maintains adequate perfusion and stable graft fixation	
[30]	Higgins et al.	Histopathological study	7	VBG vs. NVBG	6 m	Vascularized osteochondral grafts performed in the medial femoral trochlea provide synovial nutrition and generous surrounding subchondral bone beds for graft perfusion and survival.	
[31]	Ross et al.	III	4177	VBG vs. NVBG	12 m	Scaphoid non-union is treated more often with an NVBG vs. VBG (91.4% vs. 8.6%); however, the use of VBG results in a greater likelihood of receiving a CT scan in follow-up and more X-rays (mean 5.3 X-rays vs. 4.7, $p < 0.001$). Higher family income results in a greater likelihood of receiving a VBG.	Other important clinical outcomes are not considered. Potential errors in coding leading to a sampling bias. Individual surgeon indications, patient preference, the exact reasons for reoperations are not determined.
[17]	Ferguson et al.	II	5464	VBG vs. NVBG	12 m	Union was achieved in 81% of the included cases. The mean union rates between VBG and NVBG were 84% and 80%, respectively. When avascular necrosis of the proximal pole of the scaphoid was identified, the mean rate was 74% with VBG, compared with 62% with NVBG.	
[32]	Chaudhry et al.	Prospective study	19	VBG	12 m	In conclusion, the results demonstrate that MFC vascularized free graft achieved excellent results in a subgroup of scaphoid non-unions with one or more poor prognostic factors (union rate 88.5%; union rate with the presence of AVN 85%).	Small sample size and short follow-up.

Table 1. Cont.

Ref	Author	Level of Evidence/Type of Paper	N of Patients	Surgery	FU	Results	Limit of the Study
[33]	Malizos et al.	Prospective study		VBG		The study highlights some key points: smoking cessation (pre- and post-operative) to reduce its negative effects on the union; dorsal grafts (based on 1,2 or 2,3 ICSRA) are more used for proximal non-unions, while volar grafts are preferred for non-unions to the middle segment of the scaphoid. A technical tip common to both approaches is to take a larger graft based on pre-operative measurements and adapt it to the size of the defect.	Use of the MRI instead of CT scan for the follow-up protocol.
[34]	Tsantes et al.	Review	825	VBG	12 m	According to the results of the study, the consolidation rate was 86.3% for the 1.2 ICSRA graft, 93.9% for the volar bone graft (preferentially used for correction of hump deformity) and 88.8% for the free MFC graft (allows replacement of the proximal articular portion in cases of difficult non-union of the proximal pole of scaphoid).	
[35]	Sgromolo et al.	Review		VBG		VBG allows for healing, improved vascularity, and correction of humped deformity in AVN or premature failure of an NVBG.	
[2]	Talal Al-Jabr et al.	Review	245	VBG	12 m	In this study, the mean union rate for patients undergoing free VBG is 93.65%: using a VBG from the MFC, the union rate was 100% (56 pts), while from the iliac crest, it was 87.3% (188 pts).	
[36]	Kawamura et al.	Review		VBG vs. NVBG		This study suggests that vascularized bone grafting may improve the healing of scaphoid non-unions with proximal pole AVN.	
[37]	Pinder et al.	Review	1602	VBG vs. NVBG	12 m	The union incidence rate for NVBG was 88% (84–92; 95% CI), for VBG was 92% (85–96; 95% CI). In the presence of AVN, the incidence with a vascularized bone graft from the MFC and distal radius was 100% and 96%, respectively, whereas, with the use of NVBG from the iliac crest, the union rate was 27%.	
[18]	Merrell et al.	Meta-analysis	1827	VBG vs. NVB	24 m	Results show that in scaphoid non-unions with AVN, the union was achieved more often in patients who received a VBG combined with screw or K-wire fixation than NVBG and screw fixation (88% vs. 47% union; $p < 0.0005$).	Subject to detection and publication bias. Lack of foreign-language articles is a limitation Effort to control for quality by setting predetermined standards for inclusion and exclusion
[38]	Derby et al.	Review		VBG	12 m	When initial failure of an NVBG is present or if there is an AVN of the proximal pole, the use of a VBG should be considered. For the correction of DISI/carpal collapse, radial volar grafts and CFM-free grafts have good outcomes.	
[15]	Elgammal et al.	Retrospective study	30	VBG	12 m	MFC-free vascular graft allowed union in 24 of 30 patients. It is considered an appropriate treatment in cases of non-union of the scaphoid with humpback deformity and/or AVN to the proximal pole with the substantial post-operative improvement of the scapholunate and lateral interscaphoid angles ($p < 0.05$; $p < 0.001$).	Small sample size and short follow-up

Table 1. Cont.

Ref	Author	Level of Evidence/Type of Paper	N of Patients	Surgery	FU	Results	Limit of the Study
[39]	Pokorny et al.	Review		VBG		This study affirms that the main indications for VBG in non-union of the scaphoid are any non-union with proximal pole avascular necrosis and non-union that has failed a previous conventional bone graft attempt.	
[40]	Elzinga et al.	Review		VBG		The volar carpal artery and pronator quadratus VBFs are the most used volar VBFs for scaphoid non-union: they provide flaps with minimal donor site morbidity. The pisiform VBF is an option for replacing the proximal pole of the scaphoid but is often too small for humpback deformity. Volar distal ulnar VBF is not a first-line option for treating scaphoid non-unions due to the morbidity of ulnar artery harvesting.	

3. Results

3.1. Studies Included

A total of 271 articles were identified. After the exclusion of duplicates, 151 articles were selected. At the end of the first screening, we selected 56 articles eligible for reading the whole text following the selection criteria described above. Finally, after checking the reference list, we selected 25 articles, consisting of meta-analyses, systematic reviews, case studies, cohort studies, or prospective and retrospective series, following the criteria described above. A PRISMA flow chart of the selection and screening method is provided (Figure 1).

The main results of the articles included were summarized (Table 1).

3.2. Non-Vascular Bone Graft (NVBG)

A total of 11 articles included in our study focused on treating scaphoid non-union treated using non-vascular bone graft (NVBG).

In a case study by Moon et al. [29] on a non-union in a 26-year-old patient who presented constant pain 9 months after undergoing open reduction and internal fixation (ORIF) with a mini screw, the patient was treated with NVBG-treated scaphoid body fracture. It appears that 12 weeks after surgery, the fracture showed a 40% recovery at the CT scan, and during the successive evaluation, 7 months after surgery, there was a loss of 10° volar bending in terms of range of motion (ROM), a grip force of 94% compared to the healthy contralateral limb, and a union confirmed by X-ray.

Some studies in the literature compare both types of bone graft in the treatment of non-union scaphoid: Ross et al. [31], in their case studies involving 4177 patients, concluded that both techniques produce low failure rates (6.1% for NVBG vs. 5% for VBG); the difference in the probabilities of failure was not statistically significant ($p = 0.425$). The union rate was 94% for the non-union of scaphoid treated with NVBG, similar results to those shown in Pinder et al. [37]: in 35 examined subgroups, the use of non-vascularized bone grafts was reported with a union rate of 88%.

Union rates are reduced considerably when non-vascularized bone grafts are applied in the presence of avascular necrosis of the proximal pole of the scaphoid: in 144 studies examined in a review by Ferguson et al. [17], when the AVN of the proximal pole of the scaphoid is identified, the average union rate varies from 74% with VBG compared to 62% with NVBG.

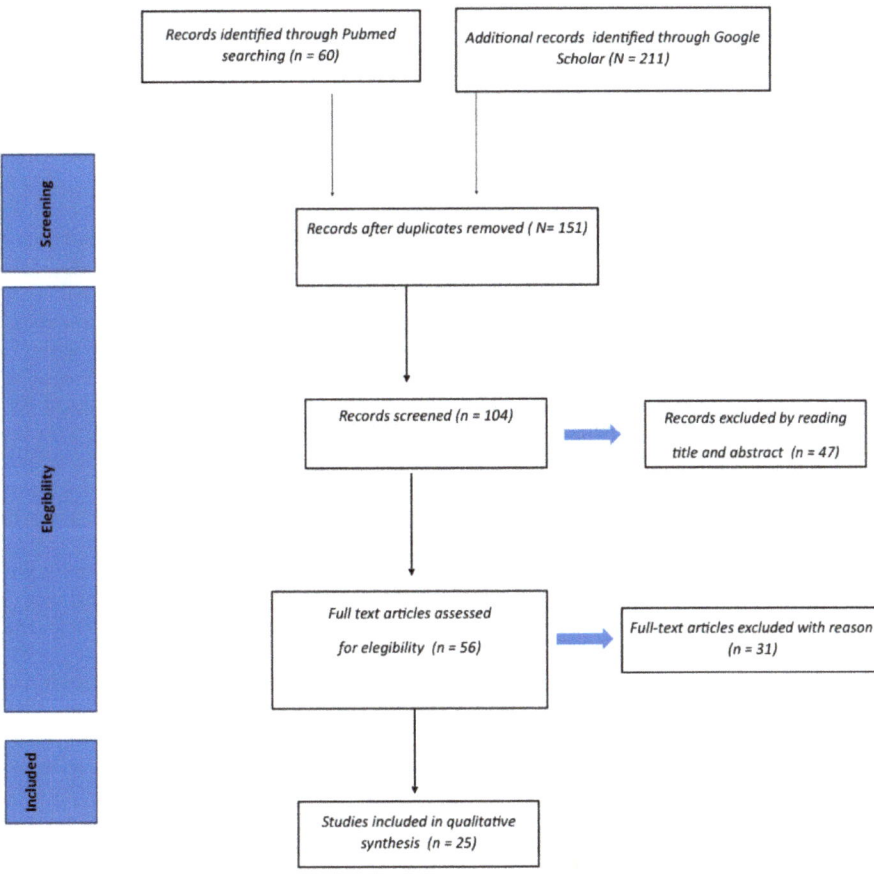

Figure 1. PRISMA (Preferred Reporting Items for Systematic Reviews and Meta-Analysis); flow diagram of the systematic review of the literature.

There were no statistically significant differences in the union rate when comparing the use of an additional internal fixation to non-vascularized bone grafts in the work of Munk et al. [13]: examining the first group of patients treated with NVBG without internal fixation after a period of immobilization of 15 weeks, a union rate of 80% was found, while in the second group, with the use of the NVBG with internal fixation, after a period of immobilization of 7 weeks, the union rate was 84%. In contrast to these results, in a metanalysis made by Merrel et al. [18], it is clear how the union was reached more often in those patients who received a vascularized graft combined with the fixation with screws or K wires compared to the non-vascularized wedge grafts combined with the fixation with screws (88% union in 34 patients vs. 47% union in 30 patients, $p < 0.0005$).

Concerning the techniques describing the use of NVBG for the treatment of non-union of the scaphoid with necrosis of the proximal pole, only three sets of cases were recovered in the analysis of Severo et al. [24]. Matsuki et al. [41] assessed the rate of consolidation of fractures of the proximal pole of the scaphoid in which NVBG was associated with the fixation of a Herbert screw; 11 patients were assessed, and consolidation was observed in all. Using the same technique, Robbins et al. [42] studied 17 patients with a 1-year follow-up and observed a consolidation rate of 52%. Ribak et al. [43] estimated the consolidation rate using NVBG in 40 patients; of these, 16 had proximal pole necrosis and 11 reached consolidation (68%).

The comparison between cartilage quality in non-vascular osteochondral grafts with vascular osteochondral flaps in an animal pig model is interesting [30]. In the NVGB, cartilage development is reduced compared to vascularized grafts; chondrocytes reside in gaps. The cartilage matrix is not well developed compared to the VBG group. The basophilic matrix cartilage is reduced due to the inadequate synthesis of collagen fibers and the amorphous extracellular matrix.

We also observe the narrowing of chondrocytes, large gaps between chondrocytes and the capsular matrix, and intra-cytoplasmic vacuolization in some chondrocytes. In the group of vascularized flaps, all the phases of development of the cartilage are observed under the optical microscope. Chondromites with clearly visible nuclei and basophile cytoplasm reside in the gaps of the cartilaginous matrix and are distributed individually or in groups. The cartilaginous matrix shows a distinct basophilia around chondrocytes, although reduced in inter-lacunar areas. All cytoplasmic characteristics and chondrocyte nuclei in the gaps retain their normal structure. The visual morphological assessment of cartilage in the vascular group revealed a smooth and continuous surface in all samples ($n = 7$) with a predominantly viable cell population ($n = 6$; 85.7%). The score for the viability of chondrocytes and surface morphology of cartilage morphology is significantly higher in the VBG group ($p < 0.05$). The distribution of chondrocytes is predominantly columnar ($n = 6$; 85.7%) in vascular cartilage compared to a disorganized or cluster distribution in non-vascularized grafts ($p < 0.05$).

Capo et al. [26] presented an interesting case concerning a non-chronic union (28 years) of scaphoid treated with NVBG and internal fixation with a screw and K-wire. The objective pre-surgery test showed tenderness above the scaphoid and the dorsally radio-scaphoid articulation. The wrist range of motion (ROM) showed an extension of 45°, a bending of 40°, and pronation and supination of 80° degrees. Its grip strength was limited to about 50% relative to the other healthy contralateral side. Six months after the surgery, the X-rays showed complete recovery with the remodeling of the bone callus near the failure to join the scaphoid. The patient had a slight tenderness around the anatomical snuffbox at the physical examination. Sensitivity was intact in all nervous distributions. The DASH score (arm, shoulder and hand disability) was 36, and the grip force of the hand was 64% compared to the healthy side counter, with a slight increase over the previous values.

3.3. Vascular Bone Graft (VBG)

A total of 23 studies examined by us consider the use of vascularized bone grafts (VBG) to treat non-union scaphoids. In Korompilias et al. [21], union was reached in 100% of patients treated with vascular bone graft by distal radius after an average of 10 weeks: the DASH scores and the degree of post-surgery satisfaction showed significant improvement in all patients. No patient suffered pain after a follow-up of at least 2 years. Consistent results can also be observed in a prospective cohort study of 32 patients [23]: 6 months after surgery, complete bone healing with vascularized periosteal flaps was observed in all patients except 1. An overall gain of 20 in ROM was observed compared to pre-surgery control and 3 months of follow-up; there were no significant differences between treated and untreated (healthy) wrists.

Regarding the data on force measurements, from before to after the surgery, a significant improvement was noted with an overall gain of 41% compared to the strength of the healthy contralateral side. Pain at rest and during exercise decreased significantly after surgery, measured by the Visual Analogue Scale (VAS) score; on average, 1.1 ± 1.4 (range, 0–6) at rest and 2.4 ± 1.7 (range, 0–8) during exercise. Significant improvements were found in the quick-DASH and the MMWS (Modified Mayo Wrist Score).

An increasing interest in indicating the use of VBG based on dorsal radio circulation has been observed, particularly with the use of the 1.2 ICSRA. In support of these data, a recent work [18] showed a consolidation rate of 88% compared to 47% using the VBG and NVBG, respectively. The effectiveness of the vascular bone graft using 1,2-ICRSA has also been proven by Rahimnia et al. [27]. Overall, 30 out of 41 patients reached the union, and 11 did not. The overall average DASH score and the average MMWS score were 26 and 78, respectively; the average follow-up was 49 months after surgery. The MMWS score improved from 60 pre-surgery to 83 at the last follow-up. Excellent results were achieved in 14 patients (46.6%), good in 10 (33.3%), discreet in 5 (16.6%) and poor results only in 1 (3.5%). The DASH score decreased from 54 to 21, and the grip force was 73% compared to the strength of the healthy contralateral hand. The pre-surgery and post-surgery radius-ulnar deviation have improved significantly, while the flexion–extension showed no significant differences. The study also included 26 patients with AVN; 20 reached the scaphoid union, and 6 did not (76.9% vs. 23.1%).

Contrasting data in the literature concern the role of smoking as a possible factor influencing failure to merge in scaphoid fractures: for many authors [24,27,31,33], smoking is regarded as a genuine risk factor with a predominant role in the emergence of the proximal pole avascular necrosis. Ferguson et al. [17] argue that it was impossible to examine the actual influence of smoking on union rates, as most studies only described the proportion of smokers at the time of patient recruitment rather than how many smokers from the population achieved union. The reported union rates ranged from 17% to 100% for non-unions treated with NVBG and 27% to 100% treated with VBG.

Different results have been reported on the treatment of non-cancered scaphoids through a VBG graft using the 1,2-ICSRA, and its usefulness for treating non-cancered scaphoid with a DISI deformity (dorsal instability of the intercalary segment) remains unclear.

In Tsumura et al. [28], there were 19 patients in whom the scaphoid failed to join with a DISI deformity: the length of the scaphoid was measured, defined as the distance from the center of the scaphoid joint to the tip of the proximal pole on Rx-graphs in AP, and inter-scaphoid lateral angle (ISA), radioulnar angle (RLA), and scafolunate angle (SLA) were also measured using CT imaging. Hump deformities have been defined as an ISA 45° or higher, DISI deformities as an RLA 15° or higher and SLA 70° or higher. The union rate at the last follow-up executed with a minimum of 6 months after the surgery was 94.7%. In the 19 patients, the post-surgery ISA was adequate in 17 and inadequate in 2. For DISI deformity, all post-surgery SLA and RLA were within the normal limit (normal SLA, 30–60°; normal RLA from −15 a + 15).

A comparison of failure rates between pedunculated VBG and free VBG was made by Ross et al. [31]: among vascularized bone grafts, 314 (87.7%) were stem grafts, and 44 (12.3%) were encoded as free micro-vascular flaps. There were no statistically significant differences between the two repair techniques for lack of union regarding age, type of insurance plan, geographical region, or comorbidity score. Among patients with vascular bone grafts, the failure rate with pedunculated grafts was 4.8% ($n = 15/314$), which was not statistically different from the rate with free grafts (6.8%, $n = 3/44$, $p = 0.499$).

Chaudhry et al. [32] focused on the free vascular graft MFC (medial femoral condyle) in a subgroup of patients with non-scaphoid unions associated with 1 or more unfavorable prognostic factors (consolidation delay >5 years, proximal pole fracture, AVN, previous surgery for lack of union). These authors reported a union rate of 88.5% (17/19 patients) with an average union time of 7.0 months (range, 2–18). For all patients with AVN, the union rate was 85% (11/13 patients). There were two confirmed non-unions reported (2/19; 10.5%).

Tsantes et al. [34] considered the treatment of scaphoid non-unions with various types of VBG grafts. These authors considered a total of 541 patients treated with VBG 1,2-ICSRA. Avascular necrosis was evident in 242 of them. Graft consolidation and scaphoid union were observed in 467 patients (86.3%). This rate was 77.9% in patients with AVN, while when avascular necrosis was not evident, the union rate was 96.2%. This difference was statistically significant ($p < 0.05$, RR = 1.23). For the graft of volar bone from the distal radius, there were 132 patients: the consolidation of the graft and the union was reached in 124 patients (93.9%). The union was significantly higher ($p < 0.05$) in patients without avascular necrosis (94.7%) than in those with necrosis (85%) (RR = 1.11).

In free grafts of the medial femoral condyle (MFC) for 143 patients with non-union of the scaphoid, the consolidation of the graft and the union was reached in 127 (88.8%) patients. In patients with avascular necrosis, this rate was 86.9%, while when avascular necrosis was not evident, the union rate was 92.3%. This difference was not statistically significant ($p < 0.05$).

In the Al-Jabri et al. [2] study, a comparison was made in 245 patients with non-union of scaphoid who had undergone iliac crest-free VBG ($n = 188$) or femoral medial condyle ($n = 56$). Free vascular bone graft from the MFC showed a significantly higher union rate than the group with iliac crest VBG (100% vs. 87.7%) ($p = 0.006$). Pain at the donor site was described in all studies, and the use of a knee brace for 2 weeks was adopted for free femoral VBG. Five patients (8.9%) suffered from ectopic bone formation, with three requiring a resection. However, no major complications, such as knee fracture or knee instability, were reported with medial femoral VBG. For vascularized bone grafts free of the iliac crest, the rate of complications was significantly higher than the medial femoral VBG, with 60 patients showing an incidence of bone deformation of the donor site of 61.37% and a 31.7% incidence of impairment of the lateral cutaneous nerve of the thigh.

Elgammal et al. [15] evaluated the effectiveness of free vascular grafting by MFC on 30 patients with scaphoid non-union: radiographic healing occurred in 24 out of 30 reconstructed scaphoids. Four patients who did not reach the union were heavy smokers with poor follow-up compliance. Twenty-four patients experienced some improvement in wrist pain, twentyt received complete relief, and four received partial relief. The average visual analog pain score improved from 6 (range 4–8; SD 1) pre-surgery to 2 after surgery (range 0–6; SD 2). The mean ranges of motion at the final follow-up were 45° extension (range 30–65°; SD 11°), 40° bending (25–55°; SD 9°), 15° radial deviation (range 10–35°; SD 7°), and 25° ulnar deviation (range 15–45°; SD 7°). The average grip force was 38 kg (range 19–65; SD 12), 74% of the healthy contralateral side. The DASH average score improved from 40 pre-surgery (range 20–80; SD 18) to 20 post-surgery (range 0–80; SD 11). Concerning the quality of life, a total of 20 patients returned to their previous work without any functional limitations, 7 with some activity limitations, and 3 patients never returned to their previous jobs.

4. Discussion

The treatment of non-scaphoid unions is quite heterogeneous; some disputes remain unresolved, but, despite this, some key concepts concerning the indications of the types of grafting have been further reiterated.

Several authors agree that non-vascular bone grafting is less technically challenging than a VBG and is mostly used as a standard treatment for simple fractures, not dislocated, in the absence of humpback deformities and avascular necrosis of the proximal pole [21,25,29,35,36]. VBG can be taken from several donor sites, but the iliac crest and the distal radius are the most used. Healing occurs by creeping replacement and resorption, which prolongs the union time and reduces mechanical stability during the healing phase. Since 1960, the Matti–Russe procedure has been the most widely used technique and was originally used to collect the donor site, the iliac crest, but similar union rates could also be obtained with grafts from the distal radius [41]. Less morbidity of the donor site is an advantage of the distal radius over the iliac crest.

In the literature, how NVBG fixation with a screw and/or K wire influences the non-union consolidation rate remains unclear: Moon et al. [29] state that high consolidation rates could be achieved when an NVBG is rigidly fixed a screw or k-wire. However, Munk et al. [13] concluded that the addition of internal fixation does not significantly increase the union rate.

Evidence supports that the arterial contribution to the proximal pole is poor compared to the two-thirds distal scaphoid: the proximal pole, being entirely intra-articular, is covered by hyaline cartilage with a single ligamentous insertion, the radio-hull-lunate ligament. Therefore, its vascularization is completely dependent on intraosseous circulation. When the continuity solution is lost due to the fracture, this circulation is compromised, favoring the non-union [42].

Vascularized bone grafts are increasingly used to treat scaphoid non-union. These grafts can be taken from different places, but they mostly come from the distal radius. The proximity of the distal radius allows the rotation of a peduncle without the need for microvascular anastomosis [29]. Kuhlmann and Zaidenberg described the first two vascular bone grafting techniques. In 1986, Kuhlmann et al. [44] described a technique in which VBG was taken from the volar portion of the distal radius (carpal volar artery), used to treat failures that occurred after the use of the Matti–Russe technique of the NVBG. Zaidenberg et al. [45] published an article describing the use of VBG removed from the dorsal-radial distal portion using the 1,2-ICSRA.

Although the use of a VBG is technically more challenging than an NVBG, several authors [17,27,29,35,36,41,45] mention several fundamental reasons for the preference of the use of VBG over NVBG: the shorter consolidation time, a high joining rate with good clinical-functional results, and a better ability to revascularize the bone.

The dorso-radial grafts are more suitable for managing non-scaphoid unions involving the proximal pole without a significant hump deformity [29]. Jones et al. [16] concluded that 1,2-ICSRA VBG was not suitable for patients with hump deformities because the graft was not large enough and the vascular peduncle was too short. For proper correction of deformities, a separate volar approach and increased dissection of soft tissues are often required, allowing an adequate restoration of carpal height [17,40].

Several bone graft fixation methodologies have been described. Rigid internal fixation with a screw has clear biomechanical advantages over immobilization with 1 or 2 Kirschner wires. In an extensive risk factors assessment study for failure after the bone graft of 1,2-ICSRA, a higher failure rate was recorded when fixation other than screws was used to immobilize the graft [33]. Korompilias et al. [21], on the other hand, are conducive to a temporary mixed immobilization of the wrist with an external fixator + K wires: this provides better support than an orthosis or a cast. In addition, the use of removable Kirschner wires has the advantage of allowing an MRI after surgery, which is crucial to assess the vascularization of the proximal pole and the vitality of the graft, if necessary.

In cases where a vascular peduncle graft has failed, in the presence of avascular necrosis and/or humpback deformities, a free vascular bone graft may be a good option. The two most widely used free vascularized bone grafts are derived from the iliac crest and medial femoral condyle. The free graft obtained from the iliac crest is based on the deep circumflex iliac artery and vein, while that obtained from the medial femoral condyle is based on the descending gene artery and vein or superomedial gene vessels. Examining the current literature, Al-Jabri et al. found a union in 88% of iliac crest cases compared to 100% of medial femoral condyle cases; this difference was significant [2].

Chaudhry et al. [32] found in their study that free vascular graft from MFC was particularly indicated in a subset of patients with non-jointed scaphoid associated with one or more unfavorable prognostic factors (presence of AVN, hump deformity, delay of non union >5 years, failure of previous surgery). In this case, the advantages include consistent arterial anatomy with few variations, blood vessels larger than 1.5 mm, and peduncle length appropriate for correcting hump deformity. This results in a high consolidation rate with lower donor site morbidity. The free grafting of the femoral condyle requires a domain of microsurgical techniques, specific training, and a long learning curve [15].

From a statistical-epidemiological point of view, it was observed by Ross et al. [31] that sex, type of insurance, comorbidity score, and region of the country did not affect the type of repair of the non-union. Income was identified as a factor influencing the probability of receiving an avascular bone graft. It has been calculated that patients in households with a higher median income have been most often associated with surgery for non-cancer scaphoids with VBG.

Evaluating all the available articles about vascular and non-vascular bone grafting in scaphoid nonunion, some limitations were highlighted. Many studies did not have a sufficient statistical analysis, some of them due to a small sample size. Furthermore, a large variability in surgical techniques, surgeons, and contexts establish a significant bias in the full comprehension of the treatment options for scaphoid nonunion.

5. Conclusions

There are several surgical treatment options for non-union scaphoid fractures. Careful evaluation and early diagnosis are crucial to establishing the best treatment option. Therefore, to exclude or confirm the presence of AVN in the treatment of non-scaphoid unions is of fundamental importance in adapting the management strategies (the presence of punctual hemorrhage displayed intra-operative to the release of the hemostatic band).

The choice of the VBG depends mainly on the defect of the scaphoid (position of the non-union, presence of AVN and/or deformity to hump, history of previous surgical operations and possible damage to the donor site). The selection of a vascular peduncle depends on the surgeon's familiarity and comfort with the technique.

For non-proximal unions, dorso-radial VBG grafts based on 1.2–2.3 ICSRA are commonly used, while for non-union scaphoid medial grafts, volar grafts are preferred: the advantages of volar flaps include the ability to come close to the scaphoid, facilitating the correction of hump deformities, while at the same time restoring height.

Free vascular graft MFC is a promising alternative to local vascularized bone grafts in difficult cases of the non-union scaphoid with one or more adverse prognostic factors. Very promising initial results were found in terms of union rates, time of union, and functional outcomes with a low incidence of donor site morbidity.

A single best surgical option for the scaphoid nonunion has not been shown so far. Further multicentric studies are necessary to fully describe a precise diagnostic algorithm and to choose the best treatment option for each case of scaphoid nonunion.

Author Contributions: Conceptualization, G.T.; methodology, M.S.; software, A.V.; validation, L.L.; formal analysis, S.D.; investigation, M.S.; resources, P.C.; data curation, S.D.; writing—original draft preparation, M.S.; writing—review and editing, G.T.; visualization, V.P.; supervision, V.P.; project administration, V.P.; funding acquisition, V.P. All authors have read and agreed to the published version of the manuscript.

Funding: This research received no external funding.

Institutional Review Board Statement: Not applicable.

Informed Consent Statement: Not applicable.

Data Availability Statement: Not applicable.

Conflicts of Interest: The authors declare no conflict of interest.

References

1. Buijze, G.A.; Ochtman, L.; Ring, D. Management of Scaphoid Nonunion. *J. Hand Surg.* **2012**, *37*, 1095–1100. [CrossRef] [PubMed]
2. Al-Jabri, T.; Mannan, A.; Giannoudis, P. The Use of the Free Vascularised Bone Graft for Nonunion of the Scaphoid: A Systematic Review. *J. Orthop. Surg. Res.* **2014**, *9*, 21. [CrossRef] [PubMed]
3. Davis, T. Prediction of Outcome of Non-Operative Treatment of Acute Scaphoid Waist Fracture. *Annals* **2013**, *95*, 171–176. [CrossRef] [PubMed]
4. Grettve, S. Arterial anatomy of the carpal bones. *Cells Tissues Organs* **1955**, *25*, 331–345. [CrossRef] [PubMed]
5. Taleisnik, J.; Kelly, P.J. The Extraosseous and Intraosseous Blood Supply of the Scaphoid Bone. *J. Bone Jt. Surg. Am.* **1966**, *48*, 1125–1137. [CrossRef]
6. Kakar, S.; Bishop, A.T.; Shin, A.Y. Role of Vascularized Bone Grafts in the Treatment of Scaphoid Nonunions Associated With Proximal Pole Avascular Necrosis and Carpal Collapse. *J. Hand Surg.* **2011**, *36*, 722–725. [CrossRef] [PubMed]
7. Bhat, M.; McCarthy, M.; Davis, T.R.C.; Oni, J.A.; Dawson, S. MRI and Plain Radiography in the Assessment of Displaced Fractures of the Waist of the Carpal Scaphoid. *J. Bone Jt. Surg. Br. Vol.* **2004**, *86B*, 705–713. [CrossRef]
8. Lucenti, L.; Lutsky, K.F.; Jones, C.; Kazarian, E.; Fletcher, D.; Beredjiklian, P.K. Antegrade Versus Retrograde Technique for Fixation of Scaphoid Waist Fractures: A Comparison of Screw Placement. *J. Wrist Surg.* **2020**, *9*, 34–38. [CrossRef]
9. El-Karef, E.A. Corrective Osteotomy for Symptomatic Scaphoid Malunion. *Injury* **2005**, *36*, 1440–1448. [CrossRef]

10. Lynch, N.M.; Linscheid, R.L. Corrective Osteotomy for Scaphoid Malunion: Technique and Long-Term Follow-up Evaluation. *J. Hand Surg.* **1997**, *22*, 35–43. [CrossRef]
11. Reigstad, O.; Grimsgaard, C.; Thorkildsen, R.; Reigstad, A.; Røkkum, M. Scaphoid non-unions, where do they come from? The epidemiology and initial presentation of 270 scaphoid non-unions. *Hand Surg.* **2012**, *17*, 331–335. [CrossRef]
12. Mack, G.R.; Bosse, M.J.; Gelberman, R.H.; Yu, E. The Natural History of Scaphoid Non-Union. *J. Bone Jt. Surg. Am.* **1984**, *66*, 504–509. [CrossRef]
13. Munk, B.; Larsen, C.F. Bone Grafting the Scaphoid Nonunion A Systematic Review of 147 Publications Including 5246 Cases of Scaphoid Nonunion. *Acta Orthop. Scand.* **2004**, *75*, 618–629. [CrossRef] [PubMed]
14. Sunagawa, T.; Bishop, A.T.; Muramatsu, K. Role of Conventional and Vascularized Bone Grafts in Scaphoid Nonunion with Avascular Necrosis: A Canine Experimental Study. *J. Hand Surg.* **2000**, *25*, 849–859. [CrossRef] [PubMed]
15. Elgammal, A.; Lukas, B. Vascularized Medial Femoral Condyle Graft for Management of Scaphoid Non-Union. *J. Hand Surg.* **2015**, *40*, 848–854. [CrossRef]
16. Jones, D.B.J.; Bürger, H.; Bishop, A.T.; Shin, A.Y. Treatment of Scaphoid Waist Nonunions with an Avascular Proximal Pole and Carpal Collapse: A Comparison of Two Vascularized Bone Grafts. *JBJS* **2008**, *90*, 2616. [CrossRef]
17. Ferguson, D.O.; Shanbhag, V.; Hedley, H.; Reichert, I.; Lipscombe, S.; Davis, T.R.C. Scaphoid Fracture Non-Union: A Systematic Review of Surgical Treatment Using Bone Graft. *J. Hand Surg.* **2016**, *41*, 492–500. [CrossRef]
18. Merrell, G.A.; Wolfe, S.W.; Slade, J.F., III. Treatment of Scaphoid Nonunions: Quantitative Meta-Analysis of the Literature. *J. Hand Surg.* **2002**, *27*, 685–691. [CrossRef]
19. Tu, Y.-K.; Bishop, A.T.; Kato, T.; Adams, M.L.; Wood, M.B. Experimental Carpal Reverse-Flow Pedicle Vascularized Bone Grafts. Part II: Bone Blood Flow Measurement by Radioactive-Labeled Microspheres in a Canine Model. *J. Hand Surg.* **2000**, *25*, 46–54. [CrossRef]
20. Page, M.J.; McKenzie, J.E.; Bossuyt, P.M.; Boutron, I.; Hoffmann, T.C.; Mulrow, C.D.; Shamseer, L.; Tetzlaff, J.M.; Akl, E.A.; Brennan, S.E.; et al. The PRISMA 2020 Statement: An Updated Guideline for Reporting Systematic Reviews. *BMJ* **2021**, *88*, 105906. [CrossRef]
21. Korompilias, A.V.; Lykissas, M.G.; Kostas-Agnantis, I.P.; Gkiatas, I.; Beris, A.E. An Alternative Graft Fixation Technique for Scaphoid Nonunions Treated With Vascular Bone Grafting. *J. Hand Surg.* **2014**, *39*, 1308–1312. [CrossRef] [PubMed]
22. Mouilhade, F.; Auquit-Auckbur, I.; Duparc, F.; Beccari, R.; Biga, N.; Milliez, P.-Y. Anatomical Comparative Study of Two Vascularized Bone Grafts for the Wrist. *Surg. Radiol. Anat.* **2007**, *29*, 15–20. [CrossRef] [PubMed]
23. Barrera-Ochoa, S.; Martin-Dominguez, L.-A.; Campillo-Recio, D.; Alabau-Rodriguez, S.; Mir-Bullo, X.; Soldado, F. Are Vascularized Periosteal Flaps Useful for the Treatment of Difficult Scaphoid Nonunion in Adults? A Prospective Cohort Study of 32 Patients. *J. Hand Surg.* **2020**, *45*, 924–936. [CrossRef] [PubMed]
24. Severo, A.L.; Lemos, M.B.; Lech, O.L.C.; Barreto Filho, D.; Strack, D.P.; Candido, L.K. Bone Graft in the Treatment of Nonunion of the Scaphoid with Necrosis of the Proximal Pole: A Literature Review. *Rev. Bras. Ortop.* **2017**, *52*, 638–643. [CrossRef]
25. Hovius, S.E.R.; de Jong, T. Bone Grafts for Scaphoid Nonunion: An Overview. *Hand Surg.* **2015**, *20*, 222–227. [CrossRef]
26. Capo, J.; Shamian, B.; Rivero, S. Chronic Scaphoid Nonunion of 28-Year Duration Treated with Non-vascularized Iliac Crest Bone Graft. *J. Wrist Surg.* **2013**, *2*, 79–82. [CrossRef]
27. Rahimnia, A.; Rahimnia, A.-H.; Mobasher-Jannat, A. Clinical and Functional Outcomes of Vascularized Bone Graft in the Treatment of Scaphoid Non-Union. *PLoS ONE* **2018**, *13*, e0197768. [CrossRef]
28. Tsumura, T.; Matsumoto, T.; Matsushita, M.; Doi, H.; Shiode, H.; Kakinoki, R. Correction of Humpback Deformities in Patients With Scaphoid Nonunion Using 1,2-Intercompartmental Supraretinacular Artery Pedicled Vascularized Bone Grafting With a Dorsoradial Approach. *J. Hand Surg.* **2020**, *45*, 160.e1–160.e8. [CrossRef]
29. Moon, E.S.; Dy, C.J.; Derman, P.; Vance, M.C.; Carlson, M.G. Management of Nonunion Following Surgical Management of Scaphoid Fractures: Current Concepts. *J. Am. Acad. Orthop. Surg.* **2013**, *21*, 548–557. [CrossRef]
30. Higgins, J.P.; Borumandi, F.; Bürger, H.K.; Benlidayi, M.E.; Vasilyeva, A.; Sencar, L.; Polat, S.; Gaggl, A.J. Non-vascularized Cartilage Grafts Versus Vascularized Cartilage Flaps: Comparison of Cartilage Quality 6 Months After Transfer. *J. Hand Surg.* **2018**, *43*, 188.e1–188.e8. [CrossRef]
31. Ross, P.R.; Lan, W.-C.; Chen, J.-S.; Kuo, C.-F.; Chung, K.C. Revision Surgery after Vascularized or Non-Vascularized Scaphoid Nonunion Repair: A National Population Study. *Injury* **2020**, *51*, 656–662. [CrossRef] [PubMed]
32. Chaudhry, T.; Uppal, L.; Power, D.; Craigen, M.; Tan, S. Scaphoid Nonunion with Poor Prognostic Factors: The Role of the Free Medial Femoral Condyle Vascularized Bone Graft. *Hand* **2017**, *12*, 135–139. [CrossRef] [PubMed]
33. Malizos, K.N.; Zachos, V.; Dailiana, Z.H.; Zalavras, C.; Varitimidis, S.; Hantes, M.; Karantanas, A. Scaphoid Nonunions: Management with Vascularized Bone Grafts from the Distal Radius: A Clinical and Functional Outcome Study. *Plast. Reconstr. Surg.* **2007**, *119*, 1513–1525. [CrossRef] [PubMed]
34. Tsantes, A.; Papadopoulos, D.; Gelalis, I.; Vekris, M.; Pakos, E.; Korompilias, A. The Efficacy of Vascularized Bone Grafts in the Treatment of Scaphoid Nonunions and Kienbock Disease: A Systematic Review in 917 Patients. *J. Hand Microsurg.* **2019**, *11*, 006–013. [CrossRef] [PubMed]
35. Sgromolo, N.M.; Rhee, P.C. The Role of Vascularized Bone Grafting in Scaphoid Nonunion. *Hand Clin.* **2019**, *35*, 315–322. [CrossRef] [PubMed]

36. Kawamura, K.; Chung, K.C. Treatment of Scaphoid Fractures and Nonunions. *J. Hand Surg.* **2008**, *33*, 988–997. [CrossRef] [PubMed]
37. Pinder, R.M.; Brkljac, M.; Rix, L.; Muir, L.; Brewster, M. Treatment of Scaphoid Nonunion: A Systematic Review of the Existing Evidence. *J. Hand Surg.* **2015**, *40*, 1797–1805.e3. [CrossRef]
38. Derby, B.M.; Murray, P.M.; Shin, A.Y.; Bueno, R.A.; Mathoulin, C.L.; Ade, T.; Neumeister, M.W. Vascularized Bone Grafts for the Treatment of Carpal Bone Pathology. *HAND* **2013**, *8*, 27–40. [CrossRef]
39. Pokorny, J.J.; Davids, H.; Moneim, M.S. Vascularized Bone Graft for Scaphoid Nonunion. *Tech. Hand Up. Extrem. Surg.* **2003**, *7*, 32–36. [CrossRef]
40. Elzinga, K.; Chung, K.C. Volar Radius Vascularized Bone Flaps for the Treatment of Scaphoid Nonunion. *Hand Clin.* **2019**, *35*, 353–363. [CrossRef]
41. Matsuki, H.; Uchiyama, S.; Kato, H.; Ishikawa, J.; Iwasaki, N.; Minami, A. Non-Vascularized Bone Graft with Herbert-Type Screw Fixation for Proximal Pole Scaphoid Nonunion. *J. Orthop. Sci.* **2011**, *16*, 749–755. [CrossRef] [PubMed]
42. Robbins, R.R.; Carter, P.R. Iliac Crest Bone Grafting and Herbert Screw Fixation of Nonunions of the Scaphoid with Avascular Proximal Poles. *J. Hand Surg.* **1995**, *20*, 818–831. [CrossRef]
43. Ribak, S.; Medina, C.E.G.; Mattar, R.; Ulson, H.J.R.; de Resende, M.R.; Etchebehere, M. Treatment of Scaphoid Nonunion with Vascularised and Nonvascularised Dorsal Bone Grafting from the Distal Radius. *Int. Orthop. (SICOT)* **2010**, *34*, 683–688. [CrossRef] [PubMed]
44. Kuhlmann, J.; Mimoun, M.; Boabighi, A.; Baux, S. Vascularized Bone Graft Pedicled on the Volar Carpal Artery for Non-Union of the Scaphoid. *J. Hand Surg.* **1987**, *12*, 203–210. [CrossRef]
45. Zaidemberg, C.; Siebert, J.W.; Angrigiani, C. A New Vascularized Bone Graft for Scaphoid Nonunion. *J. Hand Surg.* **1991**, *16*, 474–478. [CrossRef]

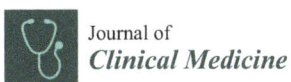

Article

Hip Fractures and Visual Impairment: Is There a Cause–Consequence Mechanism?

Gianluca Testa [1,*], Sara De Salvo [1], Silvia Boscaglia [2], Marco Montemagno [1], Antonio Longo [2], Andrea Russo [2], Giuseppe Sessa [1] and Vito Pavone [1]

[1] Department of General Surgery and Medical Surgical Specialties, Section of Orthopaedics and Traumatology, University Hospital Policlinico-San Marco, University of Catania, 95123 Catania, Italy; sarads94@hotmail.it (S.D.S.); docmontemagno@gmail.com (M.M.); giusessa@unict.it (G.S.); vitopavone@hotmail.com (V.P.)

[2] Department of General Surgery and Medical Surgical Specialties, Section of Ophthalmology, University Hospital Policlinico-San Marco, University of Catania, 95123 Catania, Italy; silviabosc@hotmail.it (S.B.); antlongo@unict.it (A.L.); andrea.russo@unict.it (A.R.)

* Correspondence: gianpavel@hotmail.com

Abstract: Background: Numerous studies have pointed out how visual impairment relates to falls in the elderly, causing dangerous consequences, such as fractures. The proximal femur fracture is one of the most frequent fracture types related to poor vision. This study investigates the link between fall-related hip fractures and visual impairment. Methods: The present is an observational monocentric case–control study. We collected the ophthalmologic anamnesis and measured the visual acuity of 88 subjects with femur neck fracture (case group), comparing it with 101 adults without fractures and a recent fall history. Results: The results showed no statistical difference between the two groups regarding visual acuity, with a p-value of 0.08 for the right eye and 0.13 for the left one. One of the major ophthalmologic morbidities found was cataracts, present in 48% of the control group and 30% of the case group. Conclusions: The data obtained suggest that visual impairment might not be crucial in determining falls in the elderly.

Keywords: aged; cataracts; elderly; falls; femur fractures; hip fractures; sight defects; vision; visual acuity; visual impairment

1. Introduction

As the population ages and becomes more fragile, the rate of falls having significant health consequences rises, creating a worldwide phenomenon. Fractures are one of these consequences, with femur neck fractures being dangerous for their association with fitness depletion and mental disorders [1,2]. When possible, surgical treatment is the preferred choice [3], with various techniques and implants used based on the fracture pattern and the patient's fitness. However, any surgery has risks, especially in the older population [4]. Particularly in well-developed countries, hip fractures are a significant cause of death and physical disability in the elderly, mainly in the postoperative period, representing a real health emergency. International and national guidelines suggest treating these patients as soon as possible, within 24–48 h, to avoid these serious consequences [5].

Why do old adults fall? Many researchers have attempted to answer this question by addressing different explanations. Among these, there is visual impairment: growing old means losing visual acuity [6]; therefore, it seems logical to expect higher chances of accidental falls. Moreover, osteoporosis, sarcopenia [7,8], arthrosis, dementia, and balance problems [9] make falls far more likely in those aged over 65 [1]. Numerous studies in the scientific literature show how visual impairment in elderly patients seems connected to a higher fall rate, often resulting in fractures, especially hip ones [10]. The present study aims to investigate the matter further. It adds different data compared to the previous literature, because it shows no significant correlation between visual impairment, falls, and femur neck fractures, widening the debate.

2. Materials and Methods

We conducted an observational monocentric study with a case–control design to compare patients' visual acuity affected by a femoral neck fracture and a cohort of randomly selected subjects.

From July 2020 to December 2021, we collected 88 patients with FNF, surgically treated at the orthopedic clinic of the University of Catania, enrolled after Ethical Committee approval. The patients admitted through the emergency department were grouped from medical records based on the following personal data: gender, age at the time of trauma, fall mechanism, fracture type. The patients selected for the study were those with femoral neck fractures classified as AO/OTA: 31A–31B, over 65 years old at the time of trauma, and referring only to accidental falls as the cause of the fractures. They were subjected to an ophthalmic examination comprehending the use of the optotype and a thorough ophthalmic anamnesis.

The control group was created by randomly contacting 101 adults aged over 65, offering them a free ophthalmologic exam. Only patients without a history of FNF and who had not experienced accidental falls in the past six months were selected. Once they reached the hospital, they were given the same exam as the case group, such as eye chart test and ophthalmic anamnesis.

We assessed 189 adults' visual acuity, for a total of 378 eyes. The results between the two groups were statistically analyzed with the t-Student test.

Moreover, we analyzed the odds ratio (OR) of the fracture population (case group), considering as cut-off 3/10 of visual acuity, as used to indicate visual impairment globally (Figure 1). According to the Italian law, in fact, mild visual impairment is attributed to those who have a visual acuity no greater than 3/10 in both eyes or in the best eye, even with the best correction, and those who have a peripheral binocular visual field residual lower than 60% [11].

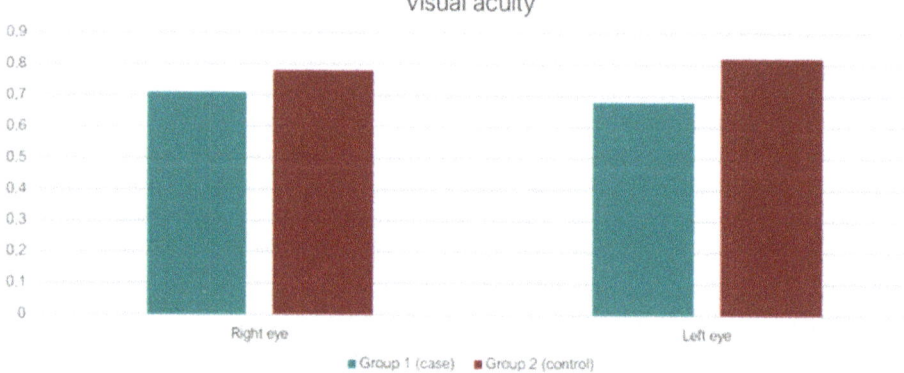

Figure 1. Visual acuity.

The case group's mean age was 84, ranging from 66 to 99. The control group's mean age was 76 (range 66–93). Despite the age gap, the visual acuity difference in these groups was not statistically significant, with a p-value of 0.09 for the right eye and 0.13 for the left one.

The odds ratio gave similar results, considering VO < 0.3 as a cut-off for the study. In fact, the OR = 0.54 with C.I. (95%) = 0.71 ± 0.05. Both measures showed no correlation between visual impairment (intended as VO < 0.3) and femur neck fractures.

One of the major ophthalmologic morbidities found was cataracts, present in 48% of the control group and 30% of the case group. Other ophthalmic conditions were glaucoma, maculopathies, and tumors. The presence of these diseases was not numerically predominant if compared to the statistical sample. The only condition that we found more frequent in the FNF group was glaucoma; the others were all more frequent in the control group. Maculopathies and cancer were found mainly in the control sample. The detailed data are displayed in Table 1.

Table 1. Study statistics.

	Case Group	Control Group	p-Value
Patients (n)	88 M/F = 0.51	101 M/F = 1.14	
Mean age	83.9 R: 66–99	76 R: 66–93	$p = 0.15$
Visual acuity mean right (std)	0.71 (±0.20)	0.78 (±0.82)	$p = 0.08$
Visual acuity mean left (std)	0.68 (±0.22)	0.82 (±0.80)	$p = 0.13$
Cataract (%)	27 30%	49 48%	

3. Discussion

Hip fractures are a major public health problem, especially in western countries. As one of the most frequent injuries in the elderly (over 65 years of age), their incidence is still rising worldwide: they are expected to reach over 6 million by 2050 [3].

This condition accounts for a high morbidity and mortality rate; throughout the years, different techniques have been developed for its treatment [12].

Conservative therapy is not advisable since it lowers the quality of life and the overall survival rate of the patients; therefore, surgery is the treatment of choice for most cases, allowing early rehabilitation and functional recovery [13]. Over time, different systems have been developed, and surgeons choose based on the fracture pattern and patients' fitness. From intramedullary nailing to hip arthroplasty, research nowadays focuses on improving mechanics and materials for the best outcomes in terms of quality and duration [14]. Hip surgery is still a high-risk surgery, especially for the elderly patients who undergo these types of procedures.

Amongst the most frequent causes of hip fracture, it is essential to cite visual impairment, osteoporosis, sarcopenia, dementia, and all other factors that make elderly subjects particularly fragile. Sight defects belong to this panorama, often neglected by patients that do not have easy access to prevention and healing facilities. Several works in the literature have tried to measure this association, with the first ones being conducted in the 1970s [15]. The majority showed some correlation, but, of course, every study has its limits and biases [16].

In fact, previous studies have used different methods to evaluate visual impairment, trying to obtain accurate data. Some used questionnaires to assess visual acuity, giving a picture of patients' perceptions rather than objective testing [17]; others studied large health insurance databases [2] to provide the highest number of cases possible. We could not find a study in the past literature on falls and sight defects that does not evidence a correlation between the two.

The data displayed for the present study were not expected. Moreover, given the different mean ages between the groups, we expected to find better visual acuity in the control group. Ageing is a risk factor for worse visual acuity [18]. When analyzing subjects' anamnesis, we found a higher rate of cataracts in the control group, where the subjects' mean age was 76 years. The case group instead had a mean age of almost 84 years. This study's results stimulate further reflections and research due to the absence of a significant difference in the groups studied. The cause–effect correlation between sight problems and falls is unclear; falls resulting in hip fractures might not be directly correlated to sight problems. It is vital to investigate how the event happened; every fall described as accidental has its peculiarities that only a scrupulous anamnesis of the patient can capture. The location in which it happened, the trigger situation, the patient's response, and their reflexes and coordination are elements that do not depend on eyesight only. Other factors probably influence these episodes more, as some studies have shown [19], such as balance disorders, gait problems, pharmaceutical use, and a history of falls. The most cited risk factor for falls is fall history [20], which indicates that patients are prone to falling, but the root of the problem remains unknown and is probably multifactorial. Regarding elderly patients, it is important to take into account the use of many different pharmaceuticals [21], often related to falls, since some active substances can alter normal reflexes and coordination. The presence of gait disorders [22] before the event, often underdiagnosed and undertreated, is another cause. Finally, fractures after these incidents happen in frail patients, and osteoporosis [23] is one of the main comorbidities associated with increasing the likelihood of fractures as a consequence of a fall.

Prevention is vital, but defining the causes of falls is essential, especially in senior patients. Since eyesight is not so reliable, other factors should be considered first. Patients with fall history should receive physicians' attention, and, after determining the main risk factors, they should be guided towards prevention strategies. Coordination and balance disorders are frequently linked to falls; recent studies have suggested that preventive physiotherapy [24] might be vital in preventing falls. Preventive strategies should also include the fall's consequences: a proper osteoporosis diagnosis and treatment can be very helpful in avoiding fractures [25].

The present study has several limitations. The collection of the control group might have been biased: subjects contacted for the ophthalmic examination might have been interested in participating due to the presence of sight defects, which they were suddenly given the opportunity to receive treatment for. Another limitation is the sample size, comparable to similar studies in Europe [26], being a monocentric study with 12 months of data collection.

Moreover, the case group could have been larger. In fact, we included a specific type of femur fracture, without considering other patients affected by different types of femur neck fractures with similar accidental traumatic events.

4. Conclusions

Amidst the risk factors correlated to accidental falls in the elderly, visual impairment has been considered one of the most important in the current literature. In contrast with this vision, the data displayed in this article underline how there are no statistically significant differences in visual acuity between fractured and non-fractured patients. Therefore, the present study questions past knowledge, underlining how sight defects might not play a critical role in this condition. For this reason, further studies are needed to investigate this matter.

Author Contributions: Conceptualization, S.D.S.; methodology, M.M.; software, S.B.; validation, G.T.; formal analysis, M.M.; investigation, A.R.; resources, S.D.S.; data curation, M.M.; writing—original draft preparation, S.D.S.; writing—review and editing, G.T.; visualization, A.L.; supervision, G.S.; project administration, V.P.; funding acquisition, V.P. All authors have read and agreed to the published version of the manuscript.

Funding: This research received no external funding.

Institutional Review Board Statement: The study was conducted according to the guidelines of the Declaration of Helsinki and approved by the Ethics Committee of University of Catania of AOUP "G. Rodolico—San Marco" (160/2020/PO).

Informed Consent Statement: Informed consent was obtained from all subjects involved in the study. Written informed consent has been obtained from the patient(s) to publish this paper.

Data Availability Statement: Study data are available from the corresponding author.

Acknowledgments: Thanks to Pia.Ce.Ri. of the University of Catania for supporting the manuscript and the research project.

Conflicts of Interest: The authors declare no conflict of interest.

References

1. Berry, S.D.; Miller, R.R. Falls: Epidemiology, Pathophysiology, and Relationship to Fracture. *Curr. Osteoporos. Rep.* **2008**, *6*, 149–154. [CrossRef] [PubMed]
2. Hamedani, A.G.; VanderBeek, B.L.; Willis, A.W. Blindness and Visual Impairment in the Medicare Population: Disparities and Association with Hip Fracture and Neuropsychiatric Outcomes. *Ophthalmic Epidemiol.* **2019**, *26*, 279–285. [CrossRef] [PubMed]
3. Kannus, P.; Parkkari, J.; Sievänen, H.; Heinonen, A.; Vuori, I.; Järvinen, M. Epidemiology of hip fractures. *Bone* **1996**, *18*, S57–S63. [CrossRef]
4. Chen, C.-L.; Chen, C.-M.; Wang, C.-Y.; Ko, P.-W.; Chen, C.-H.; Hsieh, C.-P.; Chiu, H.-C. Frailty is Associated with an Increased Risk of Major Adverse Outcomes in Elderly Patients Following Surgical Treatment of Hip Fracture. *Sci. Rep.* **2019**, *9*, 1–9. [CrossRef]
5. Saul, D.; Riekenberg, J.; Ammon, J.C.; Hoffmann, D.B.; Sehmisch, S. Hip Fractures: Therapy, Timing, and Complication Spectrum. *Orthop. Surg.* **2019**, *11*, 994–1002. [CrossRef]
6. GBD 2019 Blindness; Vision Impairment Collaborators; the Vision Loss Expert Group of the Global Burden of Disease Study. Causes of blindness and vision impairment in 2020 and trends over 30 years, and prevalence of avoidable blindness in relation to VISION 2020: The Right to Sight: An analysis for the Global Burden of Disease Study. *Lancet Glob. Health* **2021**, *9*, e144–e160, Erratum in **2021**, *9*, e408. [CrossRef]
7. Avola, M.; Mangano, G.R.A.; Testa, G.; Mangano, S.; Vescio, A.; Pavone, V.; Vecchio, M. Rehabilitation Strategies for Patients with Femoral Neck Fractures in Sarcopenia: A Narrative Review. *J. Clin. Med.* **2020**, *9*, 3115. [CrossRef]
8. Testa, G.; Vescio, A.; Zuccalà, D.; Petrantoni, V.; Amico, M.; Russo, G.I.; Sessa, G.; Pavone, V. Diagnosis, Treatment and Prevention of Sarcopenia in Hip Fractured Patients: Where We Are and Where We Are Going: A Systematic Review. *J. Clin. Med.* **2020**, *9*, 2997. [CrossRef]
9. Cuevas-Trisan, R. Balance Problems and Fall Risks in the Elderly. *Clin. Geriatr. Med.* **2019**, *35*, 173–183. [CrossRef]
10. Choi, H.; Lee, J.; Lee, M.; Park, B.; Sim, S.; Lee, S.-M. Blindness increases the risk for hip fracture and vertebral fracture but not the risk for distal radius fracture: A longitudinal follow-up study using a national sample cohort. *Osteoporos. Int.* **2020**, *31*, 2345–2354. [CrossRef]
11. The Italian Law of 3 April 2001, no. 138. Available online: https://www.gazzettaufficiale.it/eli/id/2001/04/21/001G0193/sg (accessed on 10 June 2022).
12. Johnell, O.; Kanis, J.A. An estimate of the worldwide prevalence, mortality and disability associated with hip fracture. *Osteoporos. Int.* **2004**, *15*, 897–902. [CrossRef] [PubMed]
13. Bhandari, M.; Swiontkowski, M. Management of Acute Hip Fracture. *N. Engl. J. Med.* **2017**, *377*, 2053–2062. [CrossRef] [PubMed]
14. Jamari, J.; Ammarullah, M.I.; Santoso, G.; Sugiharto, S.; Supriyono, T.; Prakoso, A.T.; Basri, H.; van der Heide, E. Computational Contact Pressure Prediction of CoCrMo, SS 316L and Ti6Al4V Femoral Head against UHMWPE Acetabular Cup under Gait Cycle. *J. Funct. Biomater.* **2022**, *13*, 64. [CrossRef] [PubMed]
15. Brocklehurst, J.C.; Exton-Smith, A.N.; Barber, S.M.L.; Hunt, L.P.; Palmer, M.K. Fracture of the Femur in Old Age: A Two-Centre Study of Associated Clinical Factors and the Cause of the Fall. *Age Ageing* **1978**, *7*, 7–15. [CrossRef]
16. Cox, A.; Blaikie, A.; MacEwen, C.J.; Jones, D.; Thompson, K.; Holding, D.; Sharma, T.; Miller, S.; Dobson, S.; Sanders, R. Visual impairment in elderly patients with hip fracture: Causes and associations. *Eye* **2005**, *19*, 652–656. [CrossRef] [PubMed]
17. Ivers, R.Q.; Norton, R.; Cumming, R.; Butler, M.; Campbell, A.J. Visual Impairment and Hip Fracture. *Am. J. Epidemiol.* **2000**, *152*, 633–639. [CrossRef]
18. Katoh, N.; Sasaki, K.; Fujisawa, K.; Sakamoto, Y.; Kojima, M.; Hatano, T. Visual acuity disturbance in subjects over 50 years of age in a population-based cataract survey. *Ophthalmic Epidemiol.* **1996**, *3*, 109–116. [CrossRef]
19. Ambrose, A.F.; Paul, G.; Hausdorff, J.M. Risk factors for falls among older adults: A review of the literature. *Maturitas* **2013**, *75*, 51–61. [CrossRef]
20. Patel, D.; Ackermann, R.J. Issues in Geriatric Care: Falls. *FP Essent.* **2018**, *468*, 18–25.
21. Zia, A.; Kamaruzzaman, S.B.; Tan, M.P. Polypharmacy and falls in older people: Balancing evidence-based medicine against falls risk. *Postgrad. Med.* **2015**, *127*, 330–337. [CrossRef]
22. Ronthal, M. Gait Disorders and Falls in the Elderly. *Med. Clin. N. Am.* **2019**, *103*, 203–213. [CrossRef] [PubMed]
23. Curtis, E.; Moon, R.J.; Harvey, N.; Cooper, C. The impact of fragility fracture and approaches to osteoporosis risk assessment worldwide. *Bone* **2017**, *104*, 29–38. [CrossRef] [PubMed]
24. Sherrington, C.; Tiedemann, A. Physiotherapy in the prevention of falls in older people. *J. Physiother.* **2015**, *61*, 54–60. [CrossRef]
25. Johnston, C.B.; Dagar, M. Osteoporosis in Older Adults. *Med. Clin. N. Am.* **2020**, *104*, 873–884. [CrossRef]
26. Loriaut, P.; Loriaut, P.; Boyer, P.; Massin, P.; Cochereau, I. Visual Impairment and Hip Fractures: A Case-Control Study in Elderly Patients. *Ophthalmic Res.* **2014**, *52*, 212–216. [CrossRef] [PubMed]

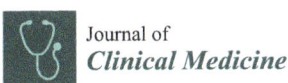

Review

Forearm Fracture Nonunion with and without Bone Loss: An Overview of Adult and Child Populations

Sara Dimartino, Vito Pavone, Michela Carnazza, Enrica Rosalia Cuffaro, Francesco Sergi and Gianluca Testa *

Department of General Surgery and Medical Surgical Specialties, Section of Orthopaedics and Traumatology, University Hospital Policlinico "Rodolico-San Marco", University of Catania, 95123 Catania, Italy; saradimartino1@gmail.com (S.D.); vitopavone@hotmail.com (V.P.); michela.carnazza@libero.it (M.C.); enricacuffaro@outlook.it (E.R.C.); fsrgbl33@gmail.com (F.S.)
* Correspondence: gianpavel@hotmail.com

Abstract: Nonunion occurs in 2–10% of all forearm fractures due to different mechanical and biological factors, patient characteristics, and surgeon-dependent causes. It is a condition that causes functional and psychosocial disability for the patient because it is a unique anatomical segment in which all the bones and structures involved embody a complex functional unit; therefore, it is a challenge for the orthopedic surgeon. The ultimate goal of the care of these patients is the restoration of function and limitations related to impairment and disability. The aim of this review is to provide an extended description of nonunion forearm fractures, related risk factors, diagnosis, classification systems, and the available evidence for different types of treatment as a tool to better manage this pathology.

Keywords: forearm; nonunion; epidemiology; risk factor; children; treatment; external fixation; bone graft

1. Introduction

Forearm nonunion represents a challenge for orthopedic surgeons both in terms of diagnosis and treatment, sometimes requiring reconstruction skills and good patient compliance because of the difficult treatment and long follow-up. The Food and Drug Administration (FDA) describes nonunion as a fractured bone that has not healed within nine months after trauma and shows no signs of progression of healing on radiographs over the course of three consecutive months [1]. In addition to this definition, nonunion has no chance of healing without additional operation. In the pediatric population, it is defined as an absence of fracture healing progression as shown on sequential radiographs or no evidence of healing by more than 10 weeks following the injury. Nonunion occurs in 2–10% of all forearm fractures, with or without infection and bone loss. A peak incidence has been observed in the age range between the ages of 35 and 44 and decreases thereafter [2], with a higher incidence in women after menopause. The most common fracture in the pediatric population is a forearm fracture [3], but nonunion is an uncommon complication after surgical treatment of displaced bones and has been described in only a few cases in the literature. Forearm nonunion is a condition that causes functional and psychosocial disability for the patient, resulting in the lowest health-related quality of life compared with other long bone nonunion and disease such as type 1 diabetes mellitus, stroke, and acquired immunodeficiency syndrome [4]. Forearm nonunion consists of different mechanical and biological factors: the type of fracture, patient characteristics, and surgeon-dependent causes. The evaluation of a suspected forearm nonunion includes medical history, laboratory tests, and clinical and instrumental factors. Successful treatment is the restoration of function and limitations related to impairment and disability. The aim of this review is to provide a correct forearm nonunion characterization with related risk factors, diagnosis, classification systems, and management with available evidence for different types of treatment.

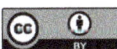

2. Evaluation

2.1. Risk Factors

Forearm nonunion is due to failure of bone healing and is caused by many factors. In clinical practice, these factors are divided into mechanical and biological ones [5,6], as shown in Table 1, and in the literature, they are divided into general and local risk factors [7,8], as shown in Table 2.

Table 1. Mechanical and biological factors.

Mechanical Factors [5,6]
- Insufficient immobilization - Nonoperative treatment - Poor internal or external fixation
- Excessive motion at the fracture site - Malreduction or an unbalanced osteosynthesis system
Biological Factors [5,6]
- Local: bone defects, open fracture, infection, soft tissue injuries, segmental fractures, pathological and comminuted fractures, and inter-fragmentary gap - Systemic: neuropathy, diabetes, chronic smoking, chronic alcoholism, drugs, and radiation therapy

Table 2. General and local risk factors.

GENERAL RISK FACTORS
- Gender [8] - Age [6] - Poor protein diet [6] - Calcium and phosphorus deficit [8] - Lack of vitamin D [7] - Osteoporosis [8] - Diabetes [7] - Low muscular mass - Alcohol [8] - Smoking [6] - Drugs (NSAIDS, opioid) [6] - Infection [7,8] - Radiation therapy [6] - Neuropathies - Genetic disorders (osteogenesis imperfecta)
LOCAL RISK FACTORS
- Fracture type [7,8] - Mechanism of injury [7,8] - Exposure [6,7] - Biological damage during the first surgery [6,8] - Surgical techniques during fracture synthesis [7,8]

2.2. History and Physical Examination

The assessment of a suspected forearm nonunion should start with the remote pathological history of the patient, together with investigation of the preliminary elements to guide the diagnostic path: the presence of risk factors, mechanism of trauma, details of prior surgical procedures, distress with weight bearing, and factors of infection. The physical examination should detect differences with the contralateral side in terms of the presence of shortening, range of movement, and lower grip strength; and assess the skin covering the nonunion and its mobility. Tenderness on palpation and preternatural mobility at the fracture site may result. The latter could represent a clinical sign of incomplete bone healing that could be associated with pain, poor functionality, and mechanical instability. The clinical examination should also assess the presence of any deformity, soft tissue, limb vascularity, and arm muscle circumference as an indicator of nutritional status. It is important to diagnose aseptic versus septic nonunion [9] because if sepsis is present, the management varies significantly.

2.3. Imaging

The diagnostic evaluation continues with radiographic aspects through the anteroposterior, lateral, and oblique views of the injured bone and adjacent joints in addition to the same view of the original fracture. Radiological signs include variable bone callus presentation, fracture stumps sclerosis with persistence of a fracture line, and the presence of a defect or a deformity. Radiography of the contralateral side may be useful as it may outline shortening and concurrent malunions or normal characteristics for the patient. In addition, computed tomography (CT) scans are frequently used in current practice (Figure 1) to identify unhealed fractures, which is useful for anticipating negative evolution of the reparative process.

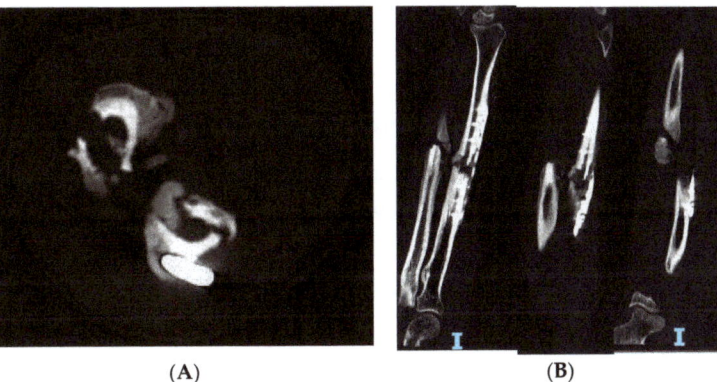

Figure 1. Forearm nonunion CT scans of a 43-year-old patient. (**A**) Coronal view, (**B**) Sagittal view.

Contrast-enhanced ultrasound (CEUS), also with the adjunct of Doppler, is helpful for investigating the presence of vessels from the perspective of vascularized flaps. Enhanced magnetic resonance with dynamic contrast (DCE-MRI) has been proposed to analyze the infection status and perfusion of a nonunion [10].

2.4. Laboratory Analysis

Additional diagnostic insights include an evaluation of inflammation markers (white blood cells, erythrocyte sedimentation rate, and C-reactive protein (CRP)); biochemical elements, such as liver function, thyroid and parathyroid, calcium, and vitamin D; in addition to multiple samples for culture examination before any antibiotic prophylaxis. Brinker et al. [11] found that the most common abnormality was vitamin D deficiency. Criteria indicative of an infection are a white blood cell count greater than $11,000 \times 10^9$, an erythrocyte sedimentation rate >30 mm/h, and a CRP level >1.0 mg/dL; three positive tests have a predictive infection value of 100% [12] These tests are useful for an initial distinction between septic and aseptic nonunion.

2.5. Characterization

The most utilized nonunion classification system was proposed by Weber and Cech, describing atrophic, oligotrophic, and hypertrophic based on callus formation as shown on the radiograph. Hypertrophic nonunion, usually resulting from insufficient fracture stabilization and showing adequate vascularization, is marked by extensive callus formation with a horse-shoe or elephant-foot radiographic configuration (Figure 2).

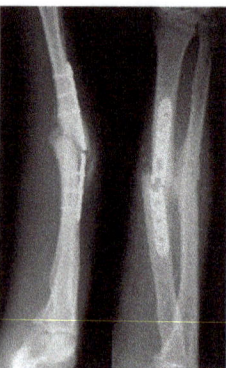

Figure 2. A 38-year-old patient presented a hypertrophic symptomatic nonunion with a broken plate after 9 months.

Atrophic nonunion, resulting from dysfunction in biological activity with insufficient vascularization but adequate fracture stabilization, typically radiologically shows minimal callus around a fibrous tissue-filled fracture gap. Oligotrophic nonunion shows some of the radiographic and biologic features of each type and typically presents biologic potential for healing with no initiation of healing and minimal to no callus formation. The AO (Arbeitsgemeinschaft für Osteosynthesefragen) classification scheme adds the concept of pseudoarthrosis in cases in which the formation of a false joint due to the persistence of movement at the site of fracture occurs [8]. Unfortunately, there is no specific classification for forearm nonunion and regarding future directions, it would be useful to create a dedicated one that is based on the following: the score obtained from the Weber and Cech, the sites of nonunion (distal, diaphysis, or proximal), whether it affects one or both bones, pediatric or adult, state of infection, with vascular deficiency, and with or without bone loss.

3. Pediatric Treatment

Forearm fractures are usual in children: 34% of cases occur in children at ages ranging from 5 to 14 years [13]. Nonunion is prevalent in children older than 10 years as compared to children under 10 years due to lesser bone remodeling potential in older children. In particular, it depends on open reduction and wide bone exposure, poor fixation, an inadequate period of immobilization (<8 weeks), and early hardware removal (<3 months). Generally, in children, the ulna is more involved than the radius [14]. Trauma in the middle third of the ulna, also called the "water-shed zone", is critical because the intraosseous circulation may be compromised, which may invalidate bone healing [15,16]. The distal third of the radius is involved due to damage of the pronator quadratus vascularization. In children's forearm fracture nonunion, it is important to evaluate the type of treatment that has been carried out previously. Ogonda et al. [17] analyzed elastic stable intramedullary nailing (ESIN) fixation in both-bone forearm fractures and showed that the frequency of ulna nonunion was higher in anterograde nailing than in retrograde, and radius nonunion was less frequent due to compression of the fracture line. However, Yaradilmis et al. [18] demonstrated that intramedullary nailing is minimally invasive and provides biological fixation. In addition, plate-screw nonunion fixation depends on wide soft tissue dissection and stripping of the bone periosteum to provide adequate exposure [19]. Metabolic disorders should be corrected to stimulate bone healing; if a lack of vitamin D is present, supplementation should be provided to promote better consolidation. Loose et al. [20] showed that a conservative approach could be adopted in asymptomatic patients; however, if a young patient is considered symptomatic when they present with an angular deformity, functional deficit or movement restriction, and pain, it is important to assess surgery. The best operative management consists of osteosynthesis with or without bone grafting (Figure 3).

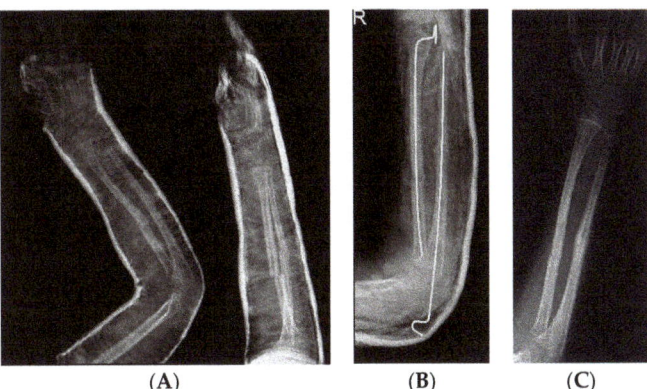

Figure 3. (**A**): Five-year-old patient treated with nonoperative treatment; after 4 months, they presented a displaced oligotrophic nonunion with pain and range of motion (ROM) deficit. (**B**): He was treated by cruentation of the fracture's sites, reduction, stabilization with k wires, and cast. (**C**): Post k-wires removal.

First, fibrous tissue is removed followed by decortication and opening of the medullary canal. In a septic nonunion, it is important to analyze bioptic samples. Second, bone grafting with an allograft or autograft has been performed. Stabilization of a nonunion is achieved with tubular plates, dynamic compression plates or locking compression plates (DCPs or LCPs), Kirschner wires, rush rods, or an external fixator. After surgery, cast immobilization is required. An algorithm from the authors is illustrated in Figure 4.

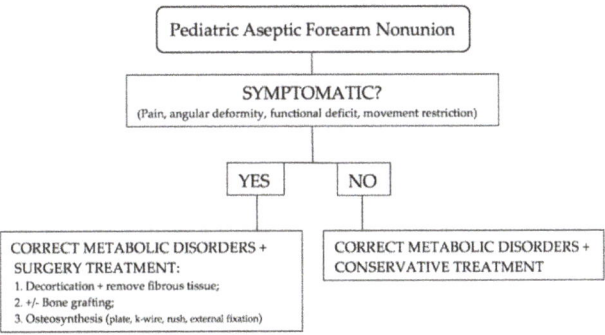

Figure 4. Treatment algorithm for pediatric aseptic forearm nonunion.

Surgical treatment of pediatric forearm nonunion provides satisfactory outcomes but is associated with sequelae and residual functional disability with several complications, such as radio-ulnar fusion, radial nerve palsy, myositis ossificans at the ulna, and olecranon bursitis with elbow stiffness.

4. Adult Forearm Nonunion Surgical Treatment

The goal of surgical management of forearm nonunion is to recover the proper bone length, anatomy, and functionality, and remove pain. Achieving a successful outcome in the management of forearm nonunion treatment requires optimization of both the patient's biological state and the stability of the nonunion site. Conservative treatment is only for special patients who are not suitable candidates for surgical treatments. The gold standard for managing septic forearm nonunion is a staged approach [21] to control infection via the use of a debridement, antibiotic spacer, and cultures followed by definitive surgery while for the aseptic situation, a single-stage treatment is used [22]. Management of nonunion forearm fracture in adults includes different types of surgical treatment such as bone grafting with compression with plates, the Masquelet technique, and external fixation. Compression plating and autologous bone grafting have mainly been regarded as the keystone of nonunion treatment. Both mechanical and biologic failure are corrected by restoring stability (by compression plating) and introducing osteoinductive and/or osteoconductive agents (by autologous bone graft). In oligotrophic or atrophic nonunion, bone grafting is necessary to fill the gap between the two ends. Ring et al. [23] obtained a 100% union rate with an autogenous iliac crest bone graft and 3.5 mm plate and screw for a forearm nonunion.

4.1. Bone Grafting

Different kinds of bone grafts exist, but autologous cancellous bone is still being considered as the gold standard to provide a biological stimulus for the consolidation process. A bone graft can be cancellous, corticocancellous, and/or vascularized. Cancellous grafts can derive from the iliac crest, distal radius, olecranon, lateral epicondyle, tibial metaphysis, or reamer/irrigator/aspirator (RIA) of the femur. A corticocancellous graft includes the tricortical iliac crest, free fibula, and medial femoral condyle. The size of the gap may be influenced by the choice of being vascularized or not. A vascularized bone graft is used for gaps greater than 5 to 6 cm; in particular, the free fibula is a great option as shown for forearm nonunion by Adani et al. [24]. An autologous graft has the advantage of being osteogenic, osteoinductive, and osteoconductive; it is biologically superior to homologous grafts. However, the disadvantages include donor site morbidity, pain, and limited supplies. For forearm nonunion, the best utilized autograft options include the iliac crest bone graft (ICBG) as shown by Regan et al. [25] and RIA of the femur. With the RIA technique, a graft of greater volume than ICBG is obtained as shown by Dawson et al. [26] and RIA is superior in improving the cost-benefit when surgical time is considered and lowering donor-site pain. On the other hand, significant blood loss may occur. Compared with an autograft, an allograft prevents donor-site morbidity and may reduce the surgical time. Allografts can contribute to bone reconstruction thanks to their osteoinductive and osteoconductive properties but require a vital environment to be effective. Moreover, the use of structural allografts can be complicated by infection, incomplete remodeling, fracture, and disease transmission. Vascularized bone grafts can be obtained from the fibula, iliac crest, rib, radius, ulna, scapula, femur, humerus, and pubic bone or metatarsals, among other sites. At present, the most frequently applied technique for bone defects > 5–6 cm in the septic non-union of one or both forearm bones is the free vascularized fibular graft (FVFG). Because of its anatomical and mechanical characteristics, it is an excellent graft for the reconstruction of forearm bone defects. The fibula has a diameter similar to that of the forearm bones, the morbidity of the donor zone is minimal, and the length available for extraction is usually sufficient [27]. One of the main advantages of FVFG is that in a single surgical intervention, it enables reconstruction of one or both forearm bones in addition to coverage of any soft tissue defects in patients with complex trauma or in infected areas with poor vascularization [28]. Vascularized bone grafts have an improved rate of survival in a poorly vascularized bed. Gan et al. [29] demonstrated for bone defects in pseudarthroses of the forearm that a vascularized fibular graft is an optimal option with fracture healing. Among its advantages, vascularized bone grafting facilitates the provision of nutrients to the deep structures of the graft and enables stable osteosynthesis, thus allowing prompt mobilization of the limb and promoting functional recovery [30]. A potential disadvantage is that the operation requires microvascular surgical skills.

4.2. Induced Membrane Technique

The induced membrane technique, also known as the Masquelet technique [31], is applicable under both aseptic and septic conditions leading to substantial bone loss and requires no advanced skills in microvascular surgery. The technique involves a two-stage procedure to restore the bone defect. Ma et al. [32] studied the induced membrane technique for infected forearm nonunion in 32 patients who haled without recurrent infection or loosening of internal fixation, finding it to be an effective solution. Walker et al. [33] demonstrated successful use of this method in forearm nonunion for defects up to 5.4 cm in size. Pachera et al. [34] reported a case of a 53-year-old patient with a left forearm deformity due to an atrophic nonunion of the ulna and a malunion of the radius, which was successfully managed with the use of the Masquelet technique associated with a corrective osteotomy of the radius, performed with the aid of a 3D model. Potential problems with the Masquelet technique include loosening of the fixation implant, infection, fracture through the graft, and bone resorption.

4.3. Ilizarov with Bone Transport

Ilizarov fixation with bone transport is a viable treatment option for atrophic forearm nonunion and is particularly indicated in cases of significant soft tissue damage or nonunion with infection. The Ilizarov methodology allows bridging of bone losses (caused by osteogenesis) with bone transport and provides stable fixation without implantation of permanent foreign bodies, thus permitting wrist and elbow movement. This technique, therefore, allows for immediate therapy of the hand, wrist, and elbow in addition to early use of the extremities during the activities of daily living. Moreover, circular systems can be used to correct complex multiplanar deformities in small areas of soft tissue defects and immediate mobilization. Its disadvantages are the long duration of external osteosynthesis materials, the frequency of pin-tract infections, and the pain accompanying the transport. Zhu et al. [35] studied the effectiveness of the Ilizarov technology for the treatment of infected forearm nonunion with satisfactory clinical results, finding radical debridement is the key to controlling bone infection. Orzechowski et al. [36] demonstrated that the Ilizarov is the method of choice in the treatment of forearm nonunion with concomitant shortening and axis deformity. Liu et al. [37] treated 12 patients with diaphyseal forearm bone defects caused by infection with bone transport using a monolateral external fixator and all patients achieved infection-free union.

5. Conclusions

Forearm nonunion is an uncommon but complex condition problem, with countless different presentations. In a future prospective, it would be useful to create a specific classification system to guide the right management. The question: "Why did the fracture not heal?" should be addressed by the surgeon to investigate risk factors, correct the metabolic abnormalities, and study the nonunion imaging characteristics to optimize the patient's biology and stability at the affected site. What kind of graft should be used? This depends on the presence of infection, patient characteristics, and the size of the defect: a cancellous graft should be used when there is cortical contact while vascularized free fibula should be preferred for defects larger than 5–6 cm. Different surgery treatments have been used successfully and future studies should investigate the role of 3D printing in the pre-operatory planning, its intraoperatory advantages, and its role in bone grafting selection. This paper presents some limitations related to its narrative nature. In fact, a quality evaluation of the literature was carried out; therefore, a statistical comparison between the references was not possible. For this reason, it appears to be difficult to confront different studies having also a low grade of evidence. Therefore, we strongly support the need to design new studies in this direction.

Author Contributions: Conceptualization, S.D.; methodology, E.R.C.; software, F.S.; validation, G.T.; formal analysis, M.C.; investigation, F.S.; resources, M.C.; data curation, S.D.; writing—original draft preparation, S.D.; writing—review and editing, G.T.; visualization, G.T.; supervision, V.P.; project administration, G.T.; funding acquisition, V.P. All authors have read and agreed to the published version of the manuscript.

Funding: This research received no external funding.

Institutional Review Board Statement: Not applicable.

Informed Consent Statement: Not applicable.

Data Availability Statement: Not applicable.

Conflicts of Interest: The authors declare no conflict of interest.

Abbreviations

Food and Drug Administration (FDA), Nonsteroidal anti-inflammatory drugs (NSAIDs), computed tomography (CT), Enhanced ultrasound with-trast (CEUS), enhanced magnetic resonance with dynamic contrast (DCE-MRI), C-reactive protein (CRP), Arbeitsgemeinschaft für Osteosynthesefragen (AO), elastic stable intramedullary nailing (ESIN), Kirschner wires (k-wires), dynamic compression plates or locking compression plate (DCP or LCP), range of motion (ROM), reamer/irrigator/aspirator (RIA), iliac crest bone graft (ICBG), free vascularized fibular graft (FVFG).

References

1. Bishop, J.A.; Palanca, A.A.; Bellino, M.J.; Lowenberg, D.W. Assessment of Compromised Fracture Healing. *J. Am. Acad. Orthop. Surg.* **2012**, *20*, 273–282. [CrossRef] [PubMed]
2. Zura, R.; Braid-Forbes, M.J.; Jeray, K.; Mehta, S.; Einhorn, T.A.; Watson, J.T.; Della Rocca, G.J.; Forbes, K.; Steen, R.G. Bone Fracture Nonunion Rate Decreases with Increasing Age: A Prospective Inception Cohort Study. *Bone* **2017**, *95*, 26–32. [CrossRef] [PubMed]
3. Caruso, G.; Caldari, E.; Sturla, F.D.; Caldaria, A.; Re, D.L.; Pagetti, P.; Palummieri, F.; Massari, L. Management of Pediatric Forearm Fractures: What Is the Best Therapeutic Choice? A Narrative Review of the Literature. *Musculoskelet. Surg.* **2021**, *105*, 225–234. [CrossRef]
4. Schottel, P.C.; O'Connor, D.P.; Brinker, M.R. Time Trade-Off as a Measure of Health-Related Quality of Life: Long Bone Nonunions Have a Devastating Impact. *J. Bone Jt. Surg. Am. Vol.* **2015**, *97*, 1406–1410. [CrossRef]
5. Rodriguez-Merchan, E.C.; Forriol, F. Nonunion: General Principles and Experimental Data. *Clin. Orthop.* **2004**, *419*, 4–12. [CrossRef]
6. Panagiotis, M. Classification of Non-Union. *Injury* **2005**, *36*, S30–S37. [CrossRef]
7. Rodriguez-Buitrago, A.F.; Mabrouk, A.; Jahangir, A. Tibia nonunion. In *StatPearls*; StatPearls Publishing: Treasure Island, FL, USA, 2022.
8. Buckley, R.E.; Moran, C.G.; Apivatthakakul, T. (Eds.) *AO Principles of Fracture Management. Volume 2: Specific Fractures*, 3rd ed.; Thieme: Stuttgart, Germany, 2017; ISBN 978-3-13-242309-1.
9. Zimmerli, W. Clinical Presentation and Treatment of Orthopaedic Implant-Associated Infection. *J. Intern. Med.* **2014**, *276*, 111–119. [CrossRef]
10. Fischer, C. Diagnostik und Klassifikation von Pseudarthrosen. *Unfallchirurg* **2020**, *123*, 671–678. [CrossRef]
11. Brinker, M.R.; O'Connor, D.P.; Monla, Y.T.; Earthman, T.P. Metabolic and Endocrine Abnormalities in Patients With Nonunions. *J. Orthop. Trauma* **2007**, *21*, 557–570. [CrossRef]
12. Stucken, C.; Olszewski, D.C.; Creevy, W.R.; Murakami, A.M.; Tornetta, P. Preoperative Diagnosis of Infection in Patients with Nonunions. *J. Bone Jt. Surg.-Am. Vol.* **2013**, *95*, 1409–1412. [CrossRef]
13. Rafi, B.M.; Tiwari, V. Forearm Fractures. In *StatPearls*; StatPearls Publishing: Treasure Island, FL, USA, 2022.
14. Fernandez, F.F.; Eberhardt, O.; Langendörfer, M.; Wirth, T. Nonunion of Forearm Shaft Fractures in Children after Intramedullary Nailing. *J. Pediatr. Orthop. B* **2009**, *18*, 289–295. [CrossRef] [PubMed]
15. Giebel, G.D.; Meyer, C.; Koebke, J.; Giebel, G. Arterial Supply of Forearm Bones and Its Importance for the Operative Treatment of Fractures. *Surg. Radiol. Anat.* **1997**, *19*, 149–153. [CrossRef] [PubMed]
16. Wright, T.W.; Glowczewskie, F. Vascular Anatomy of the Ulna. *J. Hand Surg.* **1998**, *23*, 800–804. [CrossRef]

17. Ogonda, L.; Wong-Chung, J.; Wray, R.; Canavan, B. Delayed Union and Non-Union of the Ulna Following Intramedullary Nailing in Children. *J. Pediatr. Orthop. B.* **2004**, *13*, 330–333. [CrossRef]
18. Yaradılmış, Y.U.; Tecirli, A. Successful Results Obtained in the Treatment of Adolescent Forearm Fractures with Locked Intramedullary Nailing. *Chin. J. Traumatol.* **2021**, *24*, 295–300. [CrossRef]
19. Zeybek, H.; Akti, S. Comparison of Three Different Surgical Fixation Techniques in Pediatric Forearm Double Fractures. *Cureus* **2021**, *13*, e16931. [CrossRef]
20. Loose, O.; Fernandez, F.; Morrison, S.; Schneidmüller, D.; Schmittenbecher, P.; Eberhardt, O. Treatment of Nonunion after Forearm Fractures in Children: A Conservative Approach. *Eur. J. Trauma Emerg. Surg.* **2021**, *47*, 293–301. [CrossRef]
21. Bose, D.; Kugan, R.; Stubbs, D.; McNally, M. Management of Infected Nonunion of the Long Bones by a Multidisciplinary Team. *Bone Jt. J.* **2015**, *97*, 814–817. [CrossRef]
22. Amorosa, L.F.; Buirs, L.D.; Bexkens, R.; Wellman, D.S.; Kloen, P.; Lorich, D.G.; Helfet, D.L. A Single-Stage Treatment Protocol for Presumptive Aseptic Diaphyseal Nonunions: A Review of Outcomes. *J. Orthop. Trauma* **2013**, *27*, 582–586. [CrossRef]
23. Ring, D.; Allende, C.; Jafarnia, K.; Allende, B.T.; Jupiter, J.B. Ununited Diaphyseal Forearm Fractures with Segmental Defects: Plate Fixation and Autogenous Cancellous Bone-Grafting. *J. Bone Jt. Surg. Am.* **2004**, *86*, 2440–2445. [CrossRef]
24. Adani, R.; Delcroix, L.; Innocenti, M.; Marcoccio, I.; Tarallo, L.; Celli, A.; Ceruso, M. Reconstruction of Large Posttraumatic Skeletal Defects of the Forearm by Vascularized Free Fibular Graft. *Microsurgery* **2004**, *24*, 423–429. [CrossRef] [PubMed]
25. Regan, D.K.; Crespo, A.M.; Konda, S.R.; Egol, K.A. Functional Outcomes of Compression Plating and Bone Grafting for Operative Treatment of Nonunions About the Forearm. *J. Hand Surg.* **2018**, *43*, 564.e1–564.e9. [CrossRef] [PubMed]
26. Dawson, J.; Kiner, D.; Gardner, W.; Swafford, R.; Nowotarski, P.J. The Reamer–Irrigator–Aspirator as a Device for Harvesting Bone Graft Compared With Iliac Crest Bone Graft: Union Rates and Complications. *J. Orthop. Trauma* **2014**, *28*, 584–590. [CrossRef] [PubMed]
27. Jupiter, J.B.; Gerhard, H.J.; Guerrero, J.; Nunley, J.A.; Levin, L.S. Treatment of Segmental Defects of the Radius with Use of the Vascularized Osteoseptocutaneous Fibular Autogenous Graft. *J. Bone Jt. Surg.* **1997**, *79*, 542–550. [CrossRef]
28. Yajima, H.; Tamai, S.; Ono, H.; Kizaki, K.; Yamauchi, T. Free Vascularized Fibula Grafts in Surgery of the Upper Limb. *J. Reconstr. Microsurg.* **1999**, *15*, 515–521. [CrossRef]
29. Gan, A.W.T.; Puhaindran, M.E.; Pho, R.W.H. The Reconstruction of Large Bone Defects in the Upper Limb. *Injury* **2013**, *44*, 313–317. [CrossRef]
30. Ozkaya, U. Comparison between Locked Intramedullary Nailing and Plate Osteosynthesis in the Management of Adult Forearm Fractures. *Acta Orthop. Traumatol. Turc.* **2009**, *43*, 14–20. [CrossRef]
31. Masquelet, A.C.; Fitoussi, F.; Begue, T.; Muller, G.P. Reconstruction of the long bones by the induced membrane and spongy autograft. *Ann. Chir. Plast. Esthet.* **2000**, *45*, 346–353.
32. Ma, X.-Y.; Liu, B.; Yu, H.-L.; Zhang, X.; Xiang, L.-B.; Zhou, D.-P. Induced Membrane Technique for the Treatment of Infected Forearm Nonunion: A Retrospective Study. *J. Hand Surg.* **2022**, *47*, 583.e1–583.e9. [CrossRef]
33. Walker, M.; Sharareh, B.; Mitchell, S.A. Masquelet Reconstruction for Posttraumatic Segmental Bone Defects in the Forearm. *J. Hand Surg.* **2019**, *44*, 342.e1–342.e8. [CrossRef]
34. Pachera, G.; Santolini, E.; Galuppi, A.; Dapelo, E.; Demontis, G.; Formica, M.; Santolini, F.; Briano, S. Forearm Segmental Bone Defect: Successful Management Using the Masquelet Technique with the Aid of 3D Printing Technology. *Trauma Case Rep.* **2021**, *36*, 100549. [CrossRef] [PubMed]
35. Zhu, Y.; Pan, Z.; Cui, X.; Quan, C.; Wang, J.; Zhang, W.; Zhang, Z.; Zhang, Q. Effectiveness of ilizarov technology for infected forearm nonunion. *Zhongguo Xiu Fu Chong Jian Wai Ke Za Zhi Zhongguo Xiufu Chongjian Waike Zazhi Chin. J. Reparative Reconstr. Surg.* **2016**, *30*, 1457–1461. [CrossRef]
36. Orzechowski, W.; Morasiewicz, L.; Dragan, S.; Krawczyk, A.; Kulej, M.; Mazur, T. Treatment of Non-Union of the Forearm Using Distraction-Compression Osteogenesis. *Ortop. Traumatol. Rehabil.* **2007**, *9*, 357–365. [PubMed]
37. Liu, Y.; Yushan, M.; Liu, Z.; Liu, J.; Ma, C.; Yusufu, A. Treatment of Diaphyseal Forearm Defects Caused by Infection Using Ilizarov Segmental Bone Transport Technique. *BMC Musculoskelet. Disord.* **2021**, *22*, 36. [CrossRef] [PubMed]

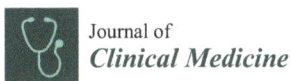

Article

Determinants of Lack of Recovery from Dependency and Walking Ability Six Months after Hip Fracture in a Population of People Aged 65 Years and Over

Enrique González Marcos [1], Enrique González García [2], Josefa González-Santos [3,*], Jerónimo J. González-Bernal [3], Adoración del Pilar Martín-Rodríguez [2] and Mirian Santamaría-Peláez [3]

1. RACA 11 Artillery Regiment, Cid Campeador Military Base, 09193 Burgos, Spain; enriquegojs@gmail.com
2. Traumatology and Orthopedic Surgery Department, Burgos University Hospital (HUBU), 09006 Burgos, Spain; egonzalezga@saludcastillayleon.es (E.G.G.); amartinro@saludcastillayleon.es (A.d.P.M.-R.)
3. Department of Health Sciences, University of Burgos, 09001 Burgos, Spain; jejavier@ubu.es (J.J.G.-B.); mspelaez@ubu.es (M.S.-P.)
* Correspondence: mjgonzalez@ubu.es

Abstract: Background: Hip fracture in the elderly means that between a quarter and a half of patients do not regain the levels of independence and walking ability that they previously had, according to the literature, after the fracture. Material and methods: Retrospective study of 537 patients aged ≥65 years who survived at the sixth month after fracturing their hip, of which the age, sex, type of fracture, surgical risk, independence (BI), walking ability, cognitive level (PS), comorbidities, indicated drugs, complications, surgical delay, hospital stay, and surgical technique are known. Using Pearson's χ^2 test, all the variables were contrasted with respect to the limitation or not, at the sixth month of the recovery of both independence and pre-admission walking ability. Multivariate analysis provides the necessary adjustment to the previous contrast. Results: We have found that age and PS ≥ 5 at admission limit recovery from both dependency and walking ability. Surgical risk, independence (BI) upon admission, anemia, and constipation during the hospital stay limit the recovery of the BI. Worsening of walking ability during the hospital stay and the type of extra-articular fracture, which was surgically treated by osteosynthesis, limit the recovery of walking ability. Conclusions: The factors previously exposed, and perhaps the fact that patients with hip fractures are not routinely referred to rehabilitation, explain the high proportion of patients who do not recover their previous independency (36%) or walking ability (45%) to the fact of fracturing.

Keywords: hip fracture; age; aging; recovery of independence; recovery of walking ability

1. Introduction

Hip fracture is the second most common fragility fracture after wrist fracture [1]. Between 28% and 35% of people aged ≥65 years have at least one fall at the same height per year that can potentially end in a fracture, and this incidence increases with age. It is called "multi-fall syndrome", which affects 30–50% of the institutionalized elderly population [2]. The incidence of hip fracture in Spain was 2.1% each year between 1997 and 2010, a year in which it was 325 cases in men and 766 in women for every 105 inhabitants, and it affects more significantly those aged 85 years or older [3].

The most pessimistic information about the percentage of elderly people who recover their previous function after suffering a hip fracture is 23% [4], but the most optimistic estimate that it can reach more than half, in which case the functional deficit baseline, 25-hydroxy-vitamin D deficiency and complication with "delirium" [5,6] are the most limiting factors for mobility recovery.

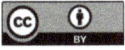

Among the instruments used to standardize the measurement of the physical health of the elderly related to the activities of daily living (ADL), the Barthel Index (BI) [7] in its Spanish version [8] has been chosen as it is widely used in geriatrics.

In previous studies, there are multiple scales used to assess mobility and gait. The Tinetti scale [9] is one of them, the "Cumulated Ambulation Score" (CAS), described by Foss N.B., et al. in 2006 [10] and used by Danish authors [11]. Other scales are gait-specific, such as the aforementioned FIM scale [12], which has a module that assesses gait function. The "Functional Ambulation Classification" (FAC) was also initially described more than three decades ago for the evaluation of walking ability in stroke patients [13,14], but it has been used in elderly patients with hip fractures, too, is used in this studio [15,16], and has the advantage of its simplicity in clinical application. It is the one that we will apply in a summarized way, as it is exposed in material and methods.

Much research studies the recovery of patients in the context of rehabilitation programs. However, the results are not conclusive and more research is required [17]. However, there are not so many who study the factors that may limit the recovery of these patients.

A greater fear of falling after a hip fracture is related to the female sex, polypharmacy, poor physical functioning and daily activities, and depressive symptoms one year after the fracture occurred [18]. Frölich et al., in a prospective cohort study, found that those who were the frailest patients were the ones who failed to return to their independent living, but they consider that the majority of the community-dwelling patients returned to independent living only with a minor increase in care needs; they also consider that standing within 24 h from hip fracture surgery was vital in maximizing short-term functional recovery [19]. One systematic review proposed the hand grip strength and frailty as emerging significant predictors of poor functional outcomes and mortality in the literature, in addition to other predictors grouped in medical factors (comorbidity, anesthesia, sarcopenia), surgical factors (delay in intervention, type of fracture), socio-economic factors (age, sex, ethnicity) and system factors including lower case-volume centers [20]. Age, male sex, trochanteric fracture, preoperative delay, postoperative drainage use, serum albumin, and ADL at discharge and internal fixation are related to functional recovery [21,22]. Some of these factors can also influence mortality after hip fracture as advanced age, male sex, living in a rural area, diabetes, tumor, preoperative delay, and postoperative drainage use [22].

This research aims to study which factors exist in our population of patients aged ≥65 years, which limit, and to what degree, the recovery of the situation of independence (BI), as well as their ability to walk prior to suffering a hip fracture.

The hypothesis of this study is based on the fact that the factors that denote poor basal functioning, as well as the presence of health problems and other complications, will be factors that may influence the recovery of the baseline situation.

2. Materials and Methods

2.1. Study Design—Participants

In a retrospective longitudinal study, all patients were treated at the University Hospital of Burgos (HUBU). Inclusion criteria: Patients aged 65 years or older who, by a low energy mechanism, suffered a hip fracture in the biennium 14 March 2019–14 March 2021. All patients admitted to the HUBU with these characteristics were included in the study, followed after discharge from the outpatient clinics of the Orthopedic Surgery and Traumatology Service of the same hospital through face-to-face and non-face-to-face consultations through interviews with the patients, their families, and/or responsible caregivers. Exclusion criteria: Patients with peri-prosthetic fractures, peri-synthesis fractures, and pathological fractures, that is, on bones affected by primary tumor or metastasis, were excluded from the study; likewise, patients who were referred to other hospitals without completing the treatment or follow-up period for any cause, except death. Data collection was carried out on all patients who were admitted to the emergency room for hip fractures and underwent surgery by the Orthopedic Surgery and Traumatology Service.

2.2. Sample Size

The sample size was estimated following the procedure for finite populations, using the formula $n = \frac{N \times (Z_\alpha = 1.96)^2 \times p \times q}{\delta^2 \times (N-1) + (1.96)^2 \times p \times q}$. The known population reported by the National Institute of Statistics (INE) (https://www.ine.es/jaxiT3/Tabla.htm?t=2852, accessed on 25 May 2022) and a similar study [23] was taken into account, establishing a proportion of hip fractures in the population of 0.389% (p = 0.000398, and its complementary q = 0.99602) and assuming a sampling error of 1% (δ^2 = 0.01). Based on this, it was concluded that the sample should be made up of 152 patients with hip fractures under care by the HUBU.

2.3. Main Outcomes—Instruments

The head of the Traumatology Section of the Orthopedic Surgery and Traumatology (OST) Service was responsible for collecting the data from each participant's electronic medical record for further analysis. In order to study variables that may influence cognitive impairment, sociodemographic data such as age (dichotomized in <85 and ≥85 years) and sex (woman/man) and clinical data such as the type of fracture (intracapsular/extracapsular), the type of treatment (surgical/conservative), the surgical technique (arthroplasty/synthesis), complications during admission such as "delirium" or constipation, the surgical risk assessed according to the American Society of Anesthesiologists Physical Status Classification (ASA) [24], prescription of different drugs before admission and after hospital discharge, and concomitant pathologies at the time of admission. The main variable refers to ambulation capacity according to the functional ambulation classification (FAC) [10,11] (categorized their levels 4–5 as "good", 3–4 as "regular", and 0–1 as "bad" walking ability).

There are multiple ways to standardize the measurement of the physical health of the elderly: the activities of daily living (ADL) index ("Activities of Daily Living" or "ADL") [7] and the instrumental activities of daily living (IADL) [8]. In specific questions of mobility, the functional independence measure (FIM) [9] is available, which is fundamentally validated for patients with neurological diseases, and its application is complex. The Barthel Index (BI) [10] in its Spanish version [11] has been chosen because it is the most widely used tool in the functional assessment of elderly patients suffering from hip fracture [12–16]. The categorization of the BI has been performed in four: "1" (BI = 100): fully independent, "2" (100 < BI ≥ 90): slightly dependent, "3" (90 < BI ≥ 60): moderately dependent and "4" (BI < 60): severely or totally dependent. "BI Recovery" is the difference between the BI (variable with four categories 1 to 4) at the income and at the sixth month, so that, if the value is negative, it is understood that they did not recover. "Walking ability recovery" is the category difference in "walking ability" at admission and at the sixth month so that "they do not recover" if said difference is a negative value. The cognitive impairment was assessed using Pfeiffer Scale (PS) [25]. It is a questionnaire that collects the number of errors of the evaluated patient when ten simple questions are posed and establishes four categories of the definition of cognitive impairment depending on the dependence of people in the intellectual area: 0–2 errors is the absence of deterioration or autonomy in the intellectual area, 3–4 errors is slight impairment and help of other people in intellectually complex matters, 5–7 errors is moderate deterioration and require help on a regular basis but not always, and 8–10 errors denote severe deterioration and continuous supervision. In the present study, cognitive impairment according to PS is expressed as a dichotomous variable: absence of cognitive impairment or mild impairment (PS ≤ 4 errors) and moderate or severe cognitive impairment (PS ≥ 5 errors). Data on FAC, BI, PS, and institutionalization prior to admission, at discharge, and at 6 months if the patient survives is collected. All clinical or sociodemographic information is obtained in the emergency department, on the hospitalization floor, or in face-to-face or telematic consultations after hospital discharge.

2.4. Statistical Analysis

To characterize the sample, the mean and standard deviation (SD) were used in the case of continuous variables and absolute frequencies and percentages if the variables were categorical. Both categorical variables from more than two categories and continuous variables were dichotomized based on previous studies and tended to obtain groups as homogeneous as possible. Bivariate analyses were performed to study the relationship between clinical features at "BI Recovery" and "Walking ability recovery", 6 months using the Pearson independence test (χ^2), as well as the likelihood ratio. In the analyses with significant results, the ratio of advantages or "odds" (OR) with its limits (lower/upper) was also obtained. In addition, in order to quantify the magnitude of relationships of bivariate analysis and identify possible predictive factors of main variables at 6 months, depending on the different clinical characteristics, an analysis was performed using binary logistic regression, where dichotomous dependent variables are "BI Recovery" and "Walking ability recovery". All the significant variables obtained in the previous bivariate analysis were included as independent in the referred multivariate study, and the OR = $e^{\beta i*(\pm \Delta i)}$ with its limits (lower/upper) was also obtained too.

Statistical analysis was performed with SPSS software version 25 (IBM-Inc., Chicago, IL, USA). For the analysis of statistical significance, a p-value < 0.05 was established.

3. Results

3.1. Recovery of the Initial Situation

The study sample consisted of 665 people, 128 of whom died during the 6 months after hip fracture. The age of the participants was between 65 and 102 years, with a mean of 86.2 years, 76.7% women (n = 510) and 23.3% men (n = 155) (Figure 1). In the group of surviving patients in the series, 36.1% did not regain independence at the sixth month, nor did 44% regain walking ability prior to the fracture.

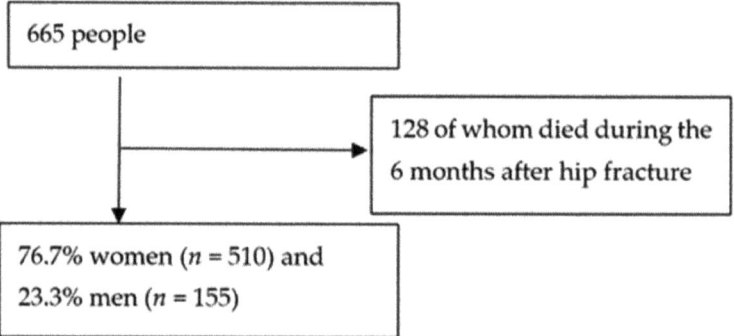

Figure 1. Participants flow.

3.2. Influence on Lack of Recovery by 6th Month of the Category of the BI Prior to Admission

3.2.1. Regarding the Previous Situation or Admission

In the bivariate analysis carried out between the BI recovery variable (yes/no) with the variables studied that take into account the situation before the patient was admitted (Table 1), an association was found with age ≥ 85 years, type of extracapsular fracture, also comorbidities such as chronic renal failure and high blood pressure, likewise the use of antihypertensive drugs, all of which are risk factors for non-recovery. There is also a relationship with independence (BI at admission ≥ 60, BI at admission ≥ 90), better cognitive status (PS at admission ≤ 4), and better gait (FAC category ≤ 2). No association was found with age, sex, or institutionalization prior to admission.

Table 1. Bivariate analysis recovery of the BI (yes/no); significant factors prior to or at admission.

Bivariate Analysis Recovery of the BI			No BI Recovery at 6th Month		
Prior to/at Admission	χ^2	p	RO	RO Limits Lower	Upper
≥85 years	34.05	<0.001	3.255	2.183	4.854
Extracapsular hip fracture	5.05	0.025	1.511	1.052	2.172
Chronic renal insufficiency prior admission	7.63	0.006	1.891	1.220	2.931
Arterial hypertension prior admission	5.03	0.025	1.543	1.071	2.224
Antihypertensive drugs prescribed before entering	4.38	0.036	1.495	1.041	2.147
BI at admission ≥ 60	45.24	<0.001	1.716	1.589	1.853
BI at admission ≥ 90	18.05	<0.001	2.293	1.570	3.350
PS at admission ≤ 4	10.19	0.001	2.148	1.355	3.404
(FAC category ≤ 2) not bad gait (good or regular)	23.81	<0.001	16.000	3.846	66.563

BI: Barthel Index; FAC: functional ambulation classification; RO: Odds Ratio; PS: Pfeiffer Scale.

Binary logistic regression (Table 2) (Nagerkelke's R^2 = 0.289) finds (in bold) age in completed years, surgical risk (ASA), independence (highest BI: 0–100), and cognitive impairment (number of errors in the EP) as risk factors for non-recovery of BI.

Table 2. Binary logistic regression of recovery of the BI (yes/no); situation prior to admission.

Prior to/at Admission	No BI Recovery at 6th Month					
R^2 = 0.294	Coef. β	χ^2 Wald	p Value	RO	L. Inf	L. Sup
Age (years)	0.107	36.506	<0.001	**1.113**	1.075	1.153
Sex male	−0.247	0.909	0.340	0.781	0.470	1.298
Extracapsular fracture	0.338	2.468	0.116	1.402	0.920	2.137
ASA III ó IV	0.478	4.923	0.026	**1.612**	1.057	2.459
BI at admission (0 a 100)	0.070	34.216	0.000	**1.073**	1.048	1.098
Walking ability (FAC categories 1–3)	−1.448	3.234	0.072	0.235	0.048	1.139
N° errors PS (0–10)	0.186	8.929	0.003	**1.204**	1.066	1.360
Arterial hypertension (yes)	0.149	0.488	0.485	1.161	0.764	1.765
Chronic renal insufficiency (yes)	0.345	1.771	0.183	1.412	0.849	2.347

BI: Barthel Index; ASA: American Society of Anesthesiologists Physical Status Classification; FAC: functional ambulation classification; PS: Pfeiffer Scale.

3.2.2. Regarding the Effect That the Fracture and Admission Exert

We obtained the bivariate analysis (Table 3), and the following risk factors were found: the use of synthesis as a surgical technique, hospital stay ≥ 11 days, BI at discharge < 90, deterioration of at least one category in the BI between hospital admission and discharge, impairment of at least one category in the ability to walk, better cognitive status at discharge (PE ≤ 4), cognitive impairment in at least one category in the PS, "de novo" institutionalization at hospital discharge it associates greater risk than staying at home, and the following events: hemoglobinemia ≤ 8.5 mg/dL, being transfused with ≥3 packed red blood cells, delirium, and constipation. The variable's type of treatment and surgical delay were not significant in this bivariate analysis.

Table 3. Bivariate analysis recovery of the BI (yes/no); significant variables—effect of the fracture and outcome.

Bivariate Analysis Recovery of the BI (Yes/No)				RO Limits	
Events during Admission	χ²	p	RO	Lower	Upper
Synthesis as a surgical technique	5.82	0.016	1.608	1.108	2.335
Hospital stay ≥ 11 days	10.12	0.001	1.907	1.293	2.812
BI at discharge < 90	11.27	0.001	1.948	1.330	2.853
Deterioration ≥ 1 category in the BI	109.22	<0.001	14.365	8.014	25.751
Impairment ≥ 1 category (FAC 1–3) in the ability to walk	17.58	<0.001	2.192	1.526	3.147
Better cognitive status at discharge (PS ≤ 4)	7.62	0.006	1.911	1.222	2.989
Cognitive impairment in at least one category in the PS	13.79	<0.001	7.102	2.323	21.716
"De novo" institutionalization at hospital discharge	23.52	<0.001	3.262	2.014	5.282
Still remain at home when discharged from hospital	9.28	0.002	1.765	1.236	2.520
Hemoglobinemia ≤ 8.5 mg/dL	15.29	<0.001	2.278	1.515	3.425
Constipation	17.29	<0.001	2.165	1.512	3.099

BI: Barthel Index; FAC: functional ambulation classification; PS: Pfeiffer Scale.

The multivariate analysis (Table 4) has estimated significant variables with adjustment for not regaining independence: older age, higher BI (0–100) at hospital discharge, but above all, deterioration of BI during admission, in addition to hemoglobinemia ≤ 8.5 mg/dL, and constipation.

Table 4. Binary logistic regression of recovery of the BI (yes/no); situation during admission.

Income Events and Effects	No Recovery of Baseline Independence					
R² = 0.503	β	χ² Wald	p	RO	L. Inf	L. Sup
Age (years)	0.115	31.046	0.000	**1.122**	1.078	1.169
Sex male	−0.120	0.161	0.688	0.887	0.495	1.592
Surgical thecnique syntesis	0.403	2.532	0.112	1.497	0.911	2.460
Hospital stay ≥ 11 days	0.507	3.622	0.057	1.661	0.985	2.801
IB (0–100) at discharge	0.025	7.886	0.0050	**1.025**	1.008	1.043
Loss of independence (BI) at least 1 category	3.236	81.737	0.000	**25.430**	12.609	51.287
Cognitive status: PS (number of errors)	0.065	0.726	0.394	1.067	0.919	1.240
Cognitive impairment at least 1 category	0.860	1.280	0.258	2.363	0.533	10.480
Walking ability at least 1 category	0.325	1.716	0.190	1.384	0.851	2.252
Institutionalization at discharge	−0.479	1.974	0.160	0.619	0.317	1.208
New institutionalization at discharge	0.320	0.638	0.424	1.378	0.628	3.022
Heglobinemia ≤ 8.5 mg/dL	0.677	4.067	0.044	**1.969**	1.019	3.803
Be transfused during admission	−0.219	0.482	0.487	0.803	0.433	1.491
"Delirium" during admission	0.388	1.665	0.197	1.474	0.818	2.657
Constipación pertinacious during admission	0.706	6.693	0.010	**2.026**	1.187	3.459

BI: Barthel Index; PS: Pfeiffer Scale.

3.3. Influence on Lack of Recovery by 6th Month of the Category of the Walking Ability Prior to Admission

3.3.1. Regarding the Previous Situation or Admission

Using Pearson's χ^2 tests and likelihood ratio ($\chi^{RV\,2}$) with the dependent variable recovering (yes/no) walking ability (Table 5), risk factors have been found for non-recovery at the sixth month, age $\geq$ 85 years, extracapsular type of fracture, ASA III or IV surgical risk, BI < 90 prior to admission, moderate or severe cognitive impairment (PS $\geq$ 5), institutionalization prior to admission, comorbidities at admission: chronic anemia, heart failure, having the patient prescribed anticoagulants and proton-pump inhibitors before the fracture. The poor ability to walk before admission has been significant as a protective factor for non-recovery at six months; this effect does not change and gains greater associative strength in the multivariate adjustment. There is no association with sex or with BI at admission < 60 points.

Table 5. Bivariate analysis recovery of the FAC (yes/no); variables significantly associated; situation prior to admission.

Bivariate Analysis Recovery of the Walking Ability (Yes/No)				RO Limits	
Prior to/at Admission	χ^2	p	RO	Lower	Upper
$\geq$85 years	53.60	<0.001	4.105	2.796	6.026
Type extracapsular of fracture	7.58	<0.001	1.657	1.168	2.351
ASA III or IV surgical risk	11.60	0.001	1.853	1.309	2.623
BI < 90 prior to admission	13.60	<0.001	1.957	1.379	2.778
Cognitive impariment PS $\geq$ 5	8.08	0.004	1.834	1.222	2.754
Institutionalization prior to admission	11.69	0.001	1.985	1.350	2.917
Chronic anemia	4.75	0.029	1.727	1.080	2.761
Heart failure	3.64	0.057	1.513	1.009	2.269
Anticoagulant drugs prescribed before admission	3.76	0.052	1.552	1.017	2.367
Proton-pump inhibitor before admission	4.22	0.04	1.587	1.042	2.419
Bad walking ability (FAC category 3)	43.23	<0.001	0.508	0.466	0.555

ASA: American Society of Anesthesiologists Physical Status Classification; BI: Barthel Index; PS: Pfeiffer Scale; FAC: functional ambulation classification.

The binary logistic regression (Table 6) has obtained the only significant results (R^2 = 0.500) for not recovering walking ability, thanks to the adjustment, in addition to older age, the extracapsular type of fracture, surgical risk, number of errors in PS, and use of proton-pump inhibitor, on or prior to admission. IB (0–100) independence and, above all, worse ambulation (FAC) prior to admission have been protective factors for the lack of recovery of gait; these two effects are found in the bivariate analysis.

Table 6. Binary logistic regression of recovery of the FAC (yes/no); situation prior to admission.

Prior to/at Admission	No Recovery of Baseline Walking Ability at 6th Month					
R^2 = 0.500	Coef. β	χ^2 Wald	p Vaule	RO	L. Inf	L. Sup
Age (years)	0.114	34.341	0.000	**1.121**	1.079	1.164
Sex male	−0.394	1.922	0.166	0.674	0.386	1.177
Extracapsular fracture	0.537	5.236	0.022	**1.710**	1.080	2.709
ASA III ó IV	0.404	2.559	0.110	**1.498**	0.913	2.457
BI prior to admission (0 a 100)	−0.043	9.946	0.002	**0.958**	0.933	0.984

Table 6. Cont.

Prior to/at Admission				No Recovery of Baseline Walking Ability at 6th Month		
Cognitive impairment prior to admission	0.258	13.024	0.000	**1.295**	1.125	1.490
Walking ability prior to admission	−3.584	79.328	0.000	**0.028**	0.013	0.061
Institutional origin prior to admission	0.574	3.403	0.065	1.776	0.965	3.269
Chronic anemia prior to admission	0.430	1.667	0.197	1.537	0.801	2.949
Chronic renal insufficiency prior to admission	0.187	0.366	0.545	1.206	0.658	2.210
Anticoagulant drugs prior admission	−0.046	0.021	0.885	0.955	0.516	1.769
Proton-pump inhibitor prior admission	0.591	4.230	0.040	**1.806**	1.028	3.172

ASA: American Society of Anesthesiologists Physical Status Classification; BI: Barthel Index.

3.3.2. Regarding the Effect That the Fracture and Admission Exert

In the bivariate analysis with variables during admission and at the end of it (Table 7), we have found that the following are risk factors for non-recovery of gait: surgical technique by synthesis, start of standing, and gait beyond the third postoperative day, BI < 90 at discharge, BI < 60 at discharge, poor walking ability at hospital discharge, impairment during admission of at least one category in ambulatory ability, cognitive impairment according to PS ≥ 5, loss during admission of at least one category according to the same PS, and new institution at discharge.

Table 7. Bivariate analysis recovery of the FAC (yes/no); variables significantly associated; effect of the fracture and outcome.

No Walking Ability Recovery at 6th Month						
Bivariate Analysis Recovery of the Walking Ability (Yes/No)					RO Limits	
Events during Admission	χ^2	p	RO	Lower	Upper	
Surgical technique by synthesis	10.00	0.002	1.809	1.263	2.589	
Start of standing and gait beyond 3rd day PI	4.36	0.037	1.525	1.044	2.227	
BI < 90 at discharge	58.85	<0.001	4.549	3.062	6.759	
BI < 60 at discharge	11.06	0.001	1.945	1.325	2.856	
Bad walking ability at discharge (FAC category 3)	13.99	<0.001	1.999	1.400	2.857	
Impairment ≥ 1 category (FAC 1–3) in the ability to walk	8.53	<0.001	1.711	1.205	2.431	
Cognitive impairment according to PS ≥ 5	9.99	0.002	1.948	1.301	2.918	
Cognitive impairment in at least one category in the PS	5.62	0.018	3.646	1.294	10.273	
New institution at discharge	15.82	<0.001	2.708	1.661	4.413	
Hemoglobinemia ≤ 8.5 mg/dL	8.46	0.004	1.771	1.217	2.577	
Being transfused ≥ 3 packed red blood cells	16.17	0.001	2.572	1.468	4.507	
Delirium	21.5	<0.001	2.429	1.675	3.523	
Constipation	22.41	<0.001	2.353	1.657	3.342	
Impaired renal function during admission	4.56	0.033	1.578	1.057	2.357	
Urinary tract infection	8.02	0.005	2.260	1.306	3.913	
Acute urine retention	10.09	0.001	2.669	1.470	4.846	
New prescription of vitamin D at discharge	13.70	<0.001	1.960	1.382	2.781	
Residential destination when discharged from hospital	36.86	<0.001	0.333	0.233	0.474	
New institutionalization at discharge	15.82	<0.001	2.708	1.661	4.413	

BI: Barthel Index; FAC: Functional Ambulation Classification; RO: Odds Ratio; PI: Post Intervention.

We have also found various complications that occurred during admission as risk factors: hemoglobinemia ≤ 8.5 mg/dL, being transfused and if performed with three or more packed red blood cells, delirium, constipation, impaired kidney function during admission, urinary tract infection (UTI), acute urine retention (AUR), need to a new prescription of vitamin D at discharge.

There are four variables: deep venous thrombosis (DVT), acute ischemic stroke (AIS) during admission, liquid thickeners, and new neuroleptics prescription at hospital discharge, which are risk factors in the analysis, but the result must be interpreted with reservation, because in the 2 × 2 table, at least one box has expected values less than 5, and therefore, despite their significance, we will not include them in the multivariate analysis.

Neither the type of treatment nor the hospital stay, nor the surgical delay influence the non-recovery of walking capacity.

Institutionalization as a residential destination (new and not new) at discharge is a protector factor in the non-recovery of walking, contrary to new institutionalization, so patients with an institutional destination at discharge have significantly greater possibilities to maintain their previous level of capacity for ambulation.

The multivariate analysis (Table 8), with binary logistic regression ($R^2 = 0.275$), only confirms as true factors associated with not recovering the ability to walk the loss of at least one category of ability to walk during admission and synthesis as a technique surgery used.

Table 8. Binary logistic regression of recovery of the FAC (yes/no); situation during admission.

Income Events and Effects	No Recovery of Baseline Walking Ability at 6th Month					
$R^2 = 0.275$	Coef. β	χ^2 Wald	*p* Value	RO	L. Inf	L. Sup
Age (years)	0.075	18.318	0.000	**1.078**	1.042	1.116
Sex male	0.239	0.937	0.333	1.269	0.783	2.058
Surgical technique synthesis	0.475	4.960	0.026	**1.609**	1.059	2.445
BI at discharge (0–100)	−0.004	0.218	0.641	0.996	0.981	1.012
Walking ability at discharge (FAC 1–3)	−0.183	0.390	0.532	0.832	0.468	1.480
Loss walking ability during admission	0.868	14.706	0.000	**2.382**	1.529	3.712
Loss ≥ 1 category PS during admission	0.219	0.133	0.715	1.245	0.383	4.047
PS (number of errors) at discharge	0.095	2.846	0.092	1.100	0.985	1.229
Residential destination when discharged	−0.433	2.694	0.101	0.648	0.386	1.088
New institutionalization at discharge	0.481	2.150	0.143	1.618	0.851	3.077
Anemia on admission	0.214	0.591	0.442	1.239	0.718	2.137
Be transfused during admission	−0.171	0.435	0.510	0.843	0.506	1.402
Delirium	0.205	0.735	0.391	1.228	0.768	1.964
Constipation	0.266	1.387	0.239	1.304	0.838	2.029
Impaired renal function	−0.075	0.095	0.758	0.928	0.575	1.497
UTI	0.347	1.105	0.293	1.415	0.741	2.701
AUR	0.259	0.526	0.468	1.295	0.644	2.605
New thickeners at hospital discharge	1.673	2.028	0.154	5.328	0.533	53.270
New vitamin D prescription at discharge	0.066	0.088	0.767	1.068	0.692	1.647

BI: Barthel Index; FAC: functional ambulation classification; PS: Pfeiffer Scale; UTI: urinary tract infection; AUR: acute urine retention.

Functional loss during admission (see Tables 9 and 10, as well as Figure 2) after hip fracture in the elderly in our series is basically related to cognitive impairment before said admission, but in a different direction. There is a direct relationship or risk factor regarding the deterioration of the ability to walk. On the other hand, there is an indirect relationship so that patients with greater cognitive impairment at admission experience less loss of independence during admission.

Table 9. Profile of patient losing independence in at least one BI category during admission according to binary logistic regression.

	Loss BI $\geq$ 1 Categories during Admission					
$R^2 = 0.168$	β	χ^2 Wald	p	OR	L. Inf	L. Sup
Age (years)	0.184	23.588	<0.001	**1.202**	1.116	1.295
Sex: male	−0.151	0.096	0.757	0.860	0.332	2.228
PS errors number (0–10)	−0.446	9.799	0.002	**0.640**	0.484	0.847
BI (0–100) at admission	−0.015	0.778	0.378	0.985	0.953	1.018
FAC (1–3) at admission	−0.237	0.299	0.585	0.789	0.338	1.844

BI: Barthel Index; PS: Pfeiffer Scale; FAC: functional ambulation classification.

Table 10. Profile of patient losing independence in at least one FAC category ($\geq$2 levels) during admission according to binary logistic regression.

	Change $\geq$ 1 Category FAC during Admission					
$R^2 = 0.293$	β	χ^2 Wald	p	OR	L. Inf	L. Sup
Age (years)	−0.005	0.124	0.725	0.995	0.970	1.021
Sex: male	−0.388	3.145	0.076	0.678	0.441	1.042
PS errors number (0–10)	0.129	5.235	0.022	**1.138**	1.019	1.270
BI (0–100) at admission	0.008	0.654	0.419	1.008	0.988	1.028
FAC (1–3) at admission	−2.284	53.251	0.000	**0.102**	0.055	0.188

FAC: functional ambulation classification; PS: Pfeiffer Scale; BI: Barthel Index.

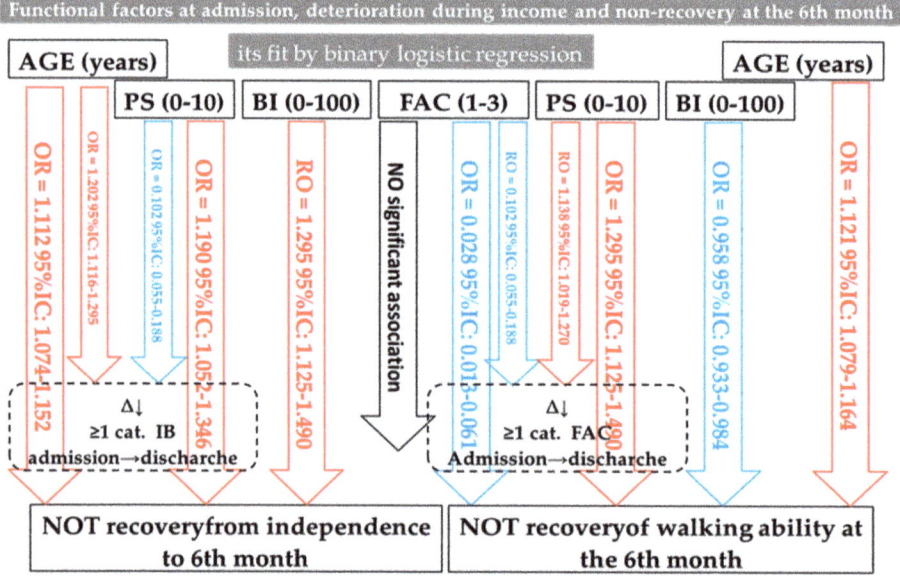

Figure 2. Summary of the interaction between functional factors in the elderly with hip fracture in our patients.

Below (Figure 2), the relationships between functional variables are exposed so that in blue, we have those that prevent and in red, those that are risk factors for non-functional recovery in the sixth month.

4. Discussion

Age is the factor that, in almost any publication, is associated with the limitation in the recovery of the previous function after a hip fracture in the elderly and in any period of time: 2 and 6 months [26]; 4 months [27], 6 months [28,29], 8 months [30], 1 year [31,32], 6 y 18 months [33], or not specifying a certain time, but when a more or less specific rehabilitation program ends [34–42]. In general, men have the worst evolution, according to much of the literature consulted [36,37,43]. According to Sylliaas et al. [44], women have a worse evolution, although there are also authors who, coincidentally with our work, do not appreciate differences [32,45]. In our study, as in the literature consulted, age, both in bivariate and multivariate analysis, is a risk factor for the non-recovery of independence and, also, for the non-recovery of ambulatory capacity.

In our investigation, the average stay is not associated with a lack of functional recovery. Martin-Martin et al. [40] associate it with worse mobility and Orive et al. [33] with BI impairment. The surgical delay in this work does not condition the functional evolution either, but there are studies in which surgical delay ≥ 48 h limits mobility [28] or the recovery of independence [33].

The pathology associated with the patient who is admitted to be treated for a hip fracture has different importance. The frailty of the elderly can be defined by the number of severe or terminal chronic diseases that the patient has [46], obtaining an index that is adjusted for age and baseline functional status. Kua J. et al. [47] have highlighted that the previously known geriatric scale [48] called Reported Edmonton Frail Scale, has a high prognostic value in all hospital admissions for acute processes in the elderly, and specifically a significant impairment (OR = 6.19, $p = 0.01$) of basic activities of daily living (ADL) [49,50] in the sixth month after hip fracture.

The number of concurrent comorbidities has been described as a factor of poor functional prognosis at four months [41] that we have not found. In fact, in our multivariate adjustment, no comorbidity influences the recovery of function at six months. Parkinson's disease has a proven relationship with ambulatory capacity in patients with hip fractures [51]. In addition, it has been described that hypertension and diabetes are co-morbidities associated with a greater limitation of functional recovery [36,41]. In addition, it has been described that hypertension and diabetes are comorbidities associated with greater limitation of functional recovery [52,53]. The greater surgical risk of our patients limits the recovery of [43] independence in terms of the BI value, not as well as the recovery of the march in our research, as other authors refer [30,33].

Several authors [51,54] associate the need for help to walk or not being able to walk alone outside the residential setting before admission with not regaining independence (IADL) [55] a year after the fracture. McGilton et al. [56] consider that poor global functional status, gait, and cognitive status at admission are limiting to recovery. Lower BI and more errors in the PS impair both the global functional status and the ability to walk Mariconda M. et al. [57] at one year. In our series, cognitive impairment prior to admission limits the recovery of both independence and gait in the sixth month after the hip fracture. The most independent patients, according to the BI before the fracture in this series, are the ones with the most limited global functional recovery (BI) in the sixth month. This phenomenon and with the same index is described in the literature [33] with prospective research at 6 and 18 months. However, in our patients, functional deterioration during admission is directly related to said previous cognitive deterioration only in the case of walking. Patients with a worse baseline cognitive situation acquire a lesser loss of their independence between admission and discharge. Similarly, patients with worse gait have at admission (higher value of the FAC variable), as occurs with dependency, with less functional reserve at admission, less loss generated by the fracture, and they maintain levels at the sixth month not as different from the previous ones. Therefore, the high value of the FAC variable prevents the non-recovery of the gait function. The essential factor so that these functions, independence and ability to walk, are not recovered is their qualitative loss during admission, especially in the case of loss of dependency (OR = 25.43, 95% CI: 12.61–51.28). Our work coincides with Dubljanin-Raspopović E. et al. [27] in that cognitive impairment is a pre-eminent factor in global functional (BI) and gait non-recovery.

Our patients from a nursing home before fracture have, after adjusting variables, a recovery of BI and gait not significantly different from those who lived at home, coinciding with Ariza-Vega P. et al. [31]. Other works instead [32,42] consider that institutionalization prior to admission limits gait recovery.

The extra-articular fracture type has, in general, a worse functional prognosis in the literature [32,40,45,52], just as we have clearly found in our multivariate analysis regarding the non-recovery of gait function. The worse prognosis in the evolution of BI can, at least in part, be explained by age since our patients with extra-articular fractures have a higher mean age, as in almost all the literature [16,53]. Di Monaco [58] does not find differences in prognosis between the types of fracture. A meta-analysis [59] showed that the use of total arthroplasty in patients with displaced intracapsular fractures gives better functional results than osteosynthesis, and total hip arthroplasty, according to prospective studies, is preferable in this type of fracture both due to its functional outcome as having fewer complications [60–62]. The synthesis, in our research, by the bivariate analysis, is followed by less recovery of both dependency (BI) and walking capacity at six months. This effect, in the multivariate analysis, is annulled in terms of non-recovery of BI; and persists as a risk factor in the non-recovery of walking. The mean age of our survivors does not differ significantly between those who underwent synthesis or arthroplasty. The only complications that we have been able to relate to the functional prognosis after multivariate adjustment have been anemia, coinciding with Foss N.B. et al. [10], and constipation; however, for other authors [63], they are ulcers by pressure and "delirium".

It is a relative limitation that the measurement of the evolution at six months is a shorter time than that of some publications, which was already mentioned that they take 12 or 18 months, although there is no lack of medium-term studies: six months like ours, even at two, and four months in some cases. It has been pointed out that most of the recovery of global independence (BI) occurs in the first trimester [51]. The scientific evidence of a retrospective observational study is less than that of a cohort study, fundamentally because it is a mere consultation of registered data, no matter how rigorous the anamnesis and record of it have been. Our hip fractures do not follow any rehabilitation program, which may be related to the high percentages of lack of functional recovery that we have; in agreement with Orive et al. [33] when they state that not referring to rehabilitation increases the possibility of deterioration of the BI prior to six months, more than two times (OR = 2.34, 95% CI: 1.31–4.16) and at 18 months more than three (OR = 3.18, 95% CI: 1.62–6.25) with respect to undergoing rehabilitation treatment.

As strengths, it should be noted that the sample is large enough. Includes all fractures treated by our hospital in relation to its health area. This minimizes potential selection biases that often accompany a retrospective study. Take all possible variables. In addition to performing statistical analysis comparing dichotomous qualitative variables, binary logistic regression, in which we also incorporate quantitative independent variables for adjustment, allows us to eliminate biases such as effect modification or interaction, especially in relation to age. Although retrospective, it is still a longitudinal study, which to a large extent allows its conclusions to be taken as a valid explanation of the knowledge of the factors that truly influence limiting functional recovery in the elderly with hip fractures in our environment.

The results of this research show the factors in our population of patients aged ≥65 years, which limit, and to what extent, the recovery of the situation of independence (IB), as well as their ability to walk before suffering a hip fracture, as established in the objective of the research.

5. Conclusions

The factors associated with both the lower recovery of the BI and the ability to walk are older age and worse cognitive status at admission. Perhaps the lack of referral to rehabilitation of our patients is a very important factor to take into account in the poor recovery from dependency and walking.

Limitations to the recovery of independence are one's own independence (high BI) on admission and discharge, the loss of it during admission, and the high surgical risk (ASA).

Both dependency (low BI) as well as impaired ambulatory capacity during admission limit recovery of gait.

Patients suffering from extracapsular fractures and surgical treatment by synthesis limit the recovery of walking in the sixth month. Likewise, patients taking proton-pump inhibitors prior to admission have less recovery from walking.

Hemoglobinemia < 8.5 mg/dL, as well as constipation, are the complications that are associated with a worse prognosis of dependence, but not "delirium".

Sex does not influence, neither have any comorbidity been found, nor the greater number of concomitant comorbid processes with hip fracture related to functional prognosis

Author Contributions: Conceptualization, E.G.M., E.G.G. and A.d.P.M.-R.; methodology, E.G.M., E.G.G. and J.J.G.-B.; software, E.G.M., E.G.G. and M.S.-P.; validation, E.G.M., E.G.G., A.d.P.M.-R. and J.J.G.-B.; formal analysis, E.G.M., E.G.G. and M.S.-P.; investigation, E.G.M. and E.G.G.; resources, E.G.M., E.G.G., A.d.P.M.-R. and J.J.G.-B.; data curation, E.G.M., E.G.G., A.d.P.M.-R. and J.J.G.-B.; writing—original draft preparation, E.G.G. and J.G.-S.; writing—review and editing, E.G.G., M.S.-P. and J.G.-S.; visualization, E.G.M., E.G.G., A.d.P.M.-R., J.J.G.-B., M.S.-P. and J.G.-S.; supervision, J.G.-S. and J.J.G.-B.; project administration, E.G.M., E.G.G. and J.J.G.-B. All authors have read and agreed to the published version of the manuscript.

Funding: This research received no external funding.

Institutional Review Board Statement: The study was conducted in accordance with the Declaration of Helsinki and approved by the Ethics Committee for Drug Research of the Health Area of Burgos and Soria (CEIm 2537, approved on 27 April 2021).

Informed Consent Statement: Informed consent was obtained from all subjects involved in the study.

Conflicts of Interest: The authors declare no conflict of interest. Official Defense Bulletin certifies that Enrique González Marcos belongs to the Military Corps of Health in the Scale of Officers.

References

1. Kanis, J.A.; McCloskey, E.V.; Johansson, H.; Cooper, C.; Rizzoli, R.; Reginster, J.-Y. European Guidance for the Diagnosis and Management of Osteoporosis in Postmenopausal Women. *Osteoporos. Int.* **2013**, *24*, 23–57. [CrossRef] [PubMed]
2. World Health Organization. *Global Age-Friendly Cities: A Guide*; World Health Organization: Geneva, Switzerland, 2007; ISBN 9241547308.
3. Azagra, R.; López-Expósito, F.; Martin-Sánchez, J.C.; Aguyé, A.; Moreno, N.; Cooper, C.; Díez-Pérez, A.; Dennison, E.M. Changing Trends in the Epidemiology of Hip Fracture in Spain. *Osteoporos. Int.* **2014**, *25*, 1267–1274. [CrossRef] [PubMed]
4. Ekegren, C.L.; Edwards, E.R.; Page, R.; Hau, R.; De Steiger, R.; Bucknill, A.; Liew, S.; Oppy, A.; Gabbe, B.J. Twelve-Month Mortality and Functional Outcomes in Hip Fracture Patients under 65 Years of Age. *Injury* **2016**, *47*, 2182–2188. [CrossRef]
5. Vochteloo, A.J.H.; Moerman, S.; Tuinebreijer, W.E.; Maier, A.B.; de Vries, M.R.; Bloem, R.M.; Nelissen, R.G.H.H.; Pilot, P. More than Half of Hip Fracture Patients Do Not Regain Mobility in the First Postoperative Year. *Geriatr. Gerontol. Int.* **2013**, *13*, 334–341. [CrossRef] [PubMed]
6. Pioli, G.; Lauretani, F.; Pellicciotti, F.; Pignedoli, P.; Bendini, C.; Davoli, M.L.; Martini, E.; Zagatti, A.; Giordano, A.; Nardelli, A.; et al. Modifiable and Non-Modifiable Risk Factors Affecting Walking Recovery after Hip Fracture. *Osteoporos. Int.* **2016**, *27*, 2009–2016. [CrossRef] [PubMed]
7. Mahoney, F.I. Functional Evaluation: The Barthel Index. *Md. State Med. J.* **1965**, *14*, 61–65.
8. Baztán, J.J.; del Molino, J.P.; Alarcón, T.; Cristóbal, E.S.; Izquierdo, G. Índice de Barthel: Instrumento Válido Para La Valoración Functional de Pacientes Con Enfermedad Cerebrovascular. *Rev. Esp. Geriatr. Gerontol.* **1993**, *28*, 32–40.
9. Tinetti, M.E. Performance-Oriented Assessment of Mobility Problems in Elderly Patients. *J. Am. Geriatr. Soc.* **1986**, *34*, 119–126. [CrossRef]
10. Foss, N.B.; Kristensen, M.T.; Kehlet, H. Prediction of Postoperative Morbidity, Mortality and Rehabilitation in Hip Fracture Patients: The Cumulated Ambulation Score. *Clin. Rehabil.* **2006**, *20*, 701–708. [CrossRef]

11. Kristensen, M.T.; Andersen, L.; Bech-Jensen, R.; Moos, M.; Hovmand, B.; Ekdahl, C.; Kehlet, H. High Intertester Reliability of the Cumulated Ambulation Score for the Evaluation of Basic Mobility in Patients with Hip Fracture. *Clin. Rehabil.* **2009**, *23*, 1116–1123. [CrossRef]
12. Ottenbacher, K.J.; Hsu, Y.; Granger, C.V.; Fiedler, R.C. The Reliability of the Functional Independence Measure: A Quantitative Review. *Arch. Phys. Med. Rehabil.* **1996**, *77*, 1226–1232. [CrossRef]
13. Holden, M.K.; Gill, K.M.; Magliozzi, M.R.; Nathan, J.; Piehl-Baker, L. Clinical Gait Assessment in the Neurologically Impaired: Reliability and Meaningfulness. *Phys. Ther.* **1984**, *64*, 35–40. [CrossRef] [PubMed]
14. Holden, M.K.; Gill, K.M.; Magliozzi, M.R. Gait Assessment for Neurologically Impaired Patients: Standards for Outcome Assessment. *Phys. Ther.* **1986**, *66*, 1530–1539. [CrossRef] [PubMed]
15. Moreno, J.A.; Garcia, I.; Serra, J.A.; Nunez, C.; Bellon, J.M.; Alvarez, A. Comparative Study of Two Rehabilitation Models in Hip Fracture. *Rehabilitación* **2006**, *40*, 123. [CrossRef]
16. Takahashi, A.; Naruse, H.; Kitade, I.; Shimada, S.; Tsubokawa, M.; Kokubo, Y.; Matsumine, A. Functional Outcomes after the Treatment of Hip Fracture. *PLoS ONE* **2020**, *15*, e0236652. [CrossRef]
17. Handoll, H.H.G.; Cameron, I.D.; Mak, J.C.S.; Panagoda, C.E.; Finnegan, T.P. Multidisciplinary Rehabilitation for Older People with Hip Fractures. *Cochrane Database Syst. Rev.* **2021**. [CrossRef] [PubMed]
18. Jaatinen, R.; Luukkaala, T.; Hongisto, M.T.; Kujala, M.A.; Nuotio, M.S. Factors Associated with and 1-Year Outcomes of Fear of Falling in a Geriatric Post-Hip Fracture Assessment. *Aging Clin. Exp. Res.* **2022**, 1–10. [CrossRef]
19. Frandsen, C.F.; Stilling, M.; Glassou, E.N.; Hansen, T.B. The Majority of Community-Dwelling Hip Fracture Patients Return to Independent Living with Minor Increase in Care Needs: A Prospective Cohort Study. *Arch. Orthop. Trauma Surg.* **2022**, 1–10. [CrossRef]
20. Xu, B.Y.; Yan, S.; Low, L.L.; Vasanwala, F.F.; Low, S.G. Predictors of Poor Functional Outcomes and Mortality in Patients with Hip Fracture: A Systematic Review. *BMC Musculoskelet. Disord.* **2019**, *20*, 568. [CrossRef]
21. Ju, J.; Zhang, P.; Jiang, B. Risk Factors for Functional Outcomes of the Elderly with Intertrochanteric Fracture: A Retrospective Cohort Study. *Orthop. Surg.* **2019**, *11*, 643–652. [CrossRef]
22. Meng, D.; Bai, X.; Wu, H.; Yao, S.; Ren, P.; Bai, X.; Lu, C.; Song, Z. Patient and Perioperative Factors Influencing the Functional Outcomes and Mortality in Elderly Hip Fractures. *J. Investig. Surg.* **2021**, *34*, 262–269. [CrossRef] [PubMed]
23. INE. Población Por Provincias y Sexo. 2852. Available online: https://www.ine.es/jaxiT3/Tabla.htm?t=2852 (accessed on 13 June 2022).
24. Johansen, A.; Tsang, C.; Boulton, C.; Wakeman, R.; Moppett, I. Understanding Mortality Rates after Hip Fracture Repair Using ASA Physical Status in the National Hip Fracture Database. *Anaesthesia* **2017**, *72*, 961–966. [CrossRef] [PubMed]
25. Pfeiffer, E. A Short Portable Mental Status Questionnaire for the Assessment of Organic Brain Deficit in Elderly Patients. *J. Am. Geriatr. Soc.* **1975**, *23*, 433–441. [CrossRef] [PubMed]
26. Cornwall, R.; Gilbert, M.S.; Koval, K.J.; Strauss, E.; Siu, A.L. Functional Outcomes and Mortality Vary among Different Types of Hip Fractures: A Function of Patient Characteristics. *Clin. Orthop. Relat. Res.* **2004**, *425*, 64–71. [CrossRef]
27. Dubljanin-Raspopović, E.; Marković-Denić, L.; Matanović, D.; Grajić, M.; Krstić, N.; Bumbaširević, M. Is Pre-Fracture Functional Status Better than Cognitive Level in Predicting Short-Term Outcome of Elderly Hip Fracture Patients? *Arch. Med. Sci. AMS* **2012**, *8*, 115. [CrossRef]
28. Maggi, S.; Siviero, P.; Wetle, T.; Besdine, R.W.; Saugo, M.; Crepaldi, G.F. A Multicenter Survey on Profile of Care for Hip Fracture: Predictors of Mortality and Disability. *Osteoporos. Int.* **2010**, *21*, 223–231. [CrossRef]
29. Ganczak, M.; Chrobrowski, K.; Korzeń, M. Predictors of a Change and Correlation in Activities of Daily Living after Hip Fracture in Elderly Patients in a Community Hospital in Poland: A Six-Month Prospective Cohort Study. *Int. J. Environ. Res. Public Health* **2018**, *15*, 95. [CrossRef]
30. Siebens, H.C.; Sharkey, P.; Aronow, H.U.; Horn, S.D.; Munin, M.C.; DeJong, G.; Smout, R.J.; Radnay, C.S. Outcomes and Weight-Bearing Status during Rehabilitation after Arthroplasty for Hip Fractures. *PM&R* **2012**, *4*, 548–555.
31. Ariza-Vega, P.; Jiménez-Moleón, J.J.; Kristensen, M.T. Non-Weight-Bearing Status Compromises the Functional Level up to 1 Yr after Hip Fracture Surgery. *Am. J. Phys. Med. Rehabil.* **2014**, *93*, 641–648. [CrossRef]
32. Pajulammi, H.M.; Pihlajamäki, H.K.; Luukkaala, T.H.; Nuotio, M.S. Pre-and Perioperative Predictors of Changes in Mobility and Living Arrangements after Hip Fracture—A Population-Based Study. *Arch. Gerontol. Geriatr.* **2015**, *61*, 182–189. [CrossRef]
33. Orive, M.; Anton-Ladislao, A.; García-Gutiérrez, S.; Las Hayas, C.; González, N.; Zabala, J.; Quintana, J.M. Prospective Study of Predictive Factors of Changes in Pain and Hip Function after Hip Fracture among the Elderly. *Osteoporos. Int.* **2016**, *27*, 527–536. [CrossRef] [PubMed]
34. Lieberman, D.; Friger, M.; Lieberman, D. Rehabilitation Outcome Following Hip Fracture Surgery in Elderly Diabetics: A Prospective Cohort Study of 224 Patients. *Disabil. Rehabil.* **2007**, *29*, 339–345. [CrossRef] [PubMed]
35. Kristensen, M.T.; Kehlet, H. Most Patients Regain Prefracture Basic Mobility after Hip Fracture Surgery in a Fast-Track Programme. *Dan. Med. J.* **2012**, *59*, A4447.
36. Semel, J.; Gray, J.M.; Ahn, H.J.; Nasr, H.; Chen, J.J. Predictors of Outcome Following Hip Fracture Rehabilitation. *PM&R* **2010**, *2*, 799–805.
37. Luk, J.K.H.; Chiu, P.K.C.; Tam, S.; Chu, L.W. Relationship between Admission Albumin Levels and Rehabilitation Outcomes in Older Patients. *Arch. Gerontol. Geriatr.* **2011**, *53*, 84–89. [CrossRef]

38. Kristensen, M.T.; Foss, N.B.; Ekdahl, C.; Kehlet, H. Prefracture Functional Level Evaluated by the New Mobility Score Predicts In-Hospital Outcome after Hip Fracture Surgery. *Acta Orthop.* **2010**, *81*, 296–302. [CrossRef]
39. Tan, A.K.H.; Taiju, R.; Menon, E.B.; Koh, G.C. Postoperated Hip Fracture Rehabilitation Effectiveness and Efficiency in a Community Hospital. *Ann. Acad. Med. Singap.* **2014**, *43*, 209–215. [CrossRef] [PubMed]
40. Martín-Martín, L.M.; Arroyo-Morales, M.; Sánchez-Cruz, J.J.; Valenza-Demet, G.; Valenza, M.C.; Jiménez-Moleón, J.J. Factors Influencing Performance-Oriented Mobility after Hip Fracture. *J. Aging Health* **2015**, *27*, 827–842. [CrossRef]
41. Gialanella, B.; Ferlucci, C.; Monguzzi, V.; Prometti, P. Determinants of Outcome in Hip Fracture: Role of Daily Living Activities. *Eur. J. Phys. Rehabil. Med.* **2015**, *51*, 253–260.
42. Cary Jr, M.P.; Pan, W.; Sloane, R.; Bettger, J.P.; Hoenig, H.; Merwin, E.I.; Anderson, R.A. Self-Care and Mobility Following Postacute Rehabilitation for Older Adults with Hip Fracture: A Multilevel Analysis. *Arch. Phys. Med. Rehabil.* **2016**, *97*, 760–771. [CrossRef]
43. Cohn, M.R.; Cong, G.-T.; Nwachukwu, B.U.; Patt, M.L.; Desai, P.; Zambrana, L.; Lane, J.M. Factors Associated with Early Functional Outcome after Hip Fracture Surgery. *Geriatr. Orthop. Surg. Rehabil.* **2016**, *7*, 3–8. [CrossRef]
44. Sylliaas, H.; Thingstad, P.; Wyller, T.B.; Helbostad, J.; Sletvold, O.; Bergland, A. Prognostic Factors for Self-Rated Function and Perceived Health in Patient Living at Home Three Months after a Hip Fracture. *Disabil. Rehabil.* **2012**, *34*, 1225–1231. [CrossRef]
45. Shakouri, S.K.; Eslamian, F.; Azari, B.K.; Sadeghi-Bazargani, H.; Sadeghpour, A.; Salekzamani, Y. Predictors of Functional Improvement among Patients with Hip Fracture at a Rehabilitation Ward. *Pak. J. Biol. Sci.* **2009**, *12*, 1516–1520. [CrossRef] [PubMed]
46. Press, Y.; Grinshpun, Y.; Berzak, A.; Friger, M.; Clarfield, A.M. The Effect of Co-Morbidity on the Rehabilitation Process in Elderly Patients after Hip Fracture. *Arch. Gerontol. Geriatr.* **2007**, *45*, 281–294. [CrossRef]
47. Kua, J.; Ramason, R.; Rajamoney, G.; Chong, M.S. Which Frailty Measure Is a Good Predictor of Early Post-Operative Complications in Elderly Hip Fracture Patients? *Arch. Orthop. Trauma Surg.* **2016**, *136*, 639–647. [CrossRef] [PubMed]
48. Hilmer, S.N.; Perera, V.; Mitchell, S.; Murnion, B.P.; Dent, J.; Bajorek, B.; Matthews, S.; Rolfson, D.B. The Assessment of Frailty in Older People in Acute Care. *Australas. J. Ageing* **2009**, *28*, 182–188. [CrossRef]
49. Katz, S.; Ford, A.B.; Moskowitz, R.W.; Jackson, B.A.; Jaffe, M.W. Studies of Illness in the Aged: The Index of ADL: A Standardized Measure of Biological and Psychosocial Function. *JAMA* **1963**, *185*, 914–919. [CrossRef]
50. Nouri, F.M.; Lincoln, N.B. An Extended Activities of Daily Living Scale for Stroke Patients. *Clin. Rehabil.* **1987**, *1*, 301–305. [CrossRef]
51. Lin, P.-C.; Chang, S.-Y. Functional Recovery among Elderly People One Year after Hip Fracture Surgery. *J. Nurs. Res. JNR* **2004**, *12*, 72–82. [CrossRef]
52. Thingstad, P.; Egerton, T.; Ihlen, E.F.; Taraldsen, K.; Moe-Nilssen, R.; Helbostad, J.L. Identification of Gait Domains and Key Gait Variables Following Hip Fracture. *BMC Geriatr.* **2015**, *15*, 150. [CrossRef] [PubMed]
53. Hagino, H.; Furukawa, K.; Fujiwara, S.; Okano, T.; Katagiri, H.; Yamamoto, K.; Teshima, R. Recent Trends in the Incidence and Lifetime Risk of Hip Fracture in Tottori, Japan. *Osteoporos. Int.* **2009**, *20*, 543–548. [CrossRef] [PubMed]
54. Ingemarsson, A.H.; Frandin, K.; Mellstrom, D.; Moller, M. Walking Ability and Activity Level after Hip Fracture in the Elderly–a Follow-Up. *J. Rehabil. Med.* **2003**, *35*, 76–83. [CrossRef] [PubMed]
55. Lawton, M.P.; Brody, E.M. Assessment of Older People: Self-Maintaining and Instrumental Activities of Daily Living. *Gerontologist* **1969**, *9*, 179–186. [CrossRef] [PubMed]
56. McGilton, K.S.; Chu, C.H.; Naglie, G.; van Wyk, P.M.; Stewart, S.; Davis, A.M. Factors Influencing Outcomes of Older Adults after Undergoing Rehabilitation for Hip Fracture. *J. Am. Geriatr. Soc.* **2016**, *64*, 1601–1609. [CrossRef]
57. Mariconda, M.; Costa, G.G.; Cerbasi, S.; Recano, P.; Orabona, G.; Gambacorta, M.; Misasi, M. Factors Predicting Mobility and the Change in Activities of Daily Living after Hip Fracture: A 1-Year Prospective Cohort Study. *J. Orthop. Trauma* **2016**, *30*, 71–77. [CrossRef]
58. Di Monaco, M.; Castiglioni, C.; De Toma, E.; Gardin, L.; Giordano, S.; Tappero, R. Handgrip Strength Is an Independent Predictor of Functional Outcome in Hip-Fracture Women: A Prospective Study with 6-Month Follow-Up. *Medicine* **2015**, *94*, e542. [CrossRef] [PubMed]
59. Rogmark, C.; Johnell, O. Primary Arthroplasty Is Better than Internal Fixation of Displaced Femoral Neck Fractures: A Meta-Analysis of 14 Randomized Studies with 2289 Patients. *Acta Orthop.* **2006**, *77*, 359–367. [CrossRef]
60. Tidermark, J.; Ponzer, S.; Svensson, O.; Söderqvist, A.; Törnkvist, H. Internal Fixation Compared with Total Hip Replacement for Displaced Femoral Neck Fractures in the Elderly: A Randomised, Controlled Trial. *J. Bone Jt. Surg. Br.* **2003**, *85*, 380–388. [CrossRef] [PubMed]
61. Blomfeldt, R.; Törnkvist, H.; Ponzer, S.; Söderqvist, A.; Tidermark, J. Displaced Femoral Neck Fracture: Comparison of Primary Total Hip Replacement with Secondary Replacement after Failed Internal Fixation: A 2-Year Follow-up of 84 Patients. *Acta Orthop.* **2006**, *77*, 638–643. [CrossRef]
62. Blomfeldt, R.; Törnkvist, H.; Eriksson, K.; Söderqvist, A.; Ponzer, S.; Tidermark, J. A Randomised Controlled Trial Comparing Bipolar Hemiarthroplasty with Total Hip Replacement for Displaced Intracapsular Fractures of the Femoral Neck in Elderly Patients. *J. Bone Jt. Surg. Br.* **2007**, *89*, 160–165. [CrossRef] [PubMed]
63. Uriz-Otano, F.; Uriz-Otano, J.I.; Malafarina, V. Factors Associated with Short-Term Functional Recovery in Elderly People with a Hip Fracture. Influence of Cognitive Impairment. *J. Am. Med. Dir. Assoc.* **2015**, *16*, 215–220. [CrossRef] [PubMed]

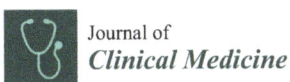

Article

Sarcopenia Is an Independent Risk Factor for Subsequent Osteoporotic Vertebral Fractures Following Percutaneous Cement Augmentation in Elderly Patients

Shira Lidar †, Khalil Salame †, Michelle Chua, Morsi Khashan, Dror Ofir, Alon Grundstein, Uri Hochberg, Zvi Lidar and Gilad J. Regev *

Department of Neurosurgery, Tel-Aviv Sourasky Medical Center, Sackler Faculty of Medicine, Tel Aviv University, Tel Aviv 6423906, Israel
* Correspondence: giladre@tlvmc.gov.il; Tel.: +972-3-697-4134
† These authors contributed equally to this work.

Abstract: Introduction: Subsequent osteoporotic vertebral fractures (SOVF) are a serious complication of osteoporosis that can lead to spinal deformity, chronic pain and disability. Several risk factors have been previously identified for developing SOVF. However, there are conflicting reports regarding the association between sarcopenia and multiple vertebral compression fractures. As such, the goal of this study was to investigate whether sarcopenia is an independent risk factor of SOVF. **Methods:** This was a retrospective case–control study of elderly patients who underwent percutaneous vertebral augmentation (PVA) due to a new osteoporotic vertebral compression fracture (OVCF). Collected data included: age, sex, BMI, steroid treatment, fracture level and type, presence of kyphosis at the level of the fracture and bone mineral density (BMD). Identification of SVOFs was based on clinical notes and imaging corroborating the presence of a new fracture. Sarcopenia was measured using the normalized psoas muscle total cross-sectional area (nCSA) at the L4 level. **Results:** Eighty-nine patients that underwent PVA were followed for a minimum of 24 months. Average age was 80.2 ± 7.1 years; 58 were female (65.2%) and 31 male (34.8%). Psoas muscle nCSA was significantly associated with age ($p = 0.031$) but not with gender ($p = 0.129$), corticosteroid treatment ($p = 0.349$), local kyphosis ($p = 0.715$), or BMD ($p = 0.724$). Sarcopenia was significantly associated with SOVF ($p = 0.039$) after controlling for age and gender. **Conclusions:** Psoas muscle nCSA can be used as a standalone diagnostic tool of sarcopenia in patients undergoing PVA. In patients undergoing PVA for OVCF, sarcopenia is an independent risk factor for SOVF.

Keywords: sarcopenia; osteoporosis; recurrent fractures; psoas; cross-sectional area

1. Introduction

Osteoporosis is a chronic bone disease characterized by a decrease in bone mass and increased risk of pathological fractures. Osteoporotic vertebral compression fractures (OVCF) are the most common complication of osteoporosis due to the high mechanical load of the spine [1]. Previous studies have found that the risk of fractures increases due to different causes such as the degree of osteopenia (loss of bone mass), presence of previous pathological fractures, and female gender [2,3].

As the population ages, osteoporotic fractures are becoming more common and identification of patients that are at increased risk of developing recurrent OVCF has gained importance. Osteoporotic vertebral compression fractures are an increasingly prevalent cause of intractable back pain, decreased mobility and prolonged bed riddance, carrying a significant socioeconomic burden [4].

Sarcopenia is a process of depletion of muscle mass in the body. Similar to osteoporosis, the incidence of this condition increases in geriatric populations and depends on various systemic conditions and diseases [5,6].

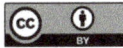

The diagnosis of sarcopenia is typically based on a combination of low handgrip strength, slow gait speed and decreased appendicular skeletal muscle mass in the upper and lower extremities as measured by dual X-ray absorptiometry (DEXA) [7,8]. Sarcopenia can also be estimated using measurement of paraspinal muscle cross sectional area (CSA) which closely correlates to the total body muscle mass [7,9–12]. Previous studies have used computed-tomography (CT) or magnetic resonance imaging (MRI) modalities to assess the total psoas CSA (tCSA) at the level of either the L3 or the L4 vertebra [13,14]. The psoas tCSA of patients can be normalized against the vertebral body area or body height. [12,15,16]. Sarcopenia can thus be estimated by low values of the normalized psoas CSA (nCSA) [16,17].

Previous studies have found that sarcopenia and frailty are correlated with increased complication rates, prolonged postoperative hospitalizations and an increase in overall mortality following major medical events such as oncological disease and major surgeries [16,17]. However, other studies did not find a clear association between poor clinical outcomes and sarcopenia following spine surgeries. [18]. Hida et al. reported that sarcopenia, measured as decreased leg skeletal mass index, was a risk factor for vertebral fractures in elderly Japanese women. In this study, the prevalence of sarcopenia was 42% and 25% in fracture and non-fracture groups, respectively [19]. On the contrary, Ashish et al. did not find that sarcopenia was an independent risk factor for recurrent fractures. However, they did find that sarcopenia was more prevalent in a subgroup of patients with previous OVCF [20]. A major complication of OVCF is subsequent osteoporotic vertebral fractures (SOVF) at adjacent levels. Development of multiple compression fractures can lead to spinal deformity, chronic pain and disability [2,21,22]. SOVFs after percutaneous vertebral augmentation are common, with an incidence of 12% to 52% of patients [23]. Therefore, the identification of risk factors may help in developing adjuvant interventions to improve clinical outcomes.

Refs. [5–17]. As such, the goal of this study was to investigate whether sarcopenia can be correlated to an increased risk of SOVFs following percutaneous vertebral augmentation.

2. Materials and Methods

2.1. Patient Population

This was a retrospective case–control study. The database of our tertiary hospital was searched for elderly patients who underwent percutaneous vertebral augmentation (PVA) due to VOFs of the thoracolumbar junction between the years 2007 and 2017 with a post-operative clinical follow-up of at least 24 months. Patients who developed SOVF and underwent a repeat single level PVA for their fracture formed the study group. Patients who did not suffer from SOVF following their first PVA formed the control group. Exclusion criteria included (1) age younger than 55 years, (2) high-energy trauma, (3) previous PVA before their enrollment to this study, (4) spinal deformities due to previous VCFs (i.e., local kyphosis), (5) pathological fractures (due to malignancy or infection), and (6) lack of preoperative CT or clinical follow-up. Data collected included: age, sex, BMI, corticosteroid treatment, fracture level, presence of kyphosis at the level of the fracture and degree of osteoporosis as measured using mean Hounsfield units (HU) values for L4 and L5 vertebrae. Identification of SVOFs was based on clinical notes and imaging corroborating the presence of a new fracture (X-rays, CT, magnetic resonance imaging or bone scintigraphy).

The study received institutional review board approval and informed consent was waived due to its retrospective nature.

2.2. Radiological Analysis

Subsequent osteoporotic vertebral fractures were assessed on preoperative thoracolumbar CT scans according to AO Spine thoracolumbar injury classification system [24]. Preoperative sagittal plane computer tomography (CT) images were used to measure local kyphosis at the level of the fracture by measuring the angle between the upper-endplate of the caudal vertebra and the lower-endplate of the superior vertebra adjacent to the facture.

Bone mineral density (BMD) on CT has been described as a tool for assessment of the risk of biomechanical complications in spinal surgery [25]. CT machines with automatic exposure control allow for easy measurement of tissue density (its linear attenuation coefficient), expressed by Hounsfield units (HU). Similar to the technique described by Schreiber et al. using HU in the cancellous bone of the vertebral body [26]. The images were analyzed using Centricity Universal Viewer, Next-gen Picture Archiving and Communications System (PACS), (GE Healthcare, Wood Dale, IL, USA). HU measurements were performed for all vertebrae included in the CT scan, at the L4 and L5 levels, using 5 mm elliptical range of interest (ROIs). The ROIs defined were restricted to cancellous bone and avoided obvious bony lesions (such as hemangiomas) and the posterior venous plexus. Average HU values were than calculated from three ROI measurements per patient in the axial plane.

Psoas measurements were obtained from axial CT images using Image J software, (U.S. National Institutes of Health, Bethesda, MD, USA) [9]. Muscles were measured bilaterally at the midlevel of the L4–5 facet. Psoas muscle tCSA was calculated as the sum of the right and left psoas muscles CSA. Vertebral body CSA was measured at the inferior endplate of L4. Psoas nCSA was then calculated as the ratio of bilateral psoas CSA to vertebral body CSA to normalize for body habitus [12,14,15,27]. Sarcopenia was defined as psoas nCSA less than the sex specific median in accordance with previous studies [15,16,28].

2.3. Statistical Methods

Statistical analysis was performed using R version 3.6.3 (R Foundation for Statistical Computing, Vienna, Austria) (http://www.r-project.org, accessed on 10 January 2022). The dependent variable is the occurrence of subsequent osteoporotic vertebral fracture. The independent variables were age, gender, fracture classification, primary PVA procedure, use of corticosteroids, local kyphosis, BMD, and psoas CSA. In univariable analysis, variables were compared between groups by Fisher's exact test for categorical variables and the Wilcoxon signed-rank test for numerical variables. Statistical significance was defined as $p < 0.05$. Multivariable analysis was performed using multiple logistic regression. Parameters were included in multivariable analysis based on clinical significance and statistical significance in univariable analysis.

3. Results

In total, 287 patients were initially identified, and 89 suitable patients remained following application of the exclusion criteria. Mean age was 80.2 ± 7.1 years; 58 were female (65.2%) and 31 male (34.8%). Patient demographics and clinical variables are presented in Table 1.

Table 1. Patient demographics and baseline characteristics.

	No Adjacent Level Fracture	Adjacent Level Fracture	p
	N = 63	N = 26	
Age (years)	80.2 ± 7.2	80.1 ± 7.1	0.986
Male	26 (41.3%)	5 (19.2%)	0.054
Female	37 (58.7%)	21 (80.8%)	
Use of corticosteroids	3 (4.8%)	2 (8.0%)	0.62

Patients' post-operative follow-up time following the first PVA ranged between 1 and 79 months. During this period, SOVFs were diagnosed in 26 (29.2%) of the patients. Sarcopenia was diagnosed in 65.4% (17) of patients with SOVF compared to 38.1% (24) of the non-sarcopenic patients. ($p = 0.5$).

In patients diagnosed with SOVF, both psoas tCSA and nCSA were lower compared to the control group. Although both parameters did not reach statistical significance, this difference was much more prominent for the nCSA ($p = 0.06$) compared to the tCSA ($p = 0.6$). No significant differences were found between the groups when comparing age, fracture classification, PVA technique, local kyphosis at the level of the fracture or chronic steroid use. Table 2

Table 2. Univariable analysis for associations between patient characteristics and adjacent level fracture.

	No Adjacent Level Fracture N = 63	Adjacent Level Fracture N = 26	p
PVA Procedure			
Kyphoplasty	38	20	
Vertboplasty	9	4	0.99
Not Available	16	2	
AO Spine Thoracolumbar Injury Classification System			
A0	10	2	
A1	27	12	
A2	2	1	0.51
A3	8	4	
Not Available	0	1	
Psoas tCSA (cm^2)	8.3 ± 2.5	7.6 ± 1.8	0.435
Psoas nCSA	0.75 ± 0.20	0.67 ± 0.14	0.064
Psoas nCSA < Q2	24 (38.1%)	17 (65.4%)	0.054
Psoas nCSA ≥ Q2	39 (61.9%)	9 (34.6%)	
Local kyphosis (degrees)	8.6 (2.0–15.6)	6.4 (−2.0–16.5)	0.642
BMD (HU)	71.9 ± 35.7	71.0 ± 41.0	0.875

PVA: percutaneous vertebral augmentation; BMD: bone mineral density; tCSA: total cross-sectional area; nCSA: normalized cross sectional area.

Psoas tCSA was significantly associated with gender ($p = 0.017$) but not with age ($p = 0.216$), use of corticosteroids ($p = 0.685$), local kyphosis ($p = 0.219$), or BMD ($p = 0.420$), whereas Psoas nCSA was significantly associated with age ($p = 0.031$) but not with gender ($p = 0.129$), use of corticosteroids ($p = 0.349$), local kyphosis ($p = 0.715$), or BMD ($p = 0.724$).

In multivariable analysis, sarcopenia was significantly associated with SOVF ($p = 0.039$) after controlling for age and gender. No other independent predictors of adjacent level fracture were identified (see Table 3).

Table 3. Multivariable analysis for independent predictors of adjacent level fracture.

	Predictor	OR (95% CI)	p
Adjacent level fracture	Psoas nCSA < Q2	2.79 (1.05–7.41)	0.039
	Age	1.00 (0.93–1.07)	0.986
	Male gender	0.35 (0.11–1.08)	0.068

nCSA normalized cross sectional area.

4. Discussion

Our study establishes sarcopenia as an independent risk factor for subsequent vertebral fragility fractures in individuals who had previous PVA for a first osteoporotic fracture. Furthermore, we found that low psoas muscle nCSA can be used as a standalone diagnostic tool for risk assessment of SOVF in patients undergoing PVA. The associations found between the psoas muscle CSA, older age and female gender reflect the higher prevalence of sarcopenia in these subgroups of patients, which is similar to findings of previous studies [27,29,30].

Several possible mechanisms can be proposed to explain why sarcopenia increases the risk of SVOF. The first is that bone and muscle interconnect not only because of their adjacent surfaces but due to their chemical and metabolic properties [30]. As such, sarcopenic patients may have relatively weaker bones that are more susceptible to fracture compared to non-sarcopenic patients. Additionally, weakness of the paraspinal and core muscles may decrease the ability of the spinal column to manage external loads of daily activities, which in turn exposes it to repeated fractures.

Previous studies have found that low bone density and alterations in the spinal sagittal balance due to an increase in kyphosis are independent risk factors for SOVF. Thus, the main strategies for preventing SOVF to date have included medications to improve bone density, correction of spinal deformity and improvement of the surgical techniques for PVA. In a recent meta-analysis, female gender, lower T-score, thoracolumbar junction fracture, intravertebral cleft, higher injected cement volume, and intradiscal cement leakage were identified as independent risk factors for adjacent level fracture, whereas BMI, use of corticosteroids and Cobb angle change were not [31]. Similarly, we did not find an association between postoperative Cobb angle or the use of corticosteroids with SOVF. Female gender was more prevalent in the SOVF group compared to the control group, nearly reaching statistical significance ($p = 0.054$). In contrast, the degree of osteopenia, as measured on CT scans, was not associated with an increased risk of SOVF. This may be explained by the fact that our measurements were not normalized for large populations, as is the case with DEXA scans measurements, in order to calculate the T-score value.

Wang et al. have previously studied the association between sarcopenia and SOVF [27]. Similar to our results, they too found that sarcopenia was an independent risk factor of SOVF in their patient cohort. This risk was further associated with lower BMD, advanced age and female sex. These authors used a patients cohort consisted solely of Chinese ethnicity who similarly underwent PVA for an osteoporotic vertebral fracture. Although the rate of SVOF in both cohorts was similar to our results (29% vs. 27%), the diagnosis of sarcopenia was two-fold more prevalent in our study population (65.4% vs. 32.8%).

This difference may be attributed to several factors, the most important of which is the method chosen for the assessment of sarcopenia. In our study, we used a simple and approachable measurement for the diagnosis of sarcopenia focusing only on the psoas muscle and adjacent vertebral body CSA, whereas Wang et al. utilized much more complex and cumbersome diagnostic criteria that used measurements of both the psoas and the posterior paraspinal muscles CSA coupled with functional parameters measured by grip strength and gait speed.

Age and sex distribution between the cohorts are additional factors that may have contributed to the large discrepancy in the prevalence of sarcopenia between the two studies. Our patients were a decade older than the patients included in Wang's study (80.2 ± 7.1 vs. 70.61 ± 8.87). Additionally, in Wang's study, the sarcopenic cohort consisted of a vast majority of females compared to the percentage of female patients in our cohort (85% vs. 65%). Lastly, the population ethnicities included in each study were different. While our population is Middle Eastern/Caucasian, Wang at al. included patients of Asian origin, who are renowned for having low bone mineral density, which may have contributed to the recurrent osteoporotic vertebral fractures more than the sarcopenia [32,33]. It may therefore be deduced that the addition of functional assessment to the imaging-based diagnosis of sarcopenia would reduce the sensitivity and enhance the specificity of the diagnosis. However, we were able to establish that, even with the use of a simpler and straightforward diagnostic tool, a clinically relevant diagnosis of sarcopenia can be achieved. This significantly increases the useability for routine preoperative assessment of patients treated for OVCF.

There are some limitations to this study. First this is a retrospective study in which some additional factors that could influence the risks for SOVF, such as body mass index (BMI), other medical conditions and routine medical treatments, were unavailable. Although we based our measurement techniques for diagnosing sarcopenia and osteoporosis on previous studies, there is still disagreement in the literature regarding the optimal method and cutoff values for the diagnosis of these conditions. As such, comparing our results to previous studies may be misleading. Lastly, our patient cohort was composed of a relatively small number of patients of Caucasian ethnicity.

Further research is required in order to validate our results with larger patient cohorts and different ethnic groups, as well as to investigate whether specific treatment strategies aimed to increase body lean mass can additionally reduce the risk of recurrent osteoporotic fractures.

5. Conclusions

The result of our study further solidified the role of sarcopenia as a risk factor for recurring fracture in osteoporotic patients. Clinical estimation of this risk assessment could be reached using a straightforward analysis of the patients' psoas muscle nCSA, without the need for additional functional tests. We recommend that this technique be used routinely in the preoperative evaluation of patients diagnosed with OVCF.

Author Contributions: Conceptualization, G.J.R.; data curation, M.C., K.S., M.K. and A.G.; formal analysis, M.C.; investigation, S.L., K.S. and D.O.; methodology, U.H.; supervision, Z.L. and K.S.; writing—original draft, S.L., Z.L., K.S. and G.J.R.; writing—review and editing, K.S. and Z.L. All authors have read and agreed to the published version of the manuscript.

Funding: This research received no external funding.

Institutional Review Board Statement: The study was conducted in accordance with the Declaration of Helsinki, and approved by the Institutional Review Board (protocol code TLV-0008-21, 16 December 2021).

Informed Consent Statement: Informed consent was obtained from all subjects involved in the study.

Data Availability Statement: Not applicable.

Conflicts of Interest: The authors declare no conflict of interest.

References

1. Lane, J.M.; Russell, L.; Khan, S.N. Osteoporosis. *Clin. Orthop. Relat. Res.* **2000**, *372*, 139–150. [CrossRef] [PubMed]
2. Park, S.-M.; Ahn, S.H.; Kim, H.-Y.; Jang, S.; Ha, Y.-C.; Lee, Y.-K.; Chung, H.-Y. Incidence and mortality of subsequent vertebral fractures: Analysis of claims data of the Korea National Health Insurance Service from 2007 to 2016. *Spine J.* **2020**, *20*, 225–233. [CrossRef] [PubMed]
3. Lu, K.; Liang, C.-L.; Hsieh, C.-H.; Tsai, Y.-D.; Chen, H.-J.; LiLiang, P.-C. Risk Factors of Subsequent Vertebral Compression Fractures after Vertebroplasty. *Pain Med.* **2012**, *13*, 376–382. [CrossRef] [PubMed]
4. Lin, H.; Bao, L.-H.; Zhu, X.-F.; Qian, C.; Chen, X.; Han, Z.-B. Analysis of recurrent fracture of a new vertebral body after percutaneous vertebroplasty in patients with osteoporosis. *Orthop. Surg.* **2010**, *2*, 119–123. [CrossRef]
5. Santilli, V.; Bernetti, A.; Mangone, M.; Paoloni, M. Clinical definition of sarcopenia. *Clin. Cases Miner Bone Metab.* **2014**, *11*, 177–180. [CrossRef]
6. Tsekoura, M.; Kastrinis, A.; Katsoulaki, M.; Billis, E.; Gliatis, J. Sarcopenia and Its Impact on Quality of Life. *GeNeDis 2017*, *2016*, 213–218. [CrossRef]
7. Cooper, C.; Dere, W.; Evans, W.; Kanis, J.A.; Rizzoli, R.; Sayer, A.A.; Sieber, C.C.; Kaufman, J.-M.; Van Kan, G.A.; Boonen, S.; et al. Frailty and sarcopenia: Definitions and outcome parameters. *Osteoporos. Int.* **2012**, *23*, 1839–1848. [CrossRef]
8. Cruz-Jentoft, A.J.; Baeyens, J.P.; Bauer, J.M.; Boirie, Y.; Cederholm, T.; Landi, F.; Martin, F.C.; Michel, J.-P.; Rolland, Y.; Schneider, S.M.; et al. Sarcopenia: European consensus on definition and diagnosis: Report of the European Working Group on Sarcopenia in Older People. *Age Ageing* **2010**, *39*, 412–423. [CrossRef]
9. Fortin, M.; Battié, M.C. Quantitative Paraspinal Muscle Measurements: Inter-Software Reliability and Agreement Using OsiriX and ImageJ. *Phys. Ther.* **2012**, *92*, 853–864. [CrossRef]
10. Zuckerman, J.; Ades, M.; Mullie, L.; Trnkus, A.; Morin, J.-F.; Langlois, Y.; Ma, F.; Levental, M.; Morais, J.A.; Afilalo, J. Psoas Muscle Area and Length of Stay in Older Adults Undergoing Cardiac Operations. *Ann. Thorac. Surg.* **2017**, *103*, 1498–1504. [CrossRef]
11. Zakaria, H.M.; Schultz, L.; Mossa-Basha, F.; Griffith, B.; Chang, V. Morphometrics as a predictor of perioperative morbidity after lumbar spine surgery. *Neurosurg. Focus* **2015**, *39*, E5. [CrossRef] [PubMed]
12. Bokshan, S.L.; Han, A.L.; DePasse, J.M.; Eltorai, A.E.M.; Marcaccio, S.E.; Palumbo, M.A.; Daniels, A.H. Effect of Sarcopenia on Postoperative Morbidity and Mortality after Thoracolumbar Spine Surgery. *Orthopedics* **2016**, *39*, e1159–e1164. [CrossRef] [PubMed]

13. Druckmann, I.; Yashar, H.; Schwartz, D.; Schwartz, I.F.; Goykhman, Y.; Ben-Bassat, O.K.; Baruch, R.; Tzadok, R.; Shashar, M.; Cohen-Hagai, K.; et al. Presence of Sarcopenia before Kidney Transplantation Is Associated with Poor Outcomes. *Am. J. Nephrol.* **2022**, *53*, 427–434. [CrossRef] [PubMed]
14. Gakhar, H.; Dhillon, A.; Blackwell, J.; Hussain, K.; Bommireddy, R.; Klezl, Z.; Williams, J. Study investigating the role of skeletal muscle mass estimation in metastatic spinal cord compression. *Eur. Spine J.* **2015**, *24*, 2150–2155. [CrossRef]
15. Ebbeling, L.; Grabo, D.J.; Shashaty, M.; Dua, R.; Sonnad, S.S.; Sims, C.A.; Pascual, J.L.; Schwab, C.W.; Holena, D.N. Psoas:lumbar vertebra index: Central sarcopenia independently predicts morbidity in elderly trauma patients. *Eur. J. Trauma Emerg. Surg.* **2013**, *40*, 57–65. [CrossRef]
16. Chua, M.; Hochberg, U.; Regev, G.; Ophir, D.; Salame, K.; Lidar, Z.; Khashan, M. Gender differences in multifidus fatty infiltration, sarcopenia and association with preoperative pain and functional disability in patients with lumbar spinal stenosis. *Spine J.* **2021**, *22*, 58–63. [CrossRef]
17. Zhang, S.; Tan, S.; Jiang, Y.; Xi, Q.; Meng, Q.; Zhuang, Q.; Han, Y.; Sui, X.; Wu, G. Sarcopenia as a predictor of poor surgical and oncologic outcomes after abdominal surgery for digestive tract cancer: A prospective cohort study. *Clin. Nutr.* **2018**, *38*, 2881–2888. [CrossRef]
18. Flexman, A.M.; Street, J.; Charest-Morin, R. The impact of frailty and sarcopenia on patient outcomes after complex spine surgery. *Curr. Opin. Anaesthesiol.* **2019**, *32*, 609–615. [CrossRef]
19. Hida, T.; Shimokata, H.; Sakai, Y.; Ito, S.; Matsui, Y.; Takemura, M.; Kasai, T.; Ishiguro, N.; Harada, A. Sarcopenia and sarcopenic leg as potential risk factors for acute osteoporotic vertebral fracture among older women. *Eur. Spine J.* **2015**, *25*, 3424–3431. [CrossRef]
20. Anand, A.; Shetty, A.P.; Renjith, K.R.; KS, S.V.A.; Kanna, R.M.; Rajasekaran, S. Does Sarcopenia Increase the Risk for Fresh Vertebral Fragility Fractures?: A Case-Control Study. *Asian Spine J.* **2020**, *14*, 17–24. [CrossRef]
21. Van Der Jagt-Willems, H.C.; De Groot, M.H.; Van Campen, J.P.C.M.; Lamoth, C.J.C.; Lems, W.F. Associations between vertebral fractures, increased thoracic kyphosis, a flexed posture and falls in older adults: A prospective cohort study. *BMC Geriatr.* **2015**, *15*, 34. [CrossRef] [PubMed]
22. Kim, M.-H.; Lee, A.S.; Min, S.-H.; Yoon, S.-H. Risk Factors of New Compression Fractures in Adjacent Vertebrae after Percutaneous Vertebroplasty. *Asian Spine J.* **2011**, *5*, 180–187. [CrossRef]
23. Bae, J.S.; Park, J.H.; Kim, K.J.; Kim, H.-S.; Jang, I.-T. Analysis of Risk Factors for Secondary New Vertebral Compression Fracture Following Percutaneous Vertebroplasty in Patients with Osteoporosis. *World Neurosurg.* **2017**, *99*, 387–394. [CrossRef]
24. Vaccaro, A.R.; Oner, F.; Kepler, C.K.; Dvorak, M.; Schnake, K.; Bellabarba, C.; Reinhold, M.; Aarabi, B.; Kandziora, F.; Chapman, J.; et al. AOSpine Thoracolumbar Spine Injury Classification System. *Spine* **2013**, *38*, 2028–2037. [CrossRef] [PubMed]
25. Schmidt, T.; Ebert, K.; Rolvien, T.; Oehler, N.; Lohmann, J.; Papavero, L.; Kothe, R.; Amling, M.; Barvencik, F.; Mussawy, H. A retrospective analysis of bone mineral status in patients requiring spinal surgery. *BMC Musculoskelet. Disord.* **2018**, *19*, 53. [CrossRef] [PubMed]
26. Schreiber, J.J.; Hughes, A.P.; Taher, F.; Girardi, F.P. An Association Can Be Found between Hounsfield Units and Success of Lumbar Spine Fusion. *HSS Journal®: Musculoskelet. J. Hosp. Spéc. Surg.* **2013**, *10*, 25–29. [CrossRef]
27. Wang, W.-F.; Lin, C.-W.; Xie, C.-N.; Liu, H.-T.; Zhu, M.-Y.; Huang, K.-L.; Teng, H.-L. The association between sarcopenia and osteoporotic vertebral compression refractures. *Osteoporos. Int.* **2019**, *30*, 2459–2467. [CrossRef]
28. Kim, Y.-Y.; Rhyu, K.-W. Recompression of vertebral body after balloon kyphoplasty for osteoporotic vertebral compression fracture. *Eur. Spine J.* **2010**, *19*, 1907–1912. [CrossRef]
29. Iolascon, G.; Giamattei, M.T.; Moretti, A.; Di Pietro, G.; Gimigliano, F. Sarcopenia in women with vertebral fragility fractures. *Aging Clin. Exp. Res.* **2013**, *25*, 129–131. [CrossRef]
30. Hirschfeld, H.P.; Kinsella, R.; Duque, G. Osteosarcopenia: Where bone, muscle, and fat collide. *Osteoporos. Int.* **2017**, *28*, 2781–2790. [CrossRef]
31. Zhang, Z.-L.; Yang, J.-S.; Hao, D.-J.; Liu, T.-J.; Jing, Q.-M. Risk Factors for New Vertebral Fracture after Percutaneous Vertebroplasty for Osteoporotic Vertebral Compression Fractures. *Clin. Interv. Aging* **2021**, *ume16*, 1193–1200. [CrossRef] [PubMed]
32. Wang, W.; Sun, Z.; Li, W.; Chen, Z. The effect of paraspinal muscle on functional status and recovery in patients with lumbar spinal stenosis. *J. Orthop. Surg. Res.* **2020**, *15*, 1–6. [CrossRef] [PubMed]
33. Morin, S.N.; Berger, C.; Liu, W.; Prior, J.C.; Cheung, A.M.; Hanley, D.A.; Boyd, S.K.; Wong, A.K.O.; Papaioannou, A.; Rahme, E.; et al. Differences in fracture prevalence and in bone mineral density between Chinese and White Canadians: The Canadian Multicentre Osteoporosis Study (CaMos). *Arch. Osteoporos.* **2020**, *15*, 1–14. [CrossRef] [PubMed]

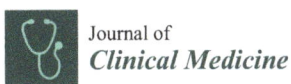

Article

Prevalence of Sleep Disturbance and Its Risk Factors in Patients Who Undergo Surgical Treatment for Degenerative Spinal Disease: A Nationwide Study of 106,837 Patients

Jihye Kim [1], Min Seong Kang [2] and Tae-Hwan Kim [2,*]

[1] Division of Infection, Department of Pediatrics, Kangdong Sacred Heart Hospital, Hallym University College of Medicine, 150 Seongan-ro, Seoul 05355, Korea
[2] Spine Center, Department of Orthopedics, Hallym University Sacred Heart Hospital, Hallym University College of Medicine, 22 Gwanpyeong-ro, Anyang 14068, Korea
* Correspondence: paragon0823@gmail.com; Tel.: +82-31-380-6000; Fax: +82-31-380-6008

Abstract: Spinal surgeons have not yet considered sleep disturbance an area of concern; thus, a comprehensive study investigating the epidemiology of sleep disturbance in patients with degenerative spinal disease is yet to be conducted. This study aimed to fill this research gap by investigating the epidemiology of sleep disturbance in patients who underwent spinal surgery for degenerative spinal disease and identifying the associated risk factors. This nationwide, population-based, cohort study, used data from January 2016 and December 2018 from the Korea Health Insurance Review and Assessment Service database. This study included 106,837 patients older than 19 years who underwent surgery for degenerative spinal disease. Sleep disorder was initially defined as a diagnosis of a sleep disorder made within one year before the index surgery and identified using the International Classification of Diseases, 10th revision, codes F51 and G47 (main analysis). We also investigated the use of sleep medication within 90 days prior to the index surgery, which was the target outcome of the sensitivity analysis. The prevalence of sleep disturbance was precisely investigated according to various factors, including demographics, comorbidities, and spinal region. Logistic regression analysis was performed to identify the independent factors associated with sleep disturbance. The results of the statistical analysis were validated using sensitivity analysis and bootstrap sampling. The prevalence of sleep disorder was 5.5% (n = 5847) in our cohort. During the 90 days before spinal surgery, sleep medication was used for over four weeks in 5.5% (n = 5864) and over eight weeks in 3.8% (n = 4009) of the cohort. Although the prevalence of sleep disturbance differed according to the spinal region, the spinal region was not a significant risk factor for sleep disorder in multivariable analysis. We also identified four groups of independent risk factors: (1) Age, (2) other demographic factors and general comorbidities, (3) neuropsychiatric disorders, and (4) osteoarthritis of the extremities. Our results, including the prevalence rates of sleep disturbance in the entire patient population and the identified risk factors, provide clinicians with a reasonable reference for evaluating sleep disturbance in patients with degenerative spinal disease and future research.

Keywords: sleep disturbance; sleep disorder; sleep medication; epidemiology; prevalence; surgery; spine; degenerative spinal disease; risk factors

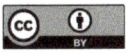

1. Introduction

Sleep plays an essential role in both cognitive and physiologic function [1,2]. Therefore, sleep disturbance can not only have detrimental effects on quality of life, but also potentially cause mental and physical illness, eventually increasing the risk of mortality [3,4]. Sleep disturbance is prevalent globally, and nationwide studies have revealed that more than 20% of the general population suffers from sleep disturbance [5–7].

Chronic pain is one of the major risk factors associated with sleep disturbance [8,9], and sleep disturbance has been reported to be prevalent in patients with degenerative joint diseases of the extremities [10,11]. Recent studies have revealed that sleep disturbance is also prevalent in patients with degenerative spinal disease, with a reported prevalence ranging from 11 to 74% [12–15]. Interestingly, studies have identified that in patients with degenerative spinal disease, the radiologic severity of degeneration is a stronger predictor of sleep disturbance than overall pain intensity [12,13]. In addition, the radiologic indices associated with sleep disturbance differed according to the spinal regions. For example, in patients with lumbar stenosis, sleep disturbance was more associated with foraminal-type stenosis than central-type stenosis [13]. In contrast, in patients with cervical myelopathy, central-type stenosis was more closely associated with sleep disturbance than foraminal-type stenosis [12]. From these results, the authors deduced that the mechanisms of sleep disturbance may differ according to the spinal regions and that sleep disturbance in patients with cervical myelopathy might be caused by the same factors causing sleep disturbance in patients with spinal cord injury, such as symptoms associated with cord injury, including pain, sleep breathing disorder, and sleep movement disorder, as well as inhibition of the neural pathway for endogenous melatonin production passing through the cervical spinal cord.

Considering that the radiologic degree of spinal degeneration is closely associated with sleep disturbance, sleep disturbance is expected to be particularly prevalent in patients who are considering surgical treatment for degenerative spinal disease, which could have influenced their choice to undergo surgical treatment. However, sleep disturbance has hitherto not been a matter of concern to spinal surgeons, and few studies have investigated the epidemiology of sleep disturbance in patients who underwent spinal surgery. Although several recent studies have been conducted for this purpose, they had the following limitations [12–14,16,17]. First, most of these studies are single-center studies with a limited number of patients. Thus, the prevalence rates of sleep disturbance and the estimates for their risk factors can be biased, reflecting the skewness of their study samples. Second, because of the small sample size, a comprehensive epidemiologic analysis including all spinal regions and considering various morbidities that are prevalent in patients with degenerative spinal disease could not be performed. This information would be very useful not only for clinicians, but also for researchers to understand the etiology or mechanisms of sleep disturbance in patients with degenerative spinal disease.

Our study has two distinct research purposes. First, by using a nationwide database that included the entire population, we aimed to investigate the epidemiology of sleep disturbance in patients who underwent spinal surgery for degenerative spinal disease. Based on the large dataset, the epidemiology of sleep disturbance was precisely investigated according to various clinical profiles, including demographics, various comorbidities, and spinal regions. We particularly focused on investigating the prevalence of sleep disturbance according to spinal regions, which has not been reported in previous studies due to the limited number of cases. Second, using this information, we attempted to identify independent risk factors for their sleep disturbance.

2. Patients and Methods

2.1. Database

In this nationwide population-based cohort study, data were obtained from the Korea Health Insurance Review and Assessment Service (HIRA) database. The HIRA database contains all inpatient and outpatient data from hospitals and community clinics in Korea, allowing for a nationwide cohort study that includes the entire population. Diagnostic codes were assigned according to the modified version of the 10th revision of the International Classification of Diseases (ICD-10) and the seventh revision of the Korean Classification of Diseases. Drug use under diagnosis was identified using anatomical therapeutic chemical (ATC) codes and the HIRA general name codes. This study was approved by the Institutional Review Board of our hospital (IRB No. 2020-03-009-001).

2.2. Study Patients

We included patients aged >19 years who underwent surgical treatment (index surgery) for degenerative spinal disease between 1 January 2016 and 31 December 2018 (Figure 1). Degenerative spinal diseases were identified using the following codes: Spinal stenosis (M48.0), spondylolisthesis (M43.1), spondylolysis (M43.0), other spondylosis (M47.1 and M47.2), and cervical disc disorder (M50).

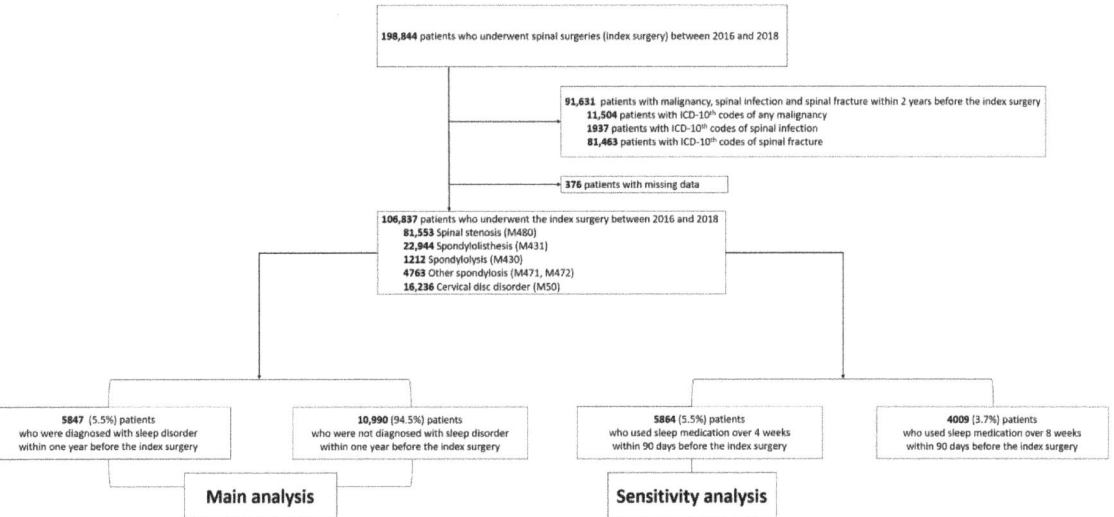

Figure 1. Enrollment of study patients.

The spinal region of surgical treatment was identified using the following electronic data interchange codes: Cervical surgery including cervical decompressive (N2491, N2492, N0491, N1491, N1497, N2497) and fusion (N2461, N0464, N2463, N2467, N2468, N0467, N2469) surgery; thoracic surgery including thoracic decompressive (N1492, N1498, N2498) and fusion surgery (N0465, N2464, N2465, N2466, N0468), and lumbar surgery including lumbar decompressive (N0492, N1493, N1499, N2499) and fusion (N0466, N1466, N0469, N1460, N1469, N2470) surgery. We excluded patients who were treated under the ICD-10 codes of spinal infection (A18.00, M46, M49, G06, and T814), spine fractures (S1, S2, S3, T02.0, T02.1, T02.7, T08, T09, T91, M48.3, M48.4, and M48.5), or malignancy (C) within two years before the index surgery (Figure 1).

2.3. Definitions of Sleep Disturbance

Sleep disturbance in the cohort was identified using the following two methods (Figure 2). First, sleep disturbance was primarily defined as a diagnosis of sleep disorder within one year before the index surgery. Preoperative sleep disorder was identified using the following diagnostic codes: Nonorganic sleep disorders (F51), and sleep disorders (G47). This was then used as the target outcome in the main analysis. Second, in the sensitivity analysis performed to internally validate our results, sleep disturbance was additionally defined by the use of sleep medication during the 90 days before the index surgery. Sleep medication was defined as drugs currently available for insomnia approved by the Korean Food and Drug Administration, including flurazepam, triazolam, flunitrazepam, brotizolam, zolpidem, eszopiclone, doxepin, doxylamine, and diphenhydramine [18]. Among them, antihistamines, including doxylamine and diphenhydramine, were excluded. The ATC and HIRA general name codes for sleep medication are presented in Supplementary Table S1. Data regarding preoperative sleep medication were used as the target outcome in the sensitivity analysis.

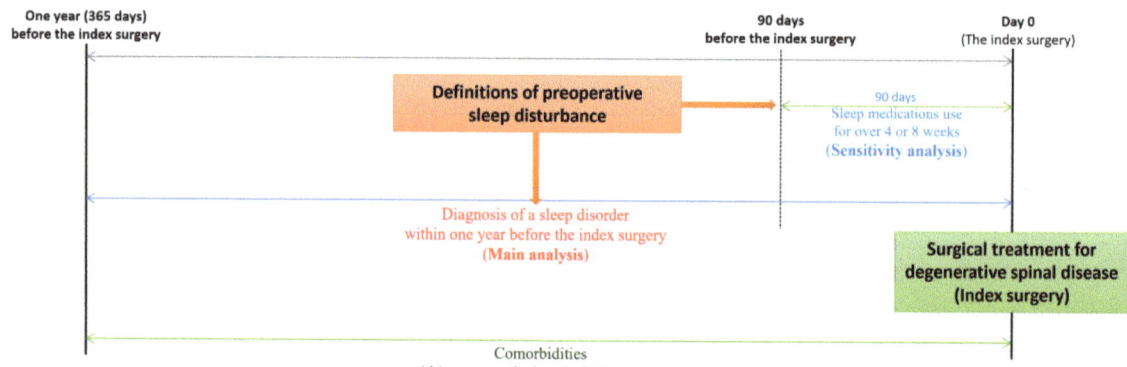

Figure 2. Definitions of sleep disturbance in the main and sensitivity analyses. The term "sleep disorder" has been used when sleep problems were identified using International Classification of Diseases, tenth revision (ICD-10) codes alone. The term "sleep disturbance" has been used when sleep problems were identified using the following two criteria: Diagnosis of a sleep disorder using ICD-10 codes and the use of sleep medication.

2.4. Factors Associated with Sleep Disturbance

Demographic data at the time of surgery were retrieved. Medical conditions diagnosed in the year before the index surgery were identified using ICD-10 codes (Supplementary Table S2) and evaluated using the Charlson comorbidity index (CCI) [19–21]. We also investigated neuropsychiatric disorders that were possibly associated with sleep disturbance using ICD-10 codes (Supplementary Table S2). The diagnosis of depression was confirmed using the ATC codes for the use of antidepressants (N06A, Supplementary Table S3).

We also evaluated osteoarthritis of the extremities using a validated method in our database [22]. Patients with osteoarthritis of the extremities were identified using the ICD-10 codes for osteoarthritis (M15 to M19) with corresponding radiographs of the extremities. The HIRA electronic data interchange codes for X-rays of the extremities are presented in Supplementary Table S4.

2.5. Statistical Analysis

Data are reported as the mean ± standard deviation for numerical variables, and as numbers and frequencies (%) for categorical variables. The prevalence of sleep disturbance was precisely presented according to the factors associated with sleep disturbance and the spinal regions. For the main analysis, sleep disturbance, defined as the diagnosis of a sleep disorder within one year before the index surgery, was chosen as the dependent variable. Logistic regression analysis was performed to identify independent factors associated with sleep disturbance, with adjustment for variables identified to be significant in the univariable analysis ($p < 0.05$).

Our statistical model was validated using the following procedures. First, a sensitivity analysis was performed to validate risk factors. Sleep disturbance was defined according to the use of sleep medication during the 90 days before the index surgery and was used as the dependent variable for the sensitivity analysis. Second, all estimates from the main and sensitivity analyses were validated using the bootstrap method. All estimates were internally validated with relative bias based on 1000 bootstrapped samples. Relative bias was estimated as the difference between the mean bootstrapped regression coefficient estimates and the mean parameter estimates of multivariable model divided by the mean parameter estimates of the multivariable model.

Multicollinearity between covariates was tested using a variance inflation factor. Data extraction and statistical analysis were performed using the SAS Enterprise Guide 6.1 (SAS Institute, Cary, NC, USA).

3. Results

Between 2016 and 2018, 198,844 patients underwent spinal surgery (index surgery) for degenerative spinal disease (Figure 1). Among them, we excluded patients who were treated under the ICD-10 codes of malignancy (n = 11,504), spinal infection (n = 1937), and spinal fracture (n = 81,463) within two years before the index surgery, and those who had missing data (n = 376).

A total of 106,837 patients were included in this study, with a mean age of 62.9 years and 52% (n = 55,595) being women.

3.1. Annual Prevalence of Sleep Disturbance According to the Three Definitions

Among the 106,837 patients, sleep disorders were diagnosed within one year before the index surgery in 5.5% (n = 5847, Table 1). During the 90 days before spinal surgery, sleep medication was used for over four weeks in 5.5% of the cohort (n = 5864) and over eight weeks in 3.8% (n = 4009) of the cohort. During the study period, the number of patients with preoperative sleep disorders and those who used sleep medications continuously increased (Table 1).

Table 1. Annual prevalence of sleep disturbance according to the three definitions.

Year	Spinal Surgery (n)	Patients Diagnosed with Sleep Disorder within One Year from the Index Surgery			Prevalence According to Sleep Medication during the Preexisting 90 Days					
					Over 4-Week Sleep Medication			Over 8-Week Sleep Medication		
		(n)	Incidence (%)	95% CI	(n)	Incidence (%)	95% CI	(n)	Incidence (%)	95% CI
2016	35,507	1866	5.3%	[5.0–5.5]	1839	5.2%	[4.9–5.4]	1229	3.5%	[3.3–3.7]
2017	35,459	1912	5.4%	[5.2–5.6]	1932	5.4%	[5.2–5.7]	1319	3.7%	[3.5–3.9]
2018	35,871	2069	5.8%	[5.5–6.0]	2093	5.8%	[5.6–6.1]	1461	4.1%	[3.9–4.3]
All	106,837	5847	5.5%	[5.3–5.6]	5864	5.5%	[5.4–5.6]	4009	3.8%	[3.6–3.9]

3.2. Prevalence of Sleep Disturbance According to the Baseline Characteristics and Comorbidities

Sleep disorders were common in patients of older age, female sex, urban residence, and surgery at a tertiary hospital (Table 2). The difference was most pronounced by age, and patients aged over 80 years had approximately three-fold higher chances of having sleep disturbance than those between 20 and 49 years (8.8% vs. 2.7%).

Table 2. Prevalence of sleep disturbance according to the baseline characteristics.

Variables	Categories	All	Patients Diagnosed with Sleep Disorder within One Year from the Index Surgery		Prevalence according to Sleep Medication during the Preexisting 90 days			
					Over 4-Week Sleep Medication		Over 8-Week Sleep Medication	
Number of Patients		106,837	5847	5.5%	5864	5.5%	4009	3.8%
Age	Mean ± SD	62.9 ± 11.8	66.7 ± 10.5		66.9 ± 10.3		66.6 ± 10.4	
	20–49	14,014	378	2.7%	358	2.6%	266	1.9%
	50–69	58,533	2857	4.9%	2881	4.9%	2007	3.4%
	70–79	28,671	2115	7.4%	2116	7.4%	1393	4.9%
	80+	5619	497	8.8%	509	9.1%	343	6.1%
Sex	Male	51,242	2298	4.5%	2203	4.3%	1503	2.9%
	Female	55,595	3549	6.4%	3661	6.6%	2506	4.5%
Region	Urban	88,826	4953	5.6%	4903	5.5%	3323	3.7%
	Rural	18,011	894	5.0%	961	5.3%	686	3.8%
Hospital	Tertiary	18,442	1154	6.3%	1169	6.3%	814	4.4%
	General	20,772	1257	6.1%	1537	7.4%	1072	5.2%
	Others	67,623	3436	5.1%	3158	4.7%	2123	3.1%

Patients with a sleep disorder had a slightly higher CCI score than those without it (1.56 ± 1.44 vs. 1.12 ± 1.26). However, the prevalence of sleep disorders did not show an increasing trend according to categorized CCI scores (Table 3). Conversely, patients with CCI scores ≥ 6 points had approximately one-half lower chances of having sleep disturbance than those with CCI scores ≤ 2 points (2.9% vs. 6.0%). Patients with specific comorbidity had a higher prevalence of sleep disorder than the overall prevalence (5.5%, Table 3). Sleep disorder was especially frequent in patients with neuropsychiatric comorbidities, including depressive disorder (11.8%), dementia (12.0%), Parkinson's disease (11.4%), migraine (11.9%), tension-type headache (11.4%), and other-type headache (10.9%). Diagnosis of sleep disorder was also frequent in patients with concurrent osteoarthritis of the extremities, especially in the ankle (9.1%), wrist (8.1%), and shoulder (7.9%).

Table 3. Prevalence of sleep disturbance according to comorbidities.

Variables	Categories	All		Patients Diagnosed with Sleep Disorder within One Year from the Index Surgery		Prevalence According to Sleep Medication during the Preexisting 90 Days			
						Over 4-Week Sleep Medication		Over 8-Week Sleep Medication	
Number of patients		106,837		5847	5.5%	5864	5.5%	4009	3.8%
Charlson comorbidity index score	Mean ± SD	1.14 ± 1.28		1.56 ± 1.44		1.67 ± 1.52		1.66 ± 1.54	
	0–2	75,632		4551	6.0%	4423	5.8%	3028	4.0%
	3–5	27,691		1195	4.3%	1310	4.7%	887	3.2%
	≥6	3514		101	2.9%	131	3.7%	94	2.7%
Comorbidities	Myocardial infarction	967		72	7.4%	73	7.5%	51	5.3%
	Congestive heart failure	3394		286	8.4%	314	9.3%	217	6.4%
	Peripheral vascular disease	12,062		969	8.0%	934	7.7%	644	5.3%
	Chronic pulmonary disease	24,116		1867	7.7%	1825	7.6%	1227	5.1%
	Rheumatologic disease	4010		292	7.3%	298	7.4%	198	4.9%
	Peptic ulcer disease	17,189		1341	7.8%	1331	7.7%	905	5.3%
	Liver disease Mild	6686		485	7.3%	496	7.4%	341	5.1%
	Moderate to severe	83		7	8.4%	9	10.8%	5	6.0%
	Diabetes Uncomplicated	23,105		1492	6.5%	1660	7.2%	1137	4.9%
	Complicated	6733		434	6.4%	559	8.3%	362	5.4%
	Hemiplegia or paraplegia	849		50	5.9%	70	8.2%	42	4.9%
	Renal disease	2053		179	8.7%	211	10.3%	157	7.6%
	End stage renal disease	379		39	10.3%	57	15.0%	39	10.3%
	Osteoporosis	15,495		1185	7.6%	1189	7.7%	813	5.2%
Concurrent neuropsychiatric disorders	Depressive disorder	23,921		2818	11.8%	3740	15.6%	2806	11.7%
	Cerebrovascular disease	9502		808	8.5%	971	10.2%	695	7.3%
	Dementia	1388		167	12.0%	160	11.5%	109	7.9%
	Parkinson disease	875		100	11.4%	175	20.0%	152	17.4%
	Migraine	3222		384	11.9%	356	11.0%	242	7.5%
	Tension type headache	3011		343	11.4%	329	10.9%	219	7.3%
	Other-type headache	4304		469	10.9%	449	10.4%	303	7.0%
Concurrent osteoarthritis of extremities	Shoulder	8503		674	7.9%	648	7.6%	450	5.3%
	Elbow	2276		141	6.2%	121	5.3%	86	3.8%
	Wrist	2268		183	8.1%	192	8.5%	135	6.0%
	Hip	7104		542	7.6%	531	7.5%	357	5.0%
	Knee	24,338		1828	7.5%	1898	7.8%	1274	5.2%
	Ankle	4024		368	9.1%	353	8.8%	239	5.9%

The proportions of patients who had over 4- or 8-week sleep medication during the 90 days before the index surgery were generally concordant with the proportions of those who were diagnosed with sleep disorders (Tables 2 and 3).

3.3. Prevalence of Sleep Disturbance According to Spinal Regions

The prevalence of sleep disorders was 6.9%, 5.7%, and 4.4% in patients with thoracic, lumbar, and cervical spinal lesions, respectively (Figure 3). Prevalence rates of sleep disturbance defined by the use of sleep medication were also concordant with the proportions of those who were diagnosed with a sleep disorder, and the patients who underwent thoracic spine surgery consistently showed the highest prevalence rates according to all three definitions of sleep disturbance (Figure 3).

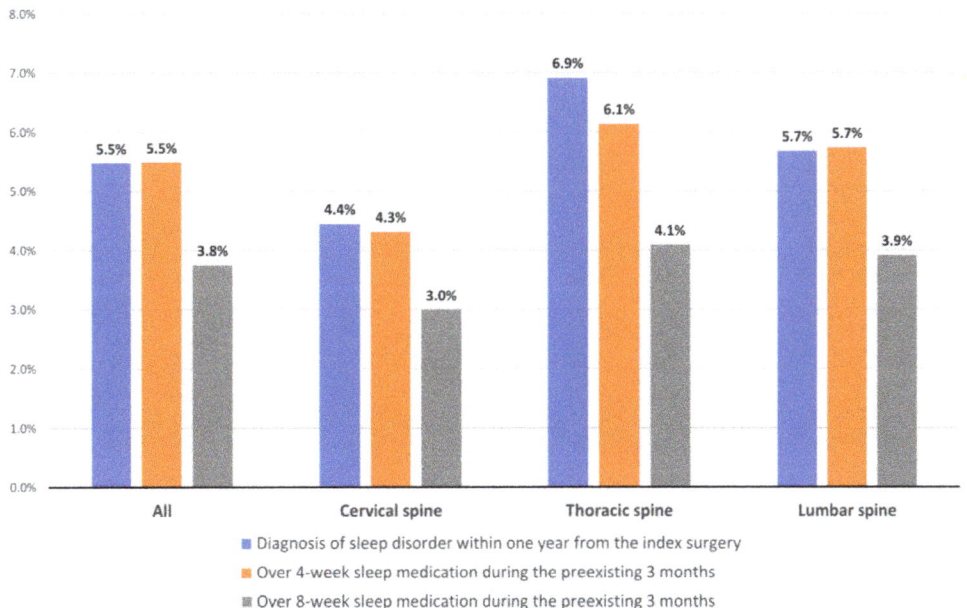

Figure 3. Prevalence of sleep disturbance by spinal region according to the three definitions.

3.4. Prevalence of Sleep Disturbance According to Concurrent Neuropsychiatric Disorders and Osteoarthritis of Extremities

The two most common types of concurrent neuropsychiatric disorders in our cohort were depressive disorder (21.8%, n = 23,921) and cerebrovascular disease (8.9%, n = 9502; Table 3), which were more common in patients with thoracic or lumbar lesions (Table 4). The prevalence of the three types of sleep disturbance according to the spinal region and concurrent neuropsychiatric disorders are presented in Table 4. The prevalence of sleep disorder in patients with a specific neuropsychiatric disorder was higher in those with a lumbar lesion than in those with a cervical lesion.

The three most common regions of concurrent osteoarthritis in our cohort were the knee (22.8%, n = 24,338), shoulder (8.0%, n = 8503), and hip (6.6%, n = 7104; Table 3). Osteoarthritis of the upper extremities was the most common in patients with a cervical lesion, and that of the lower extremities was common in patients with thoracic or lumbar lesions (Table 5). We present the prevalence of three types of sleep disturbance according to spinal region and concurrent osteoarthritis of the extremities in Table 4. The prevalence of sleep disorder in patients with concurrent osteoarthritis of the upper extremities was higher in those with lumbar lesions than in those with cervical lesions.

Table 4. Prevalence of sleep disturbance according to spinal regions and concurrent neuropsychiatric disorders.

Spinal Regions	According to Concurrent Neuropsychiatric Disorders	Cases (n) with Its Proportion (%)		Patients Diagnosed with Sleep Disorder within one Year from the Index Surgery		Prevalence According to Sleep Medication during the Preexisting 90 Days			
						Over 4-Week Sleep Medication		Over 8-Week Sleep Medication	
Cervical	All cases	18,819	(100)	837	4.4%	812	4.3%	563	3.0%
	Depressive disorder	3660	19.4%	372	10.2%	526	14.4%	403	11.0%
	Cerebrovascular disease	1380	7.3%	107	7.8%	136	9.9%	97	7.0%
	Dementia	103	0.5%	10	9.7%	14	13.6%	11	10.7%
	Parkinson disease	88	0.5%	8	9.1%	20	22.7%	17	19.3%
	Migraine	566	3.0%	60	10.6%	54	9.5%	37	6.5%
	Tension type headache	513	2.7%	49	9.6%	45	8.8%	29	5.7%
	Other-type headache	742	3.9%	71	9.6%	59	8.0%	37	5.0%
Thoracic	All cases	1027	(100)	71	6.9%	63	6.1%	42	4.1%
	Depressive disorder	271	26.4%	30	11.1%	36	13.3%	24	8.9%
	Cerebrovascular disease	127	12.4%	16	12.6%	12	9.4%	7	5.5%
	Dementia	18	1.8%	1	5.6%	0	0.0%	0	0.0%
	Parkinson disease	6	0.6%	1	16.7%	2	33.3%	2	33.3%
	Migraine	24	2.3%	2	8.3%	3	12.5%	2	8.3%
	Tension type headache	31	3.0%	3	9.7%	2	6.5%	1	3.2%
	Other-type headache	45	4.4%	3	6.7%	3	6.7%	1	2.2%
Lumbar	All cases	86,991	(100)	4939	5.7%	4989	5.7%	3404	3.9%
	Depressive disorder	19,990	23.0%	2416	12.1%	3178	15.9%	2379	11.9%
	Cerebrovascular disease	7995	9.2%	685	8.6%	823	10.3%	591	7.4%
	Dementia	1267	1.5%	156	12.3%	146	11.5%	98	7.7%
	Parkinson disease	781	0.9%	91	11.7%	153	19.6%	133	17.0%
	Migraine	2632	3.0%	322	12.2%	299	11.4%	203	7.7%
	Tension type headache	2467	2.8%	291	11.8%	282	11.4%	189	7.7%
	Other-type headache	3517	4.0%	395	11.2%	387	11.0%	265	7.5%

Table 5. Prevalence of sleep disturbance according to concurrent osteoarthritis of extremities.

Spinal Regions	Categories	Extremities	Cases (n) with Its Proportion		Patients Diagnosed with Sleep Disorder within One Year from the Index Surgery		Prevalence According to Sleep Medication during the Preexisting 90 Days			
							Over 4-Week Sleep Medication		Over 8-Week Sleep Medication	
Cervical	All cases		18,819	(100)	837	4.4%	812	4.3%	563	3.0%
	Upper extremities	Shoulder	2214	11.8%	156	7.0%	142	6.4%	101	4.6%
		Elbow	568	3.0%	25	4.4%	24	4.2%	18	3.2%
		Wrist	532	2.8%	39	7.3%	42	7.9%	27	5.1%
	Lower extremities	Hip	446	2.4%	38	8.5%	45	10.1%	29	6.5%
		Knee	2283	12.1%	155	6.8%	173	7.6%	123	5.4%
		Ankle	459	2.4%	46	10.0%	38	8.3%	31	6.8%
Thoracic	All cases		1027	(100)	71	6.9%	63	6.1%	42	4.1%
	Upper extremities	Shoulder	94	9.2%	8	8.5%	4	4.3%	2	2.1%
		Elbow	27	2.6%	3	11.1%	3	11.1%	2	7.4%
		Wrist	25	2.4%	2	8.0%	3	12.0%	2	8.0%
	Lower extremities	Hip	94	9.2%	8	8.5%	10	10.6%	5	5.3%
		Knee	334	32.5%	31	9.3%	34	10.2%	23	6.9%
		Ankle	68	6.6%	6	8.8%	9	13.2%	8	11.8%
Lumbar	All cases		86,991	(100)	4939	5.7%	4989	5.7%	3404	3.9%
	Upper extremities	Shoulder	6195	7.1%	510	8.2%	502	8.1%	347	5.6%
		Elbow	1681	1.9%	113	6.7%	94	5.6%	66	3.9%
		Wrist	1711	2.0%	142	8.3%	147	8.6%	105	6.1%
	Lower extremities	Hip	6564	7.5%	496	7.6%	476	7.3%	323	4.9%
		Knee	21,721	25.0%	1642	7.6%	1691	7.8%	1128	5.2%
		Ankle	3497	4.0%	316	9.0%	306	8.8%	200	5.7%

3.5. Risk Factors for Sleep Disorder: Main Analysis

Multivariable analysis identified the following variables as significant risk factors for sleep disturbance in patients who underwent surgical treatment for degenerative spinal diseases: (Table 6): Age of 50–69 years (odds ratio, OR [95% confidence interval] = 1.40 [1.25–1.57]), age of 70–79 years (OR = 1.80 [1.60–2.03]), age over 80 years (OR = 2.22 [1.92–2.58]), female sex (OR = 1.14 [1.07–1.21]), urban residence (OR = 1.18 [1.09–1.27]), surgery at a tertiary hospital (OR = 1.08 [1.00–1.16]), peripheral vascular disease (OR = 1.22 [1.13–1.32]), chronic pulmonary disease (OR = 1.31 [1.23–1.40]), peptic ulcer disease (OR = 1.26 [1.17–1.35]), mild liver disease (OR = 1.27 [1.14–1.41]), depressive disorder (OR = 2.86 [2.70–3.02]), cerebrovascular disease (OR = 1.12 [1.10–1.20]), dementia (OR = 1.49 [1.26–1.78]), Parkinson's disease' (OR = 1.51 [1.22–1.88]), migraine (OR = 1.61 [1.44–1.82]), other-type headache (OR = 1.25 [1.03–1.52]), shoulder arthritis (OR = 1.15 [1.06–1.26]), knee arthritis (OR = 1.11 [1.04–1.18]), and ankle arthritis (OR = 1.32 [1.17–1.48]). All the results from the main statistical analysis are presented in Supplementary Table S5.

Table 6. Risk factors for sleep disorder: Main analysis.

Variables	Categories	Model 1 (Univariable)		Model 2 (Fully Adjusted)		Model 3 (Bootstrap Validation after Fully Adjusted)	
		Odds Ratio (95% Confidence Interval)	p-Value	Adjusted Odds Ratio (95% Confidence Interval)	p-Value	Adjusted Odds Ratio (95% Confidence Interval)	Relative Bias (%)
Age	50–69 vs. 20–49 years	1.85 [1.66–2.06]	<0.001	1.40 [1.25–1.57]	<0.001	1.41 [1.29–1.56]	2.21
	70–79 vs. 20–49 years	2.87 [2.57–3.21]	<0.001	1.80 [1.60–2.03]	<0.001	1.81 [1.64–2.04]	0.89
	80+ vs. 20–49 years	3.50 [3.05–4.02]	<0.001	2.22 [1.92–2.58]	<0.001	2.23 [1.96–2.55]	0.80
Sex	Female vs. male	1.45 [1.38–1.53]	<0.001	1.14 [1.07–1.21]	<0.001	1.13 [1.08–1.20]	−4.45
Region	Urban vs. rural	1.13 [1.05–1.22]	0.001	1.18 [1.09–1.27]	<0.001	1.17 [1.11–1.24]	−2.97
Hospital	Tertiary vs. others	1.25 [1.16–1.34]	<0.001	1.08 [1.00–1.16]	0.047	1.08 [1.00–1.15]	−3.33
Comorbidities	Peripheral vascular disease	1.61 [1.50–1.73]	<0.001	1.22 [1.13–1.32]	<0.001	1.22 [1.13–1.31]	0.68
	Chronic pulmonary disease	1.66 [1.57–1.76]	<0.001	1.31 [1.23–1.40]	<0.001	1.30 [1.23–1.38]	−1.42
	Peptic ulcer disease	1.60 [1.50–1.70]	<0.001	1.26 [1.17–1.35]	<0.001	1.26 [1.19–1.34]	−0.91

Table 6. Cont.

Variables	Categories	Model 1 (Univariable)		Model 2 (Fully Adjusted)		Model 3 (Bootstrap Validation after Fully Adjusted)	
		Odds Ratio (95% Confidence Interval)	p-Value	Adjusted Odds Ratio (95% Confidence Interval)	p-Value	Adjusted Odds Ratio (95% Confidence Interval)	Relative Bias (%)
	Mild liver disease	1.38 [1.26–1.52]	<0.001	1.27 [1.14–1.41]	<0.001	1.26 [1.17–1.37]	−1.68
Comorbidities associated neuropsychiatric disorders	Depressive disorder	3.52 [3.34–3.72]	<0.001	2.86 [2.70–3.02]	<0.001	2.86 [2.72–3.00]	0.03
	Cerebrovascular disease	1.70 [1.58–1.84]	<0.001	1.12 [1.10–1.20]	0.040	1.10 [1.02–1.19]	−16.00
	Dementia	2.41 [2.04–2.83]	<0.001	1.49 [1.26–1.78]	<0.001	1.50 [1.32–1.71]	0.96
	Parkinson disease	2.25 [1.83–2.78]	<0.001	1.51 [1.22–1.88]	<0.001	1.50 [1.21–1.83]	−1.63
	Migraine	2.43 [2.18–2.71]	<0.001	1.61 [1.44–1.82]	<0.001	1.62 [1.45–1.79]	1.76
	Other-type headache	2.21 [2.00–2.44]	<0.001	1.25 [1.03–1.52]	0.023	1.24 [1.06–1.44]	−2.75
Concurrent osteoarthritis	Shoulder	1.55 [1.43–1.69]	<0.001	1.15 [1.06–1.26]	0.002	1.15 [1.08–1.24]	1.17
	Knee	1.59 [1.50–1.68]	<0.001	1.11 [1.04–1.18]	0.002	1.11 [1.05–1.17]	−1.40
	Ankle	1.79 [1.60–2.00]	<0.001	1.32 [1.17–1.48]	<0.001	1.32 [1.18–1.46]	0.67

Relative bias was estimated as the difference between the mean bootstrapped regression coefficient estimates (model 3) and the mean parameter estimates of multivariable model (model 2) divided by the mean parameter estimates of multivariable model (model 2).

3.6. Validation of Risk Factors: Sensitivity Analysis

During the study period, the annual prevalence of sleep disorder in the year before the index surgery (main analysis) was similar to the proportions of patients who used sleep medication for over four weeks during the 90 days before the index surgery (Table 1): 5.3% vs. 5.2% in 2016, 5.4% vs. 5.4% in 2017, and 5.8% vs. 5.8% in 2018. Therefore, the target outcome for the sensitivity analysis was determined as the use of sleep medication for over four weeks during the 90 days before the index surgery. Except for region of residence and other-type headaches, most variables in the main analysis remained significant in the sensitivity analysis (Table 7). In addition, congestive heart failure, uncomplicated diabetes, and renal disease, including end-stage renal disease, were newly identified as significant variables in the sensitivity analysis. All the results from the sensitivity analysis are presented in Supplementary Table S6.

Table 7. Risk factors for over 4-week sleep medication during the preoperative 90 days: Sensitivity analysis.

Variables	Categories	Univariable		Model 2 (Fully Adjusted)		Model 3 (Bootstrap Validation after Fully Adjusted)	
		Odds Ratio (95% Confidence Interval)	p-Value	Adjusted Odds Ratio (95% Confidence Interval)	p-Value	Adjusted Odds Ratio (95% Confidence Interval)	Relative Bias (%)
Age	50–69 vs. 20–49 years	1.97 [1.77–2.21]	<0.001	1.32 [1.17–1.49]	<0.001	1.31 [1.19–1.44]	−2.60
	70–79 vs. 20–49 years	3.04 [2.71–3.41]	<0.001	1.54 [1.36–1.75]	<0.001	1.53 [1.37–1.71]	−0.78
	80+ vs. 20–49 years	3.80 [3.31–4.37]	<0.001	1.95 [1.68–2.27]	<0.001	1.94 [1.71–2.22]	−0.69
Sex	Female vs. male	1.57 [1.49–1.66]	<0.001	1.20 [1.13–1.27]	<0.001	1.19 [1.14–1.26]	−3.96
Hospital	Tertiary vs. others	1.38 [1.29–1.48]	<0.001	1.17 [1.08–1.15]	<0.001	1.16 [1.09–1.24]	−4.46
	General vs. others	1.63 [1.53–1.74]	<0.001	1.38 [1.29–1.47]	<0.001	1.38 [1.30–1.46]	−0.34
Comorbidities	Congestive heart failure	1.80 [1.60–2.03]	<0.001	1.16 [1.02–1.33]	0.023	1.17 [1.06–1.32]	6.99
	Peripheral vascular disease	1.53 [1.42–1.65]	<0.001	1.09 [1.00–1.18]	0.040	1.09 [1.01–1.18]	−0.67
	Chronic pulmonary disease	1.60 [1.51–1.69]	<0.001	1.21 [1.13–1.29]	<0.001	1.20 [1.13–1.27]	−4.26
	Peptic ulcer disease	1.58 [1.48–1.68]	<0.001	1.20 [1.11–1.29]	<0.001	1.20 [1.13–1.29]	−0.34
	Mild liver disease	1.42 [1.29–1.56]	<0.001	1.27 [1.14–1.40]	<0.001	1.27 [1.17–1.39]	−0.13
	Uncomplicated diabetes	1.46 [1.38–1.55]	<0.001	1.12 [1.04–1.20]	0.002	1.11 [1.05–1.19]	−4.17
	Renal disease	2.01 [1.74–2.32]	<0.001	1.23 [1.01–1.49]	0.042	1.22 [1.01–1.48]	−5.03
	End stage renal disease	3.07 [2.31–4.07]	<0.001	1.97 [1.39–2.79]	<0.001	1.96 [1.45–2.71]	−0.76
Comorbidities associated neuropsychiatric disorders	Depressive disorder	7.05 [6.67–7.45]	<0.001	5.84 [5.51–6.18]	<0.001	5.84 [5.57–6.16]	0.01
	Cerebrovascular disease	2.15 [2.00–2.31]	<0.001	1.28 [1.18–1.39]	<0.001	1.28 [1.19–1.38]	0.54
	Dementia	2.28 [1.93–2.69]	<0.001	1.33 [1.11–1.59]	0.002	1.32 [1.13–1.55]	−1.68
	Parkinson disease	4.41 [3.73–5.21]	<0.001	2.80 [2.34–3.36]	<0.001	2.83 [2.46–3.32]	1.00
	Migraine	2.21 [1.98–2.48]	<0.001	1.30 [1.15–1.47]	<0.001	1.31 [1.18–1.44]	1.88
Concurrent osteoarthritis	Shoulder	1.47 [1.35–1.60]	<0.001	1.08 [1.02–1.17]	0.013	1.08 [1.01–1.17]	3.82
	Knee	1.68 [1.58–1.77]	<0.001	1.14 [1.06–1.21]	<0.001	1.13 [1.07–1.19]	−5.13
	Ankle	1.70 [1.52–1.90]	<0.001	1.19 [1.06–1.35]	0.004	1.20 [1.09–1.32]	5.14

Relative bias was estimated as the difference between the mean bootstrapped regression coefficient estimates (model 3) and the mean parameter estimates of multivariable model (model 2) divided by the mean parameter estimates of multivariable model (model 2).

3.7. Validation of Estimates: Bootstrap Sampling

In the main analysis, the relative bias of the estimates for the risk factors was very low at between −4.45 and 2.21%, except for that of cerebrovascular disease (−16%). In the sensitivity analysis, the relative bias of the estimates was also very low between −5.13 and 6.99%. Bootstrap-adjusted odds ratios and 95% confidence intervals for the multivariable model are also displayed in Figure 4 (main analysis) and Figure 5 (sensitivity analysis). Multicollinearity among covariates was low, and all variance inflation factors were less than 1.9.

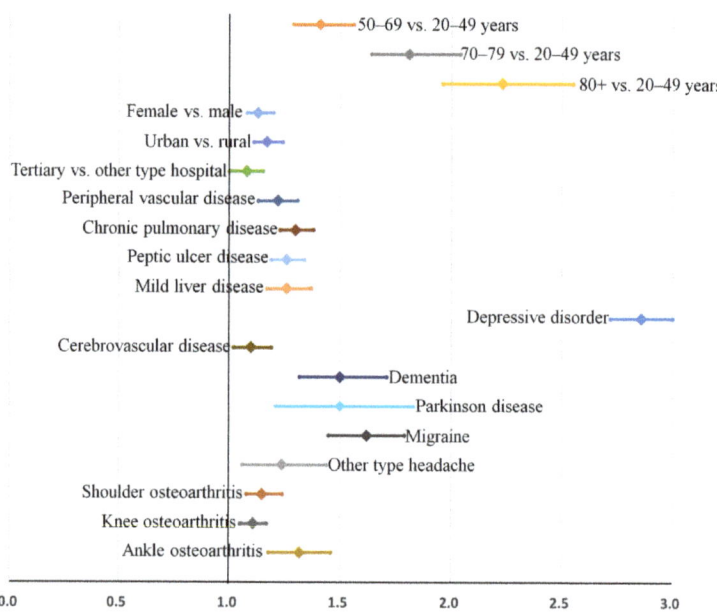

Figure 4. Risk factors for sleep disorder (main analysis). Bootstrap-adjusted odds ratios and their 95% confidence intervals have been presented. Risk factors can be categorized into four groups: (1) Age, (2) other demographic factors and general comorbidities, (3) neuropsychiatric disorders, and (4) osteoarthritis of the extremities.

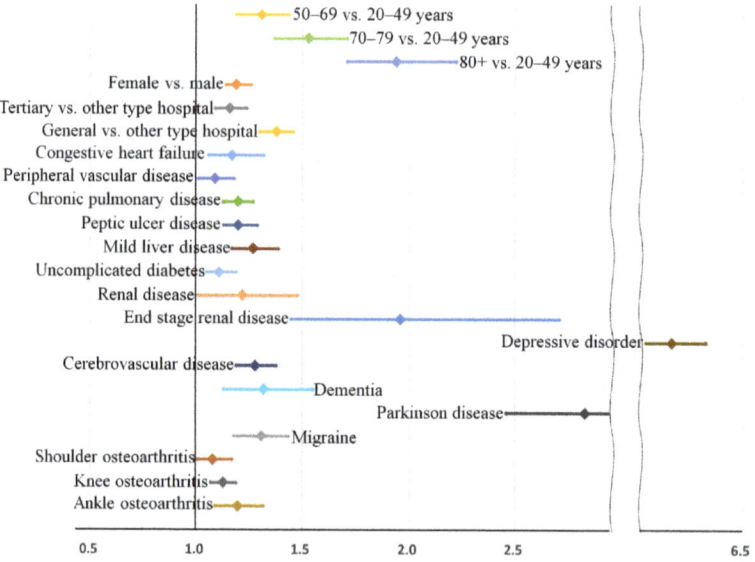

Figure 5. Risk factors for sleep medication use for over 8 weeks during the preoperative 90 days (subgroup analysis). Bootstrap-adjusted odds ratios and their 95% confidence intervals have been presented. Risk factors can be categorized into four groups: (1) Age, (2) other demographic factors and general comorbidities, (3) neuropsychiatric disorders, and (4) osteoarthritis of the extremities.

4. Discussions

To the best of our knowledge, this is the largest study to investigate the epidemiology of preoperative sleep disturbance in patients who underwent surgery for degenerative spinal disease. Among the 106,837 patients, the prevalence of sleep disorder was 5.5% (n = 5847), and during the 90 days before the spinal surgery, sleep medication was used over four weeks in 5.5% of the cohort (n = 5864) and over eight weeks in 3.8% (n = 4009) of the cohort. The prevalence of sleep disturbance differed according to the spinal regions, and sleep disorder was present in 6.9%, 5.7%, and 4.4% of patients with thoracic, lumbar, and cervical lesions, respectively. However, the spinal region was not a significant risk factor for sleep disorders in the multivariable analysis (Supplementary Tables S5 and S6). The presence of sleep disorder in patients who underwent surgery for degenerative spinal disease was significantly associated with the following factors: Older age; female sex; urban residence; surgery at a tertiary hospital; general comorbidities, including peripheral vascular disease, chronic pulmonary disease, peptic ulcer disease, and mild liver disease; neuropsychiatric disorders, including depressive disorder, cerebrovascular disease, dementia, Parkinson's disease, migraine, and other-type headache; and arthritis of the shoulder, knee, and ankle joints.

Compared with the prevalence of sleep disturbance in recent studies in the general population (1.6 to 18.6%) [23], and in patients with degenerative spinal disease (11 to 74%) [12–17], the prevalence of sleep disturbance in our cohort (3.8 to 5.5%, Table 3) is quite low. This difference results from the different methods used to evaluate sleep disturbance. Most previous studies used self-administered questionnaire-based surveys without objective clinical evidence to evaluate sleep disturbance, and the prevalence could have been overestimated. In contrast, in our study, sleep disturbance was only defined as present when the sleep disorder was diagnosed by doctors after a hospital visit or when sleep medication was prescribed for a sufficient period. Therefore, the prevalence of sleep disturbance in our cohort could have been underestimated.

The core results of our analysis identifying the independent factors associated with sleep disturbance are presented in Figure 4. In Figure 4, the bootstrap-adjusted ORs and 95% confidence intervals of individual factors can be evidently divided into four groups: (1) Age, (2) other demographic factors and general comorbidities, (3) neuropsychiatric disorders, and (4) osteoarthritis of the extremities. While older age is a strong risk factor for sleep disturbance in our cohort, other demographic variables including sex and region of residence, various general comorbidities, and osteoarthritis of the extremities did not show comparable risks for sleep disturbance (all their adjusted ORs are below 1.4). In contrast, most neuropsychiatric disorders showed higher ORs for sleep disturbance than general comorbidities, and depressive disorder was the most prominent risk factor for sleep disturbance (OR = 2.86 [2.72–3.00]).

Interestingly, the prevalence of sleep disturbance differed according to the location of the spinal lesion (Figure 3), and univariable analysis identified significant differences according to spinal regions, especially between the cervical and lumbar regions ($p < 0.001$, Supplementary Table S5). However, the location of the spinal lesion was not an independent risk factor for sleep disturbance in the multivariable analysis (Tables 6 and 7). Based on the results of our study, we suggest that regional differences in the prevalence of sleep disturbance in the unadjusted analysis (Figure 3 and Supplementary Table S5) result from regional differences in factors associated with sleep disturbance, such as neuropsychiatric disorders (Table 4) and degenerative joint diseases of the extremities (Table 5).

The major advantage of our study is that we could precisely present the prevalence of sleep disturbance according to four groups of factors (Tables 2–5). Our database represents the entire Korean population, and these prevalence rates can be used as the base rates for sleep disturbance in patients with specific risk factors. It is well known that the accuracy of prediction by a simple 'base rate' of the entire population can be comparable to that obtained from a complex statistical analysis [24]. Although our prediction model (Tables 6 and 7) for sleep disturbance could be inevitably biased by unknown confounders due to the study's limitations, our prevalence rates of sleep disturbance presented by four groups of factors can be used as a reasonable source of the base rates.

This study has some limitations. First, the HIRA database is a claims database not originally designed for clinical research. Although we used validated data retrieval methods for the HIRA database, possible discrepancies between the diagnostic codes in the database and the actual diseases may be potential sources of bias. However, the HIRA system is based on our compulsory national health insurance system, and the control policy for high-revenue spinal surgeries has been the object of priority. Therefore, therapeutic information about drug and device use, as well as precise surgical approaches, is thoroughly reviewed by government officials and is thus considered very accurate. Second, information possibly related to sleep disturbance, including the radiologic degree of spinal degeneration such as disc degeneration or canal stenosis, or the degree of neurological impairment, could not be included in the study. In particular, information regarding the radiologic degree or types of degeneration could have influenced our results as a confounder [12,13], although most patients who underwent surgical treatment have an end-stage degenerative spinal disease. To reduce the influence of such unknown confounders, we performed a two-step validation procedure, and the results were consistent. Third, we could not include patients with degenerative spinal deformities because of the limited data capacity for analysis. Finally, we particularly focused on investigating the sleep disturbance according to spinal regions, and multivariable analysis showed that the prevalence of sleep disturbance was not significantly different among spinal regions. However, due to the lack of important information, including the presence of various symptoms or signs depending on spinal regions and their severity, our results could be biased. Previous studies have suggested different mechanisms of sleep disturbance according to spinal regions, and further studies including such important clinical information would be interesting and helpful to understand the actual mechanisms of sleep disturbance in patients with degenerative spinal disease.

In conclusion, our population-based study using a nationwide database identified that the prevalence of sleep disturbance in patients undergoing surgery for degenerative spinal disease was 5.5% (5847 of 106,837 patients). Although the prevalence of sleep disturbance differed according to spinal regions, the spinal region was not a significant risk factor for sleep disorder in the multivariable analysis. In addition, we identified four groups of independent risk factors: (1) Age, (2) other demographic factors and general comorbidities, (3) neuropsychiatric disorders, and (4) osteoarthritis of the extremities. Our results, including the prevalence rates of sleep disturbance based on the entire population and the identified risk factors, provide clinicians with a reasonable reference for evaluating sleep disturbance in patients with degenerative spinal diseases and future research.

Supplementary Materials: The following supporting information can be downloaded at: https://www.mdpi.com/article/10.3390/jcm11195932/s1, Table S1: Types of the used sleep medication; Table S2. ICD-10 codes for comorbidities including Charlson comorbidities index items and scores; Table S3. ATC and HIRA codes for the used antidepressant; Table S4. HIRA codes for the x-rays of the extremities; Table S5. Risk factors for sleep disorder (main analysis): all the results from statistical analysis; Table S6. Risk factors for over 8-week sleep medication during the preoperative 90 days (sensitivity analysis): all the results from statistical analysis.

Author Contributions: Conceptualization, J.K. and T.-H.K.; Data curation, M.S.K.; Formal analysis, J.K.; Investigation, M.S.K.; Methodology, J.K., M.S.K. and T.-H.K.; Resources, M.S.K.; Software, J.K. and M.S.K.; Validation, T.-H.K.; Visualization, T.-H.K.; Writing—original draft, J.K.; Writing–review & editing, T.-H.K. All authors have read and agreed to the published version of the manuscript.

Funding: This research received no external funding.

Institutional Review Board Statement: This study was approved by the Institutional Review Board of our hospital (IRB No. 2020-03-009-001).

Informed Consent Statement: Patient consent was waived due to the retrospective study design and anonymity of the HIRA database.

Data Availability Statement: The datasets generated for the current study are not publicly available due to Data Protection Laws and Regulations in Korea, but the analyzing results are available from the corresponding authors on reasonable request.

Conflicts of Interest: The authors declare no conflict of interest.

References

1. Dattilo, M.; Antunes, H.K.; Medeiros, A.; Mônico Neto, M.; Souza, H.S.; Tufik, S.; de Mello, M.T. Sleep and muscle recovery: Endocrinological and molecular basis for a new and promising hypothesis. *Med. Hypotheses* **2011**, *77*, 220–222. [CrossRef] [PubMed]
2. Cirelli, C.; Tononi, G. Is sleep essential? *PLoS Biol.* **2008**, *6*, e216. [CrossRef] [PubMed]
3. Luyster, F.S.; Strollo, P.J., Jr.; Zee, P.C.; Walsh, J.K. Sleep: A health imperative. *Sleep* **2012**, *35*, 727–734. [CrossRef] [PubMed]
4. Cappuccio, F.P.; Elia, L.; Strazzullo, P.; Miller, M.A. Sleep duration and all-cause mortality: A systematic review and meta-analysis of prospective studies. *Sleep* **2010**, *33*, 585–592. [CrossRef]
5. Stranges, S.; Tigbe, W.; Gómez-Olivé, F.X.; Thorogood, M.; Kandala, N.B. Sleep problems: An emerging global epidemic? Findings from the INDEPTH WHO-SAGE study among more than 40,000 older adults from 8 countries across Africa and Asia. *Sleep* **2012**, *35*, 1173–1181. [CrossRef]
6. Sutton, D.A.; Moldofsky, H.; Badley, E.M. Insomnia and health problems in Canadians. *Sleep* **2001**, *24*, 665–670. [CrossRef]
7. Hossain, J.L.; Shapiro, C.M. The prevalence, cost implications, and management of sleep disorders: An overview. *Sleep Breath* **2002**, *6*, 85–102. [CrossRef]
8. Burgess, H.J.; Burns, J.W.; Buvanendran, A.; Gupta, R.; Chont, M.; Kennedy, M.; Bruehl, S. Associations between sleep disturbance and chronic pain intensity and function: A test of direct and indirect pathways. *Clin. J. Pain* **2019**, *35*, 569–576. [CrossRef]
9. Onen, S.H.; Onen, F. Chronic medical conditions and sleep in the older adult. *Sleep Med. Clin.* **2018**, *13*, 71–79. [CrossRef]
10. Sasaki, E.; Tsuda, E.; Yamamoto, Y.; Maeda, S.; Inoue, R.; Chiba, D.; Okubo, N.; Takahashi, I.; Nakaji, S.; Ishibashi, Y. Nocturnal knee pain increases with the severity of knee osteoarthritis, disturbing patient sleep quality. *Arthritis Care Res.* **2014**, *66*, 1027–1032. [CrossRef]
11. Khazzam, M.S.; Mulligan, E.P.; Brunette-Christiansen, M.; Shirley, Z. Sleep quality in patients with rotator cuff disease. *J. Am. Acad. Orthop. Surg.* **2018**, *26*, 215–222. [CrossRef]
12. Kim, J.; Oh, J.K.; Kim, S.W.; Yee, J.S.; Kim, T.H. Risk factors for sleep disturbance in patients with cervical myelopathy and its clinical significance: A cross-sectional study. *Spine J.* **2021**, *21*, 96–104. [CrossRef]
13. Kim, J.; Park, J.; Kim, S.W.; Oh, J.K.; Park, M.S.; Kim, Y.W.; Kim, T.H. Prevalence of sleep disturbance in patients with lumbar spinal stenosis and analysis of the risk factors. *Spine J.* **2020**, *20*, 1239–1247. [CrossRef]
14. Kim, H.J.; Hong, S.J.; Park, J.H.; Ki, H. Sleep disturbance and its clinical implication in patients with adult spinal deformity: Comparison with lumbar spinal stenosis. *Pain Res. Manag.* **2020**, *2020*, 6294151. [CrossRef]
15. Artner, J.; Cakir, B.; Spiekermann, J.-A.; Kurz, S.; Leucht, F.; Reichel, H.; Lattig, F. Prevalence of sleep deprivation in patients with chronic neck and back pain: A retrospective evaluation of 1016 patients. *J. Pain Res.* **2013**, *6*, 1–6. [CrossRef]
16. Kim, J.; Kim, G.; Kim, S.W.; Oh, J.K.; Park, M.S.; Kim, Y.W.; Kim, T.H. Changes in sleep disturbance in patients with cervical myelopathy: Comparison between surgical treatment and conservative treatment. *Spine J.* **2021**, *21*, 586–597. [CrossRef]
17. Kim, J.; Lee, S.H.; Kim, T.H. Improvement of sleep quality after treatment in patients with lumbar spinal stenosis: A prospective comparative study between conservative versus surgical treatment. *Sci. Rep.* **2020**, *10*, 14135. [CrossRef]
18. Choi, H.; Youn, S.; Um, Y.H.; Kim, T.W.; Ju, G.; Lee, H.J.; Lee, C.; Lee, S.D.; Bae, K.; Kim, S.J.; et al. Korean Clinical Practice Guideline for the Diagnosis and Treatment of Insomnia in Adults. *Psychiatry Investig.* **2020**, *17*, 1048–1059. [CrossRef]
19. Kim, J.; Ryu, H.; Kim, T.-H. Early reoperation rates and its risk factors after instrumented spinal fusion surgery for degenerative spinal disease: A nationwide cohort study of 65,355 patients. *J. Clin. Med.* **2022**, *11*, 3338. [CrossRef]
20. Lim, J.S.; Kim, T.-H. Recurrence rates and its associated factors after early spinal instrumentation for pyogenic spondylodiscitis: A nationwide cohort study of 2148 patients. *J. Clin. Med.* **2022**, *11*, 3356. [CrossRef]
21. Kim, J.; Kim, T.-H. Risk factors for postoperative deep infection after instrumented spinal fusion surgeries for degenerative spinal disease: A nationwide cohort study of 194,036 patients. *J. Clin. Med.* **2022**, *11*, 778. [CrossRef]
22. Park, H.-R.; Im, S.; Kim, H.; Jung, S.-Y.; Kim, D.; Jang, E.; Sung, Y.-K.; Cho, S.-K. Validation of algorithms to identify knee osteoarthritis patients in the claims database. *Int. J. Rheum. Dis.* **2019**, *22*, 890–896. [CrossRef]
23. Koyanagi, A.; Stickley, A. The association between sleep problems and psychotic symptoms in the general population: A global perspective. *Sleep* **2015**, *38*, 1875–1885. [CrossRef]
24. Kahneman, D. *Thinking, Fast and Slow*; Farrar, Straus and Giroux: New York, NY, USA, 2017.

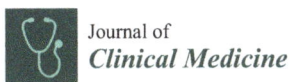

Article

Reliability of the Spanish Version of the Movement Imagery Questionnaire-3 (MIQ-3) and Characteristics of Motor Imagery in Institutionalized Elderly People

Manuel Enrique Suárez Rozo [1], Sara Trapero-Asenjo [2,3,*], Daniel Pecos-Martín [2,4], Samuel Fernández-Carnero [2,4], Tomás Gallego-Izquierdo [2,4], José Jesús Jiménez Rejano [5] and Susana Nunez-Nagy [2,3,4]

1. Amavir Torrejón de Ardoz Nursing Home, 28850 Torrejón de Ardóz, Spain
2. Department of Nursing and Physiotherapy, Faculty of Medicine and Health Sciences, University of Alcalá, 28805 Alcalá de Henares, Spain
3. Humanization in the Intervention of Physiotherapy for the Integral Attention to the People (HIPATIA) Research Group, Physiotherapy Department, Faculty of Medicine and Health Sciences, University of Alcalá, 28801 Alcalá de Henares, Spain
4. Physiotherapy and Pain Group, Physiotherapy Department, University of Alcalá, 28871 Alcalá de Henares, Spain
5. Department of Physiotherapy, University of Seville, 41009 Seville, Spain
* Correspondence: sara.trapero@uah.es

Abstract: Motor imagery (MI) training is increasingly used to improve the performance of specific motor skills. The Movement Imagery Questionnaire-3 (MIQ-3) is an instrument for assessing MI ability validated in Spanish although its reliability has not yet been studied in the elderly population. The main objective of this study was to test its reliability in institutionalized elderly people. Secondarily, we studied whether there are differences according to gender and age in MI ability (measured by the MIQ-3) and in temporal congruency (measured by mental chronometry of elbow and knee flexion-extension and getting up and sitting down from chair movements). The subjects were 60 elderly, institutionalized, Spanish-speaking individuals without cognitive impairment or dementia, and aged between 70 and 100 years. Cronbach's alpha showed high internal consistency in the internal visual and external visual subscales and moderate in the kinesthetic subscale. The intraclass correlation coefficient showed good test-retest reliability for all three subscales. Mixed factorial analysis of variances (ANOVAs) showed that MI ability decreased with increasing age range, the imagery time decreased concerning the execution of the same movement, and there were no gender differences in either IM ability or temporal congruence. The Spanish version of the MIQ-3 is a reliable instrument for measuring MI ability in institutionalized elderly.

Keywords: physical therapy; imagery; institutionalized persons

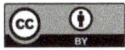

1. Introduction

Motor imagery (MI) comprises imagining a movement without executing it to optimize motor skills [1]. It is a specific cognitive process in which the planning of a movement is carried out without executing it through actual physical movement [2], and it is observed to have the same components and involve the same brain areas as when a real movement is performed [2,3]. This process can also be explained thanks to the existence of the psychoneuromuscular theory, whose foundations support the idea that MI improves motor learning based on the role played by mirror neurons when these are activated during the visualization of a movement in mental practice [2]. In turn, the motor schema involved in the actual activity is reinforced during MI so that the processes occurring during imagery aid performance, reinforcing coordination patterns for motor skill development [2].

Therefore, MI practice is a technique that is increasingly used in the therapeutic context to improve the performance of specific motor skills, and whenever possible, it is combined with physical practice [2,4,5]. Thus, MI practice has been studied in healthy subjects, athletes [6–12], as well as in multiple neurological conditions [13–16] and pain conditions [17–20], among others. It has also been used in combination with virtual reality using brain–computer-interface-based systems in people with neurological sequelae [20,21].

A recent systematic review showed improved balance, mobility, and gait speed among the therapeutic benefits of MI training in older people without neurological conditions [22]. For an MI training program to be effective, the ability to generate imagery needs to be assessed [23]. However, there are few studies on MI capacity in the elderly, specifically in institutionalized elderly people. As is well-known, the institutionalization of elderly people in nursing homes is one of the best options when they can no longer live at home. This change entails social, affective, self-esteem, and motivation losses, increasing hopelessness about old age and suffering from chronic diseases and/or disabilities [24]. Among the latter are those caused by injuries to the locomotor system, as most institutionalized older people are below average in terms of lower- and upper-limb muscle strength, which is associated with a low level of physical activity [24]. High physical activity levels have been associated with a greater capacity to generate motor mental images [20], and MI capacity must be trained in older people to obtain positive results [22].

Imagery capacity can be assessed in different ways. Studies on the elderly have pointed out that MI capacity should be carefully assessed, where MI capacity questionnaires and mental chronometry would be very appropriate, among others [25]. Thus, MI can be assessed in terms of vividness through self-reported questionnaires such as the Movement Imagery Questionnaire-3 (MIQ-3) and temporal characteristics through temporal congruency through mental chronometry. Both forms of MI assessment are complementary, as each assesses different aspects of MI.

The MIQ-3 is an instrument validated in Spanish, consisting of 12 items grouped into three subscales. It is a multidimensional measure that has been used to measure the capacity for internal, external, and kinesthetic imagery and whose psychometric properties have shown good internal consistency as well as internal reliability and predictive validity, suggesting that it is a suitable instrument for assessing MI abilities in healthy and young people of both sexes [26,27]. It is important to consider the age of the subject, as it has been shown that the capacity for imagery decreases progressively with age, affecting the development of motor skills [22]. Furthermore, scientific evidence suggests that the MI capacity of some movements is modified due to some age-related alterations, indicating that aging produces selective effects on mental imagery [28]. Nevertheless, the reliability of the MIQ-3 for use in the elderly has not been tested so far, nor have similar questionnaires been validated for use in the elderly. A recent systematic review of MI assessments suggests that more studies are needed in this context, including older populations [29].

On the other hand, temporal congruence is considered the time course of mental operations between simulated and real movements [25]. It is measured through mental chronometry, measuring the time it takes the subject to execute a movement and the time it takes to imagine that movement.

Liu et al. [30] compared MI ability among populations distributed by gender and in three age ranges. They concluded that temporal congruency is preserved with age for simple and usual movements and is impaired for limited and unusual movements. They also observed a lower capacity for internal visual and kinesthetic imagery in people over 60 years of age relative to younger people. Regarding gender, MI ability was found to be better in men than in women. However, some studies have found no significant gender differences in this population [31]. Another study found that women may overestimate the imagined task relative to actual practice, while men underestimate it [32].

Therefore, more studies are needed to support the use of the MIQ-3 and mental chronometry to assess MI ability for these groups of elderly people, paying attention to differences according to age and gender.

This study's main objective was to determine whether the Spanish version of the MIQ-3 is a reliable instrument for measuring motor imagery ability in institutionalized elderly people. The secondary objectives were to explore MI ability as a function of this population's age range, gender, and temporal characteristics (through temporal congruence). As hypotheses, it was established that the Spanish version of the MIQ-3 is a reliable instrument to measure MI capacity in this population and that MI capacity measured by this questionnaire is higher in males than in females and decreases as the age range increases. It is expected that temporal congruency is better preserved in males than in females, and it similarly decreases with age.

2. Materials and Methods

The design adopted corresponded to reliability studies. A repeated-measures cross-sectional design was carried out on the subjects in the sample. In addition, the recommendations established in the Guidelines for Reporting Reliability and Agreement Studies (GRRAS) [33] were followed.

2.1. Participants

The study sample comprised 60 institutionalized elderly people: 27 men (45%) and 33 women (55%). The 60 subjects were divided into groups according to three age ranges. The first group consisted of 16 people (26.67%) aged between 70 and 79 years (mean (M) = 72.6; standard deviation (SD) = 1.86). The second group consisted of 26 persons (43.33%) aged 80–89 years (M = 84; SD = 1.92), and the third group consisted of 18 persons (30%) aged 90–100 years (M = 92.5; SD = 2.0) (Table 1).

Table 1. Sociodemographic characteristics of the sample.

Variables	Frequency (%)
Gender	
Male	27 (45%)
Female	33 (55%)
n (%)	60 (100%)
Age (M ± SD)	83.5 ± 7.80
70–79 years	16 (26.67%)
80–89 years	26 (43.33%)
90–100 years	18 (30%)

n, sample size; M, mean; SD, standard deviation.

The inclusion criteria for the study were: Spanish-speaking, aged 70–100 years, of both genders, and without cognitive impairment or dementia as measured by Pfeiffer's Short-Portable Mental State Questionnaire (SPMSQ) [34,35] and Yesavage's Geriatric Depression Scale [36]. The exclusion criteria were having suffered traumatic processes in the last 6 months and being under treatment with central nervous system suppressant drugs. Participants were recruited from the "Residencia de mayores Amavir" social-health center in Torrejón de Ardoz after the center's medical committee granted permission. Participation was voluntary after signing the informed consent form.

2.2. Data Collection Instrument

The MIQ-3 is composed of 12 items grouped into three subscales (internal visual imagery, external visual imagery, and kinesthetic imagery), which allow for the assessment of MI in both genders about four movements involving knee elevation, jumping, arm movement, and leaning forward at the waist, all repeated in three subscales [26,27]. These movements are described in each statement to be performed under instructions that indicate the initial position, the action, the mental task, and the score using a seven-point Likert scale, indicating the difficulty or ease of "seeing" and "feeling" the movements [26]. It has been validated in different languages and different populations [27].

2.3. Variables

Gender and age were considered independent and controlled sociodemographic variables in the study. In addition, MI, measured through the MIQ-3, and temporal congruence, measured through mental chronometry, were considered dependent variables. Three movements were performed to measure mental chronometry: elbow flexion-extension, knee flexion-extension, and getting up and sitting down from a chair.

2.4. Procedure

The same researcher oversaw carrying out the two data collection sessions. To homogenize the conditions, the verbal orders given to the subjects during the sessions were standardized before the sessions and carried out in the same room and under the same environmental conditions.

In the first session, the MIQ-3 was administered, and time congruency was measured by mental chronometry of elbow flexion-extension, knee flexion-extension, and getting up and sitting down from a chair. Before performing the mental chronometry task, the experimenter gave a physical demonstration of the movements to be performed. Afterward, using previously standardized commands, they were asked to perform the different movements and then try to imagine them. The execution and imagination times were calculated employing a stopwatch, which was pressed by the researcher at the subjects' "start" and "stop" commands at the moments of both the actual execution of the movements and the imagined execution. Each movement was performed and imagined on three occasions, and each movement's mean mental chronometry value was then calculated.

In the second session (after one week), the MIQ-3 was administered again for the study of retest reliability.

2.5. Statistical Analysis

Statistical analysis was carried out using SPSS, version 26.0 for Windows (International Business Machines Corporation (IBM), Armonk, NY, USA).

First, the descriptive analysis of the results obtained in the two measurements made with the questionnaire (test and retest) was carried out as well as the mean and the difference between the measurements.

Subsequently, internal consistency was assessed by calculating Cronbach's alpha coefficient. Interpretation was based on the following values: very low (0 to 0.2); low (0.2 to 0.4); moderate (0.4 to 0.6); good (0.6 to 0.8); and high (0.8 to 1). Adequate internal consistency was between 0.7 and 0.939 since excessively high values could indicate redundant items within the questionnaire [37].

The test-retest reliability of each questionnaire item was analyzed by calculating the value of the weighted kappa coefficient, following Cicchetti's method. The weighted kappa coefficient values were interpreted following the classification established by Landis and Koch [38]. Agreement was no agreement if the Kappa index took a value of 0.00; negligible if it was between 0.01 and 0.20; medium if it was between 0.21 and 0.40; moderate between 0.41 and 0.60; substantial between 0.61 and 0.80; and near perfect between 0.81 and 1.00 [39,40]. These analyses were carried out with the statistical program Epidat 4.2. (Consellería de Sanidade, Xunta de Galicia, Spain; Pan American Health Organization (PAHO); CES University, Medellin, Colombia).

The test-retest reliability of each subscale was analyzed by calculating the intraclass correlation coefficient (ICC) using a two-factor model with mixed effects and absolute agreement. The 95% confidence interval for the ICC values was also calculated. The Weir criteria [41] were followed to interpret the ICC values, where values of 0.50 to 0.69 are considered moderate, values of 0.70 to 0.89 as high, and values of 0.90 and above as excellent.

The analysis of differences in MI ability measured by the MIQ-3 was carried out according to sex and age considering that the sample was distributed into three age groups. Two mixed factorial analysis of variances (ANOVAs) were used for this purpose. This design was used to determine whether the differences analyzed were because of the inter-subject factor (either sex or age range). In this sense, in the first mixed factorial analysis of variance (ANOVA), the inter-subject factor was the sex of the subjects, while in the second one, the age range was considered. The hypothesis of interest was the inter-subject factor interaction by time, with an a priori alpha level of 0.05. In addition, the effect size of the observed differences was estimated by calculating the partial eta-squared coefficient (η_p^2). The assumption of the sphericity hypothesis was tested using Mauchly's test. In those cases where the assumption of sphericity was not met, the Greenhouse–Geisser correction was used. In addition, the analysis was completed by employing multiple comparison tests, using the Bonferroni correction, and determining the effect size, and Cohen's d was calculated.

The data analysis for time congruence was carried out using a mixed factorial ANOVA with respect to sex and age. For differences that conformed to the normal and were homoscedastic, the Mann–Whitney U test was used for those differences that did not conform to the normal, and the effect size was determined by calculating Rosenthal's r with the formula: $r = Z/\sqrt{N}$ [42,43]. Kruskal–Wallis ANOVA was performed for comparison according to age range.

3. Results

3.1. Descriptive Analysis

The descriptive analysis of the scores obtained in each subscale of the MIQ-3 showed that in the second session, the values in the three subscales were higher than those obtained in the first session. In this regard, the differences obtained between the means between the two sessions were −2.50 in the external visual subscale, followed by −2.25 in the internal visual subscale and −2.00 in the kinesthetic scale (Table 2).

Table 2. Results of the descriptive analysis in each subscale.

Subscale		Mean	CI 95%	SD
IVS	1st S	14.42	13.63–15.21	3.055
	2nd S	16.67	15.86–17.47	3.112
EVS	1st S	18.08	17.32–18.84	2.936
	2nd S	20.58	19.90–21.27	2.651
KS	1st S	12.25	11.59–12.91	2.55
	2nd S	14.25	13.56–14.94	2.678

IVS, Internal Visual Subscale; EVS, External Visual Subscale; KS, Kinesthetic Subscale; 1st S, first session; 2nd S, second session; CI, confidence interval; SD, standard deviation.

3.2. Analysis of Internal Consistency

The Cronbach's alpha analysis showed values that allowed us to establish a high internal consistency in the case of the questionnaire. The internal and external visual subscales showed good internal consistency, while the kinesthetic subscale showed moderate consistency (Table 3).

Table 3. Results of the analysis of internal consistency and test-retest reliability of Movement Imagery Questionnaire-3 (MIQ-3).

N_o	K_w	CI (95%)	p
Item 1	0.29	0.14–0.45	<0.0001
Item 2	0.47	0.31–0.64	<0.0001
Item 3	0.36	0.20–0.52	<0.0001
Item 4	0.70	0.58–0.82	<0.0001
Item 5	0.26	0.11–0.41	<0.0001
Item 6	0.34	0.18–0.49	<0.0001
Item 7	0.30	0.15–0.45	<0.0001

Table 3. Cont.

N₀	K_w		CI (95%)	p
Item 8	0.71		0.59–0.82	<0.0001
Item 9	0.39		0.24–0.54	<0.0001
Item 10	0.40		0.24–0.55	<0.0001
Item 11	0.25		0.12–0.39	=0.001
Item 12	0.70		0.55–0.81	<0.0001
	Cronbach's Alpha	ICC	CI (95%)	p
IVS	0.615	0.611	0.02–0.83	<0.001
EVS	0.651	0.534	0.07–0.80	<0.001
KS	0.556	0.691	0.07–0.90	<0.001

N₀, item number in MIQ-3; K_W, kappa value; CI, confidence interval; p, statistical significance; IVS, Internal Visual Subscale; EVS, External Visual Subscale; KS, Kinesthetic Subscale; ICC, intraclass correlation.

3.3. Analysis of the Test-Retest Reliability

The analysis using the weighted kappa coefficient established that, of the 12 items, 8 showed a medium degree of agreement, 1 item showed a moderate degree of agreement, and 3 items showed substantial agreement (Table 3). The analysis corresponding to the test-retest reliability of each subscale by calculating the ICC made it possible to establish good reliability values (Table 3). These results are confirmed by the visual distributions of the Bland–Altman plots for the test-retest comparison of the three subscales of the MIQ-3 (Figures 1–3).

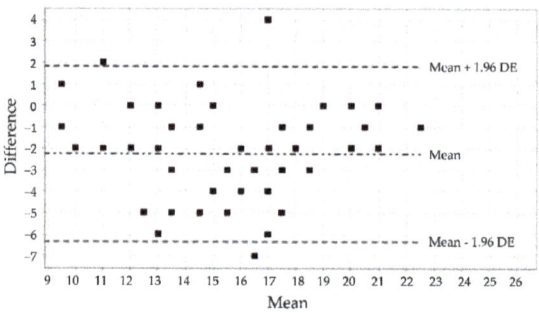

Figure 1. Bland–Altman plot of the internal visual subscale of the MIQ-3.

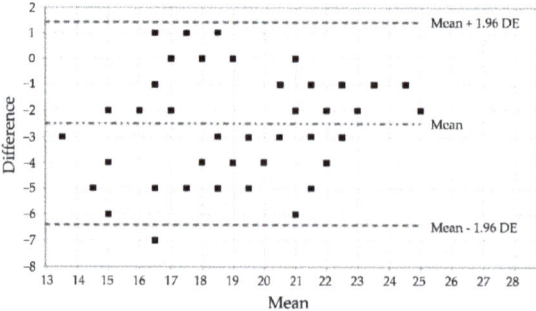

Figure 2. Bland–Altman plot of the external visual subscale of the MIQ-3.

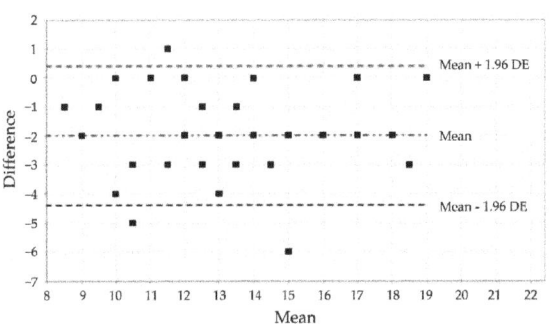

Figure 3. Bland–Altman plot of the kinesthetic subscale of the MIQ-3.

3.4. Analysis of Differences in MI Ability as Measured by the MIQ-3 Concerning Sex and Age

The mixed factorial ANOVA indicated in the case of the comparison according to sex in the three subscales, i.e., internal visual, external visual, and kinesthetic, that there was no significant interaction between the within-subjects factor (the two measurements taken) and the between-subjects factor (sex). There was also no significant effect of the inter-subject factor, but there was a significant effect of the intra-subject factor. Both sexes behaved similarly, with significantly higher values in the second session than in the first session. There were no differences between males and females in either measurement (Table 4).

Table 4. The mixed factorial analysis of variance (ANOVA) results of the differences in motor imagery (MI) ability measured through the MIQ-3, according to sex.

Inter-Subject Factor			MIQ-3	
				Mean (SD)
			First session	Second session
		Male (*n* = 27)	14.41 (2.76)	16.56 (2.91)
		Female (*n* = 33)	14.42 (3.32)	16.76 (3.31)
	Internal Visual Subscale	Time × sex interaction	$F_{(1, 58)} = 0.12$; $p = 0.736$; $\eta_p^2 = 0.002$	
		Inter-subject factor (Sex)	$F_{(1, 58)} = 0.02$; $p = 0.886$; $\eta_p^2 < 0.001$	
		Inter-group mean difference and CI (95%)	First session	−0.02 (−1.62; 1.58) $p = 0.983$ $d < 0.01$
			Second session	−0.20 (−1.84; 1.43) $p = 0.805$ $d = 0.06$
		Intra-subject factor	$F_{(1, 58)} = 67.68$; $p < 0.001$; $\eta_p^2 = 0.537$	
		Intra-group mean difference and CI (95%)	Male	−2.15 (−2.96; −1.34) $p < 0.001$
			Female	−2.33 (−3.07; −1.60) $p < 0.001$
Sex				Mean (SD)
			First session	Second session
		Male (*n* = 27)	18.41 (2.42)	20.67 (2.24)
		Female (*n* = 33)	17.82 (3.31)	20.52 (2.98)
	External Visual Subscale	Time × sex interaction	$F_{(1, 58)} = 0.71$; $p = 0.403$; $\eta_p^2 = 0.012$	
		Inter-subject factor (sex)	$F_{(1, 58)} = 0.30$; $p = 0.589$; $\eta_p^2 = 0.005$	
		Inter-group mean difference and CI (95%)	First session	0.59 (0.94; 2.12) $p = 0.444$ $d = 0.20$
			Second session	0.15 (−1.24; 1.54) $p = 0.828$ $d = 0.06$
		Intra-subject factor	$F_{(1, 58)} = 91.13$; $p < 0.001$; $\eta_p^2 = 0.611$	
		Intra-group mean difference and CI (95%)	Male	−2.26 (−3.03; −1.49) $p < 0.001$
			Female	−2.70 (−3.39; −2.00) $p < 0.001$

Table 4. Cont.

Inter-Subject Factor			MIQ-3	
				Mean (SD)
			First session	Second session
	Kinesthetic Subscale	Male (n = 27)	12.48 (2.55)	14.26 (2.68)
		Female (n = 33)	12.06 (2.59)	14.24 (2.72)
		Time × sex interaction	$F_{(1, 58)} = 1.64; p = 0.205; \eta_p^2 = 0.028$	
		Inter-subject factor (Sex)	$F_{(1, 58)} = 0.11; p = 0.743; \eta_p^2 = 0.002$	
		Inter-group mean difference and CI (95%)	First session	0.42 (−0.91; 1.75) $p = 0.530$ d = 0.16
			Second session	0.02 (−1.39; 1.42) $p = 0.981$ d < 0.01
		Intra-subject factor	$F_{(1, 58)} = 157.80. p < 0.001; \eta_p^2 = 0.731$	
		Intra-group mean difference and CI (95%)	Male	−1.78 (−2.25; −1.31) $p < 0.001$
			Female	−2.18 (−2.61; −1.76) $p < 0.001$

n, sample size; SD, standard deviation; CI, confidence interval; p, statistical significance; F, Fisher; η_p^2, partial eta-squared coefficient.

Regarding the differences according to MI age range (MIQ-3) in the three subscales, namely internal visual, external visual, and kinesthetic, it was found that there was a significant interaction between the within-subjects factor (the two measurements taken) and the between-subjects factor (age range). There was also a significant effect of the inter-subject and intra-subject factors. The three age ranges behaved similarly in the three subscales (internal visual, external, and kinesthetic), with significantly higher values in the second session compared to the first (Table 5).

Table 5. The mixed factorial ANOVA results of differences in MI ability as measured by the MIQ-3, by age range.

Inter-Subject Factor			MIQ-3	
				Mean (SD)
			First session	Second session
		70–79 years (n = 16)	18.12 (2.22)	19.25 (2.02)
		80–89 years (n = 26)	13.77 (1.93)	17.73 (1.43)
		90–100 years (n = 18)	12.06 (1.77)	12.83 (1.86)
		Time × age range interaction	$F_{(2, 57)} = 31.68; p < 0.001; \eta_p^2 = 0.526$	
		Inter-subject factor (age range)	$F_{(2, 57)} = 57.54; p < 0.001; \eta_p^2 = 0.669$	
	Internal Visual Subscale	Inter-group mean difference and CI (95%)	First session	
			70–79 vs. 80–89	4.36 (2.82; 5.89) $p < 0.001$ d = 2.13
			70–79 vs. 90–100	6.07 (4.41; 7.73) $p < 0.001$ d = 3.04
			80–89 vs. 90–100	1.71 (0.23; 3.19) $p = 0.018$ d = 0.92
			Second session	
			70–79 vs. 80–89	1.52 (0.16; 2.88) $p = 0.023$ d = 0.91
			70–79 vs. 90–100	6.42 (4.95; 7.88) $p < 0.001$ d = 3.32
			80–89 vs. 90–100	4.88 (3.59; 6.21) $p < 0.001$ d = 3.03
		Intra-subject factor	$F_{(1, 57)} = 109.86; p < 0.001; \eta_p^2 = 0.643$	
		Intra-group mean difference and CI (95%)	70–79 years	−1.13 (−1.86; −0.39) $p = 0.003$
			80–89 years	−3.96 (−4.54; −3.39) $p < 0.001$
Age range			90–100 years	−0.78 (−1.47; −0.09) $p = 0.028$

Table 5. Cont.

Inter-Subject Factor		MIQ-3		
			Mean (SD)	
			First session	Second session
External Visual Subscale	70–79 years ($n = 16$)		21.13 (2.03)	23.00 (1.55)
	80–89 years ($n = 26$)		17.62 (2.32)	21.38 (1.42)
	90–100 years ($n = 18$)		16.06 (2.24)	17.28 (1.13)
	Time × age range interaction		$F_{(2, 57)} = 14.03; p < 0.001; \eta_p^2 = 0.330$	
	Inter-subject factor (age range)		$F_{(2, 57)} = 45.60; p < 0.001; \eta_p^2 = 0.615$	
	Inter-group mean difference and CI (95%)	First session	70–79 vs. 80–89	3.51 (1.77; 5.25) $p < 0.001$ d = 1.58
			70–79 vs. 90–100	5.07 (3.19; 6.95) $p < 0.001$ d = 2.36
			80–89 vs. 90–100	1.56 (−0.12; 3.24) $p = 0.077$ d = 0.68
		Second session	70–79 vs. 80–89	1.62 (0.54; 2.69) $p = 0.001$ d = 1.10
			70–79 vs. 90–100	5.72 (4.56; 6.89) $p < 0.001$ d = 4.26
			80–89 vs. 90–100	4.11 (3.07; 5.15) $p < 0.001$ d = 3.13
	Intra-subject factor		$F_{(1, 57)} = 109.03; p < 0.001; \eta_p^2 = 0.657$	
	Intra-group mean difference and CI (95%)	70–79 years		−1.88 (−2.71; −1.04) $p < 0.001$
		80–89 years		−3.77 (−4.42; −3.12) $p < 0.001$
		90–100 years		−1.22 (−2.01; −0.44) $p = 0.003$
			Mean (SD)	
			First session	Second session
Kinesthetic Subscale	70–79 years ($n = 16$)		15.44 (1.86)	17.44 (1.63)
	80–89 years ($n = 26$)		11.62 (1.42)	14.12 (1.28)
	90–100 years ($n = 18$)		10.33 (1.61)	11.61 (1.79)
	Time × age range interaction		$F_{(2, 57)} = 6.28; p = 0.003; \eta_p^2 = 0.181$	
	Inter-subject Factor (age range)		$F_{(2, 57)} = 60.47; p < 0.001; \eta_p^2 = 0.680$	
	Inter-group mean difference and CI (95%)	First session	70–79 vs. 80–89	3.82 (2.57; 5.08) $p < 0.001$ d = 2.39
			70–79 vs. 90–100	5.10 (3.75; 5.46) $p < 0.001$ d = 2.95
			80–89 vs. 90–100	1.28 (0.07; 2.05) $p = 0.034$ d = 0.86
		Second session	70–79 vs. 80–89	3.32 (2.12; 4.53) $p < 0.001$ d = 2.34
			70–79 vs. 90–100	5.83 (4.52; 7.13) $p < 0.001$ d = 3.40
			80–89 vs. 90–100	2.50 (1.34; 3.67) $p < 0.001$ d = 1.67
	Intra-subject factor		$F_{(1, 57)} = 168.59. p < 0.001; \eta_p^2 = 0.747$	
	Intra group mean difference and CI (95%)	70–79 years		−2.00 (−2.56; −1.44) $p < 0.001$
		80–89 years		−2.50 (−2.94; −2.06) $p < 0.001$
		90–100 years		−1.28 (−1.81; −0.75) $p < 0.001$

n, sample size; SD, standard deviation; CI, confidence interval; p, statistical significance; F, Fisher; η_p^2, partial eta-squared coefficient.

On the other hand, there were statistically significant differences between the values of the three age ranges in the internal visual and kinesthetic subscales, with the 70–79 age group presenting the highest values, followed by the 80–89 age group and, finally, the 90–100 age group with the lowest values. In the external visual subscale, the group aged 70 to 79 years presented the highest values, followed by the group aged 80 to 89 years and, finally, the group aged 90 to 100 years with the lowest values, with there being significant differences between the group aged 70 to 79 years and the other two groups (80 to 89 and 90 to 100 years). However, the differences observed were not significant between the 80–89 and 90–100 age groups (Table 5).

3.5. Analysis of Temporal Congruence Concerning Sex and Age

Mixed factorial ANOVA was performed to compare, according to sex, the three movements corresponding to temporal congruency: elbow flexion-extension, knee flexion-extension, and getting up and sitting down on the chair. The results obtained indicated that in the case of the first two movements (elbow and knee flexion-extension), there was no significant interaction between the intra-subject factor in the two measurements (performed and imagined) and the inter-subject factor (sex). There was also no significant effect of the intra-subject factor, but there was a significant effect of the inter-subject factor, $F_{(1, 58)} = 5.48$; $p = 0.023$; $\eta_p^2 = 0.086$ in the elbow flexion-extension movement and $F_{(1, 58)} = 10.06$; $p = 0.002$; $\eta_p^2 = 0.148$ in the knee flexo-extension movement. Both sexes behaved differently. In men, the values of the executed measurement (elbow flexion-extension M = 3.71, SD = 0.42; knee flexion-extension M = 4.06, SD = 0.41) were higher than those of the imagined measurement in both subscales (elbow flexion-extension M = 3.64, SD= 0.33; knee flexion-extension M = 3.90, SD = 0.38). In women, the values of the executed measurement (M = 3.96, SD = 0.48) were slightly higher than those of the imagined measurement in the elbow movement (M = 3.94, SD = 0.60), and the values of the executed measurement (M = 4.06, SD = 0.41) were slightly lower than the imagined one in the knee movement. In both movements, differences ($p < 0.05$) were found between men and women in both the executed and imagined measurements, with women's values being significantly higher. In the intra-group comparison of the two movements of the two measurements carried out (the executed and the imagined), it was found that neither in men nor in women were there significant differences between the two measurements.

As for the get up and sit down on the chair movement, this mixed factorial ANOVA showed no significant interaction between the intra-subject and inter-subject (sex) factors, but there was a significant effect of the inter-subject factor $F_{(1, 58)} = 6.72$; $p = 0.012$; $\eta_p^2 = 0.104$ and the intra-subject factor $F_{(1, 58)} = 54.23$; $p < 0.001$; $\eta_p^2 = 0.483$. Both sexes behaved similarly, with higher values for the imagined measurement (male M = 5.10, SD = 0.71; female M = 5.47, SD = 0.60) than for the executed measurement (male M = 4.61, SD = 0.41; female M = 4.93, SD = 0.55). There were statistically significant differences ($p < 0.05$) between men and women in the two measurements, with women having significantly higher values. In the intra-group comparison of the two measurements carried out, we obtained that in both men and women, there were significant differences ($p < 0.05$) between the two measurements, with the imagined scores being significantly higher.

Next, the results obtained for temporal congruence were analyzed, i.e., the difference in the three movements of elbow flexion-extension, knee flexion-extension, and getting up and sitting down on the chair, comparing the two measurements (executed less imagined) concerning sex. The Mann–Whitney U-test was used for all movements. These analyses showed no gender differences in the three movements (Table 6).

Table 6. Temporal congruency concerning sex.

Inter-Subject Factor		Temporal Congruence		
		Male (*n* = 27) Median (Q1–Q3)	Female (*n* = 33) Median (Q1–Q3)	Effect Size
Sex	Elbow Flexo-Extension Difference	0.20 (−0.30; 0.35)	0.00 (−0.20; 0.30)	$p = 0.720$ $r = 0.05$
	Knee Flexo-Extension Difference	0.10 (−0.05; 0.40)	0.10 (−0.30; 0.30)	$p = 0.162$ $r = 0.02$
	Get up and Sit down Difference	−0.60 (−0.80; −0.25)	−0.60 (−0.80; −0.30)	$p = 0.905$ $r = 0.12$

Mann–Whitney U-test was used; Q1–Q3, first through third quartiles; r, Rosenthal's "r"; p, statistical significance.

Mixed factorial ANOVA was performed to analyze, according to age range (inter-subject factor), the two measurements (performed and imagined) of the three movements corresponding to temporal congruency: elbow flexion-extension, knee flexion-extension, and getting up and sitting down on the chair. These analyses showed a significant interaction between movement execution and imagery (intra-subject factor) and age range (inter-subject factor) in the elbow flexion-extension ($F_{(2, 57)} = 9.68$, $p < 0.001$; $\eta_p^2 = 0.253$) and knee flexion-extension ($F_{(2, 57)} = 5.97$, $p = 0.004$; $\eta_p^2 = 0.173$). There was also a significant effect of the inter-subject factor (elbow flexion-extension $F_{(2, 57)} = 10.36$, $p < 0.001$; $\eta_p^2 = 0.267$; knee flexion-extension $F_{(2, 57)} = 6.42$, $p = 0.003$; $\eta_p^2 = 0.184$) but no significant effect of the intra-subject factor. Thus, the three age ranges did not behave similarly in both the elbow flexion-extension movement and the knee flexion-extension movement. While the values of the imagined measurement decreased compared to the executed one in the 80–89 years and 90–100 years age groups, the values increased in the 70–79 years age group. In both movements, there were significant differences ($p < 0.05$) between the value of the executed and imagined measurement in the 70–79 years (the value of the imagined measurement being higher) and 90–100 years (the value of the executed measurement being higher in this case), while in the 80–89 years group, there were no differences between the two measurements. On the other hand, in the executed measurement in both the elbow flexion-extension and knee flexion-extension movements, there were statistically significant differences ($p < 0.05$) between the three age ranges, with the 70–79 age group showing the lowest values, followed by the 80–89 age group and, finally, the 90–100 age group showing the highest values. However, in the imagined measurement of the elbow flexion-extension movement, there were only significant differences ($p < 0.05$) between the 70–79 years and 90–100 years groups, with no significant differences between the other groups, and in the knee flexion-extension movement, there were no significant differences between any of the three age ranges.

Finally, in the movement of getting up and sitting down from a chair, there was a significant effect of the intra-subject factor $F_{(1, 57)} = 64.25$, $p < 0.001$; $\eta_p^2 = 0.530$ (the two measurements taken, executed, and imagined) and inter-subject factor $F_{(2, 57)} = 20.47$, $p < 0.001$; $\eta_p^2 = 0.418$ (the three age groups considered), but there was no significant interaction between the two factors. In the three age ranges, in this movement of standing up and sitting down, there were significant differences ($p < 0.05$) between the executed and imagined measurement, with higher values for the imagined measurement. On the other hand, in the executed measurement, there were significant differences ($p < 0.05$) between the three age ranges, with the 90–100 age group showing the highest values, followed by the 80–89 age group and, finally, the 70–79 age group with the lowest values of the three. Meanwhile, in the imagined measurement, there were only significant differences between the 70–79 age group and the 90–100 age group.

Next, the results obtained for temporal congruence were analyzed, i.e., the difference in the three movements of elbow flexion-extension, knee flexion-extension, and getting up and sitting down on a chair, comparing the two measurements (performed and imagined) according to age range by carrying out a Kruskal–Wallis ANOVA. There were no differences between the three age ranges compared in temporal congruence in standing and sitting. However, there were significant differences ($p < 0.05$) between the three age ranges in the temporal congruence in elbow flexion-extension and knee flexion-extension movements. Specifically, in elbow flexion-extension, there were significant differences ($p < 0.05$) between the 70–79 age group and the other two groups. In the knee flexion-extension movement, there were significant differences ($p < 0.05$) between the subjects aged 70–79 years and the group aged 90–100 years (Table 7).

Table 7. Temporal congruence concerning age.

Inter-Subject Factor		Temporal Congruence				
		70–79 Years Median (Q1–Q3)	80–89 Years Median (Q1–Q3)	90–100 Years Median (Q1–Q3)	Effect Size	
Age range	Elbow Flexo-Extension Difference	−0.25 (−0.30; −0.15)	0.20 (−0.10; 0.30)	0.20 (−0.10; 0.50)	Global	$p = 0.001$
					70–79 vs. 80–89	$p = 0.007$
					70–79 vs. 90–100	$p = 0.001$
					80–89 vs. 90–100	$p = 0.999$
	Knee Flexo-Extension Difference	−0.05 (−0.40; 0.10)	0.10 (−0.20; 0.40)	0.35 (0.10; 0.50)	Global	$p = 0.008$
					70–79 vs. 80–89	$p = 0.086$
					70–79 vs. 90–100	$p = 0.007$
					80–89 vs. 90–100	$p = 0.752$
	Get up and Sit down Difference	−0.65 (−1.10; −0.20)	−0.45 (−0.80; −0.20)	−0.70 (−0.90; −0.30)	Global	$p = 0.134$
					70–79 vs. 80–89	$p = 0.312$
					70–79 vs. 90–100	$p = 0.999$
					80–89 vs. 90–100	$p = 0.258$

Q1–Q3, first through third quartiles.

4. Discussion

The aim of this study was to test the reliability of the Spanish version of the Movement Imagery Questionnaire-3 in 60 institutionalized elderly people. The first translation, cultural adaptation, and validation of the Spanish version of the MIQ-3 [27] have recently been published. This work is focused on healthy young people. For older people, no work has been found that evaluates the reliability of this test or similar questionnaires for older people.

The descriptive analysis of the results obtained in the two measurements made with the questionnaire (test and retest) showed higher values in the second session in the three subscales, which suggests that the participants showed a better ability to imagine measured with the MIQ-3 the second time they took the questionnaire. This could be the result of the MI practice implicit in the development of the first session, in which subjects performed both the questionnaire itself and the imagery tasks related to temporal congruence. This is consistent with the results of the study by Rufino et al. [44], where it was observed that a single MI session already induces use-dependent brain plasticity.

Cronbach's alpha was acceptable for all the values obtained, and none of the items was redundant [37]. In this sense, these results are consistent with Trapero-Asenjo et al. [27] even though the value obtained was lower than in the study by the authors.

Concerning the subscales, the analysis revealed a good internal consistency for both the internal visual subscale (0.615) and the external visual subscale (0.651) and a moderate internal consistency (0.556) for the kinesthetic subscale. These results show that the values obtained were lower than those obtained in the study by Trapero-Asenjo et al. [27], which indicated a high internal consistency for the three subscales, with 0.849 for the internal visual subscale, 0.837 for the external visual subscale, and 0.615 for the kinesthetic subscale. These lower values in the study by Trapero-Asenjo et al. [27] coincide with the lower values obtained in validating the MIQ-3 in Portuguese by Mendes et al. [8].

The test-retest reliability analysis of each of the 12 items that make up the questionnaire by means of the weighted and interpreted kappa coefficient value showed medium, moderate, and substantial degrees of agreement in 8 items. Therefore, these correspond to adequate test-retest reliability values as established in the classification of Landis and Koch in 1977 [38]. These findings partially coincide with the results obtained by Trapero-Asenjo et al. [27], who found moderate to substantial agreement on all 12 items. In contrast, in the present investigation, items 1 and 3 of the internal visual subscale; items 1, 2, and 3 of the external visual subscale; and items 1, 2, and 3 of the kinesthetic subscale showed a medium degree of agreement, i.e., below the values obtained by Trapero-Asenjo et al. [27].

The results of the test-retest reliability analysis of each MIQ-3 subscale by calculating the ICC showed for the external visual subscale an ICC of 0.534 (95% confidence interval (CI) = 0.07, 0.80; $p < 0.001$), in the internal visual subscale a CCI of 0.611 (95% CI = 0.02, 0.83; $p < 0.001$), and the highest value was in the kinesthetic subscale, with a CCI of 0.691 (95% CI = 0.07, 0.90; $p < 0.001$). These values were interpreted according to Weir's criteria [41], showing internal consistency with moderate values in all subscales. These findings are consistent with the results presented by Trapero-Asenjo et al. [27]; however, the values obtained were lower, as the ICC of the three scales were high in the study by Trapero-Asenjo et al. [27], while in this study, the values were moderate.

All these results suggest that the Spanish version of the MIQ-3 is a reliable measure of MI capacity for use in institutionalized elderly people. The study by Suica et al. [29] showed that the questionnaires for assessing MI with the best psychometric properties were the Movement Imagery Questionnaire (MIQ) [45] as well as its versions Movement Imagery Questionnaire—Revised (MIQ-R) [46], MIQ-3, and the Vividness of Movement Imagery Questionnaire (VMIQ-2) [47]. The same study showed that most studies assessing MI had been conducted in a young population [29], thus highlighting the need to validate MI assessment tools in the elderly. On the other hand, of all these questionnaires, only the MIQ-3 and the VMIQ-2 assess MI ability and MI vividness, respectively, in the three subscales of internal visual, external visual, and kinesthetic imagery [26,47]. It has been shown that these three forms of imagery are separate but related constructs [26,46], so the assessment of all three is of particular importance for both research and clinical applicability. Thus, this is the first study to confirm that MI capacity can be reliably assessed in institutionalized elderly people using the Spanish version of the MIQ-3, which currently represents the most suitable questionnaire for assessing MI ability on all three subscales. In clinical applicability, it has been proven that the ability to image can be improved with practice [48]. The results of this study will allow the design of more effective MI programs in the elderly since they not only allow the evaluation of MI through these questionnaires at the beginning of programs with MI but also allow them to monitor changes in the capacity of MI that are happening along the program.

On the other hand, studies have been carried out in which the capacity and vividness of MI in elderly people has been explored through questionnaires and their temporal characteristics through temporal congruence studies. It has been seen that the study of both issues is important, as it was pointed out that the ability to imagine and the temporal congruence are separate constructs and should be evaluated separately because they are affected differently by age [32]. To explore those questions, the present study analyzed the scores of the three subscales of MIQ-3 and three tasks of time congruence according to sex and age in the elderly population.

Thus, regarding the secondary objectives, in the analysis of differences in MI ability measured through the MIQ-3, there were no differences between men and women in the two measurements. These results partially coincide with the findings reported by Campos et al. [31]. They assessed in a sample of adult subjects whether there are age and gender differences by using self-report and a performance-based test, reporting no significant differences between the sexes concerning MI ability even though males scored higher than females.

Regarding the differences according to MI age range (MIQ-3), the analysis of the results suggests that the three age ranges behaved similarly in the three subscales (internal visual, external, and kinesthetic), with significantly higher values in the second session compared to the first. This could be associated with a learning process derived from the execution of the movement.

On the other hand, there were statistically significant differences between the values of the three age ranges in the internal visual and kinesthetic subscales, with the group of septuagenarians presenting the highest values, followed by the group of octogenarians and, finally, the group of nonagenarians and centenarians with the lowest values. In the external visual subscale, the decrease in scores with increasing age was similar to the other two subscales. However, in this case, the significant differences were between the septuagenarian group with respect to octogenarians and nonagenarians to centenarians, but the differences observed were not significant between these last two groups. These results confirm the findings of Subirats et al. [32]. They found that MI ability (measured with the Vividness of Movement Imagery Questionnaire-2 and MI timing using the performances of the real Timed Up and Go (rTUG) test) is affected by age, with a tendency for MI to decrease with age in the present study, with no significant differences between the group of nonagenarians and centenarians with respect to the group of adults aged 70–79 years. They also confirm the results that Mulder et al. [49] obtained, which showed that older participants had slightly worse MI ability (measured with the Vividness of Movement Imagery Questionnaire) than younger participants.

Similarly, they corroborate the findings of Schott [50], whose study examined key characteristics of MI ability in three groups of healthy older men and women (measured with the Movement Imagery Questionnaire, the Controllability of Motor Imagery test, and two different chronometry tests) distributed across three age groups (60–69, 70–79, and ≥80 years) and 40 younger subjects aged 20–30 years. They found that MI ability was better in younger adults compared to older adults aged 70 years and older but not in older adults aged 60–69 years. However, as noted above, IM ability can be improved with practice, and low scores are not exclusive to IM programs [48].

Regarding the differences in temporal congruence, no significant differences were observed concerning the differences between gender. However, there were differences in the time used to perform and imagine the movements. Thus, both sexes took significantly longer to imagine than to execute the movement of sitting down and getting up from the chair, and on the other hand, the men took longer to execute than to imagine the less global movements of flexion-extension of the elbow and knee, whereas the women had very similar results in both moments of the task. Therefore, it seems that in the simplest movements, the imagery of the movement tends to have a shorter duration than the movement itself, while in more global movements, such as getting up and sitting down, the imagery of the movement is reproduced more slowly than the execution of the same movement in the elderly population. The previous study by Saimpont et al. [25] pointed out that temporal congruence in the elderly seems to be more reserved in simple and usual movements, so all these issues should be further explored in future studies.

Regarding the differences in temporal congruence with respect to age, differences were only observed in the elbow and knee flexo-extension movements. In both cases, it was seen that as age increased, the imagery time was significantly reduced compared to the execution time of the same movement. This again suggests that the ability to maintain temporal congruence varies with increasing age. In this sense, Schott et al. [50] observed that from the age of 79, the difference between the values of imagery and execution of the movement increased progressively, so this issue should be further explored in future studies.

Limitations

To conclude, for the analysis of the study's main objective, the sample of five people per item was adequate [51], and for the study of the characteristics of the imagery, the total sample was also adequate, with a size equal to 60 subjects. However, as a limitation of the study, the sample consisted of 26 participants in the 80–89 age group, 18 subjects in the 90–100 age group, and 16 subjects in the 70–79 age group. It would be desirable to carry out studies with a larger sample in each age range to obtain more representative results for each age group and validate the results in non-institutionalized elderly people.

In the study, the sample was selected based on the absence of cognitive impairment or dementia as well as depressive disorders, traumatic processes in the last 6 months, and treatment with central nervous system suppressant drugs. Thus far, no studies have explored how other health aspects may influence the ability to imagine in older people (high blood pressure, diabetes, vision, and hearing problems, among others). It is suggested that these data could be collected in future studies. Although it is not possible to establish relationships due to the design, this will help to understand the sample's characteristics better.

Finally, it should also be considered that the participants only belong to one center, so the results should not be extrapolated. Therefore, future studies should include larger samples and institutionalized and non-institutionalized elderly in different institutions.

5. Conclusions

The study allows us to conclude that the Spanish version of the MIQ-3 is a reliable instrument for measuring MI capacity in institutionalized elderly people.

The findings obtained did not demonstrate significant differences in MI ability measured with the MIQ-3 between women and men in this population. However, the results of this study support the hypothesis that MI ability decreases with the increasing age range.

In relation to temporal congruency, the analyses did not show differences between genders and observed that as age increases, the imagery time decreases with respect to the execution time of the same movement.

Author Contributions: Conceptualization, S.N.-N. and S.T.-A.; methodology, S.N.-N., S.T.-A. and T.G.-I.; software, S.T.-A. and S.F.-C.; validation, M.E.S.R., S.T.-A. and D.P.-M.; formal analysis, M.E.S.R., S.T.-A. and J.J.J.R.; investigation, M.E.S.R. and S.T.-A.; resources, M.E.S.R., S.N.-N., D.P.-M. and T.G.-I.; data curation, M.E.S.R., S.T.-A. and J.J.J.R.; writing—original draft preparation, M.E.S.R., S.T.-A. and D.P.-M.; writing—review and editing, S.T.-A., D.P.-M. and T.G.-I.; visualization, M.E.S.R., S.F.-C. and S.N.-N.; supervision, S.N.-N. and T.G.-I.; project administration, D.P.-M. All authors have read and agreed to the published version of the manuscript.

Funding: This research received no external funding.

Institutional Review Board Statement: The study was conducted following the Declaration of Helsinki and was approved by the Ethical Committee for Animal Research and Experimentation of the University of Alcalá with the number CEIM2021/2/032.

Informed Consent Statement: Informed consent was obtained from all subjects involved in the study.

Data Availability Statement: Not applicable.

Acknowledgments: We would like to thank the Amavir Torrejón de Ardoz nursing home for facilitating fieldwork with the center's users as well as every one of the residents who agreed to participate in this research.

Conflicts of Interest: The authors declare no conflict of interest.

References

1. Schack, T.; Essig, K.; Frank, C.; Koester, D. Mental representation and motor imagery training. *Front. Hum. Neurosci.* **2014**, *8*, 328. [CrossRef]
2. Fernández Gómez, E.; Sánchez Cabeza, A. Imaginería motora: Revisión sistemática de su efectividad en la rehabilitación de la extremidad superior tras un ictus. *Rev. Neurol.* **2018**, *66*, 137–146. [CrossRef] [PubMed]

3. Jeannerod, M. Mental imagery in the motor context. *Neuropsychologia* **1995**, *33*, 1419–1432. [CrossRef]
4. Campos, A.; López-Araujo, Y.; Perez-Fabello, M.J. Imágenes mentales utilizadas en diferentes actividades físicas y deportivas. *Cuad. Psicol. Deporte* **2016**, *16*, 45–50.
5. Feltz, D.L.; Landers, D.M. The effects of mental practice on motor skill learning and performance: A meta-analysis. *J. Sport Psychol.* **1983**, *5*, 25–57. [CrossRef]
6. Richardson, A. Verbalizer-visualizer: A cognitive style dimension. *J. Ment. Imag.* **1977**, *1*, 109–125.
7. de Sousa Fortes, L.; Ferreira do Carmo, Y.A.; dos Santos Felix Cruz, R.B.; Pereira de Lima, E.T.; Novais Mansur, H. Efeito do treino mental no desempenho do arremesso de lance livre em jovens basquetebolistas. *Motricidade* **2017**, *13*, 4–12. [CrossRef]
8. Mendes, P.A.; Marinho, D.A.; Petrica, J.D.; Silveira, P.; Monteiro, D.; Cid, L. Translation and validation of the Movement Imagery Questionnaire-3 (MIQ-3) with Portuguese athletes/Traducao e validacao do Movement Imagery Questionnaire-3 (MIQ-3) com atletas portugueses. *Motricidade* **2016**, *12*, 149–159. [CrossRef]
9. García Delgado, W.L. La imagen mental del movimiento para el mejoramiento de la precisión y rapidez de los grados principiantes en taekwondo. *Lect. Educ. Física Deportes* **2014**, *195*, 8.
10. Amorim, A.; Duarte-Mendes, P.; Travassos, B. Efficacy of an Imagery program training in competitive and non-competitive Boccia participants. *Cuad. Psicol. Deporte* **2018**, *18*, 205–213.
11. Marshall, B.; Wright, D.J. Layered Stimulus Response Training versus Combined Action Observation and Imagery: Effects on Golf Putting Performance and Imagery Ability Characteristics. *J. Imag. Res. Sport Phys. Act.* **2016**, *11*, 35–46. [CrossRef]
12. McNeill, E.; Ramsbottom, N.; Toth, A.J.; Campbell, M.J. Kinaesthetic imagery ability moderates the effect of an AO + MI intervention on golf putt performance: A pilot study. *Psychol. Sport Exerc.* **2020**, *46*, 101610. [CrossRef]
13. Urquiola Echeguia, A.; Sánchez Hernández, I. Rehabilitación de la Marcha Mediante el Uso de la Imagen Motora en Pacientes Hemipléjicos [Trabajo Final de Grado]. 2014. Available online: http://hdl.handle.net/20.500.13002/176 (accessed on 5 February 2022).
14. Kolbaşı, E.N.; Ersoz Huseyinsinoglu, B.; Erdoğan, H.A.; Çabalar, M.; Bulut, N.; Yayla, V. What are the determinants of explicit and implicit motor imagery ability in stroke patients? A controlled study. *Somat. Mot. Res.* **2020**, *37*, 84–91. [CrossRef]
15. Cores, E.V.; Merino, A.; Eizaguirre, M.B.; Vanotti, S.; Rodríguez Quiroga, S.A.; Arakaki, T.; Garreto, N.S. Imaginería motriz en pacientes con Parkinson: El paradigma de la cronometría mental. *Rev. Argent. Neuropsicol.* **2015**, *27*, 25–34.
16. Grande Alonso, M. Análisis Neurofisiológico y Abordaje Fisioterápico Multimodal en Pacientes con Dolor Lumbar Crónico Inespecífico. Ph.D. Thesis, Universidad Autónoma de Madrid, Madrid, España, 2020. Available online: http://hdl.handle.net/10486/693363 (accessed on 5 February 2022).
17. Daly, A.E.; Bialocerkowski, A.E. Does evidence support physiotherapy management of adult Complex Regional Pain Syndrome Type One? A systematic Review. *Eur. J. Pain* **2009**, *13*, 339–353. [CrossRef]
18. Mirela Cristina, L.; Matei, D.; Ignat, B.; Popescu, C.D. Mirror therapy enhances upper extremity motor recovery in stroke patients. *Acta Neurol. Belg.* **2015**, *115*, 597–603. [CrossRef]
19. Cuenca-Martínez, F.; Suso-Martí, L. Capacidad de Generar Imágenes Mentales Motoras y su Relación con los Niveles de Actividad Física. *NeuroRehabNews* **2019**, *3*, e0057. [CrossRef]
20. Tabernig, C.B.; Lopez, C.A.; Carrere, L.C.; Spaich, E.G.; Ballario, C.H. Neurorehabilitation therapy of patients with severe stroke based on functional electrical stimulation commanded by a brain-computer interface. *J. Rehabil. Assist. Technol. Eng.* **2018**, *5*, 1–12. [CrossRef]
21. Lovat, A.M. Las personas como sujetos de investigación. ¿Aplicación de la ingeniería genética para mejorar personas humanas y curar la vejez? *Rev. Derecho Priv.* **2021**, *9*, 559–608.
22. Nicholson, V.; Watts, N.; Chani, Y.; Keogh, J.W.L. Motor imagery training improves balance and mobility outcomes in older adults: A systematic review. *J. Physiother.* **2019**, *65*, 200–207. [CrossRef]
23. Schuster, C.; Hilfiker, R.; Amft, O.; Scheidhauer, A.; Andrews, B.; Butler, J.; Kischka, U.; Ettlin, T. Best practice for motor imagery: A systematic literature review on motor imagery training elements in five different disciplines. *BMC Med.* **2011**, *17*, 75. [CrossRef] [PubMed]
24. Muñoz Cruz, R. Diferencias en la autopercepción entre ancianos institucionalizados y no institucionalizados. *Gerokomos* **2015**, *26*, 45–47. [CrossRef]
25. Saimpont, A.; Malouin, F.; Tousignant, B.; Jackson, P.L. Motor imagery and aging. *J. Mot. Behav.* **2013**, *45*, 21–28. [CrossRef] [PubMed]
26. Williams, S.E.; Cumming, J.; Ntoumanis, N.; Nordin Bates, S.M.; Ramsey, R.; Hall, C. Further validation and development of the movement imagery questionnaire. *J. Sport Exerc. Psychol.* **2012**, *34*, 621–646. [CrossRef]
27. Trapero-Asenjo, S.; Gallego-Izquierdo, T.; Pecos-Martín, D.; Nunez-Nagy, S. Translation, cultural adaptation, and validation of the Spanish version of the Movement Imagery Questionnaire-3 (MIQ-3). *Musculoskelet. Sci. Pract.* **2020**, *51*, 102313. [CrossRef]
28. Dror, I.E.; Kosslyn, S.M. Mental imagery and aging. *Psychol. Aging* **1994**, *9*, 90. [CrossRef]
29. Suica, Z.; Behrendt, F.; Gäumann, S.; Gerth, U.; Schmidt-Trucksäss, A.; Ettlin, T.; Schuster-Amft, C. Imagery ability assessments: A cross-disciplinary systematic review and quality evaluation of psychometric properties. *BCM Med.* **2022**, *20*, 166. [CrossRef]
30. Liu, K.P.; Lai, M.; Fong, S.S.; Bissett, M. Imagery Ability and Imagery Perspective Preference: A Study of Their Relationship and Age-and Gender-Related Changes. *Behav. Neurol.* **2019**, *2019*, 7536957. [CrossRef]

31. Campos, A.; Pérez-Fabello, M.J.; Gómez-Juncal, R. Gender and age differences in measured and self-perceived imaging capacity. *Personal. Individ. Differ.* **2004**, *37*, 1383–1389. [CrossRef]
32. Subirats, L.; Allali, G.; Briansoulet, M.; Salle, J.Y.; Perrochon, A. Age and gender differences in motor imagery. *J. Neurol. Sci.* **2018**, *391*, 114–117. [CrossRef]
33. Kottner, J.; Audigé, L.; Brorson, S.; Donner, A.; Gajewski, B.J.; Hróbjartsson, A.; Roberts, C.; Shoukri, M.; Streiner, D.L. Guidelines for Reporting Reliability and Agreement Studies (GRRAS) were proposed. *J. Clin. Epidemiol.* **2011**, *64*, 96–106. [CrossRef]
34. Pfeiffer, E. A short portable mental status questionnaire for the assessment of organic brain deficit in elderly patients. *J. Am. Geriatr. Soc.* **1975**, *23*, 433–441. [CrossRef]
35. Martínez de la Iglesia, J.; Dueñas Herrero, R.; Onís Vilches, M.C.; Aguado Taberné, C.; Albert Colomer, C.; Luque, R. Adaptación y validación al castellano del cuestionario de Pfeiffer (SPMSQ) para detectar la existencia de deterioro cognitivo en personas mayores de 65 años. *Med. Clin.* **2001**, *117*, 129–134. Available online: https://www.elsevier.es/es-revista-medicina-clinica-2-articulo-adaptacion-validacion-al-castellano-del-S0025775301720404 (accessed on 15 March 2022). [CrossRef]
36. Yesavage, J.A.; Brink, T.L.; Rose, T.L.; Lung, O.; Huang, V.; Adey, M.; Leirer, V.O. Development and validation of a geriatric depression screening scale: A preliminary report. *J. Psychiatr. Res.* **1982**, *17*, 37. [CrossRef]
37. Tavakol, M.; Dennick, R. Making sense of Cronbach's alpha. *Int. J. Med. Educ.* **2011**, *2*, 53–55. [CrossRef]
38. Landis, J.R.; Koch, G.G. The measurement of observer agreement for categorical data. *Biometrics* **1977**, *33*, 159–174. [CrossRef]
39. López de Ullibarri Galparsoro, I.; Pita Fernández, S. Medidas de concordancia: El índice de Kappa. *Cad Aten Primaria* **1999**, *6*, 169–171.
40. Sim, J.; Wright, C.C. The kappa statistic in reliability studies: Use, interpretation, and sample size requirements. *Phys. Ther.* **2005**, *85*, 257–268. [CrossRef]
41. Weir, J.P. Quantifying test-retest reliability using the intraclass correlation coefficient and the SEM. *J. Strength Cond. Res.* **2005**, *19*, 231–240. [CrossRef]
42. Field, A. *Discovering Statistics Using SPSS: (And Sex, Drugs, and Rock'n'roll)*, 3rd ed.; SAGE: Thousand Oaks, CA, USA, 2009.
43. Rosenthal, R.; DiMatteo, M.R. Meta-analysis: Recent developments in quantitative methods for literature reviews. *Annu. Rev. Psychol.* **2001**, *52*, 59–82. [CrossRef]
44. Ruffino, C.; Gaveau, J.; Papaxanthis, C.; Lebon, F. An acute session of motor imagery training induces use-dependent plasticity. *Sci. Rep.* **2019**, *9*, 20002. [CrossRef]
45. Hall, C.R.; Pongrac, J.; Buckolz, E. The measurement of imagery ability. *Hum. Mov. Sci.* **1985**, *4*, 107–118. [CrossRef]
46. Hall, C.R.; Martin, K.A. Measuring movement imagery abilities: A revision of the Movement Imagery Questionnaire. *J. Ment. Imag.* **1997**, *21*, 143–154.
47. Roberts, R.; Callow, N.; Hardy, L.; Markland, D.; Bringer, J. Movement imagery ability: Development and assessment of a revised version of the vividness of movement imagery questionnaire. *J. Sport Exerc. Psychol.* **2008**, *30*, 200–221. [CrossRef]
48. Dickstein, R.; Deutsch, J.E. Motor imagery in physical therapist practice. *Phys. Ther.* **2007**, *87*, 942–953. [CrossRef]
49. Mulder, T.; Hochstenbach, J.B.; van Heuvelen, M.J.; den Otter, A.R. Motor imagery: The relation between age and imagery capacity. *Hum. Mov. Sci.* **2007**, *26*, 203–211. [CrossRef]
50. Schott, N. Age-related differences in motor imagery: Working memory as a mediator. *Exp. Aging Res.* **2012**, *38*, 559–583. [CrossRef]
51. Worthington, R.L.; Whittaker, T.A. Scale Development Research A Content Analysis and Recommendations for Best Practices. *Couns. Pyschol.* **2006**, *34*, 806–838. [CrossRef]

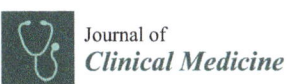

Article

Association of Body Mass Index with Long-Term All-Cause Mortality in Patients Who Had Undergone a Vertebroplasty for a Vertebral Compression Fracture

Wen-Chien Wang [1], Yun-Che Wu [1], Yu-Hsien Lin [1], Yu-Tsung Lin [1], Kun-Hui Chen [1,2,3], Chien-Chou Pan [1,4], Jun-Sing Wang [2,5,6,*] and Cheng-Hung Lee [1,2,7,*]

[1] Department of Orthopedics, Taichung Veterans General Hospital, Taichung 40705, Taiwan
[2] Department of Post-Baccalaureate Medicine, College of Medicine, National Chung Hsing University, Taichung 40227, Taiwan
[3] Department of Computer Science and Information Engineering, Providence University, Taichung 43301, Taiwan
[4] Department of Rehabilitation Science, Jenteh Junior College of Medicine, Nursing and Management, Miaoli 35664, Taiwan
[5] Division of Endocrinology and Metabolism, Department of Internal Medicine, Taichung Veterans General Hospital, Taichung 40705, Taiwan
[6] Rong Hsing Research Center for Translational Medicine, Institute of Biomedical Science, National Chung Hsing University, Taichung 40227, Taiwan
[7] Department of Food Science and Technology, Hung Kuang University, Taichung 43304, Taiwan
* Correspondence: jswang@vghtc.gov.tw (J.-S.W.); leechenghung0115@gmail.com (C.-H.L.)

Abstract: We aimed to investigate the association between preoperative body mass index (BMI) and postoperative long-term mortality in patients who underwent a vertebroplasty. We retrospectively enrolled patients with a vertebral compression fracture who underwent a vertebroplasty between May 2013 and June 2020 in a medical center in Taiwan. The survival status of the study sample was confirmed by the end of March 2021. Cox-proportional hazard models were conducted to examine the effects of being overweight/obese (≥ 25 kg/m^2 vs. <25 kg/m^2) and BMI (as a continuous variable) on all-cause mortality after adjusting for age, sex, history of smoking, diabetes, hypertension, chronic kidney disease, and osteoporosis. A total of 164 patients were analyzed (mean age 75.8 ± 9.3 years, male 25.6%, mean BMI 24.0 ± 4.1 kg/m^2) after a median follow-up of 785 days. Compared with a BMI < 25 kg/m^2, a BMI ≥ 25 kg/m^2 was associated with a significantly lower risk of all-cause mortality (HR 0.297, 95% CI 0.101 to 0.878, $p = 0.028$). These findings were consistent when BMI was examined as a continuous variable (HR 0.874, 95% CI 0.773 to 0.988, $p = 0.031$). A low BMI (<22 kg/m^2) should be considered as a risk factor for postoperative long-term mortality in this ageing population.

Keywords: body mass index; mortality; vertebral fracture; vertebroplasty

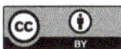

1. Introduction

The global age-standardized body mass index (BMI) has continuously increased over the past decades [1]. Despite variations in the prevalence of overweight/obese people in different regions in the world, a BMI ≥ 25 kg/m^2 has been associated with an increase in all-cause mortality [2,3]. This association may be partly attributed to the high risks of some non-communicable diseases (e.g., diabetes and cardiovascular diseases) for people who are overweight/obese. Alternatively, some studies have reported a J- or U-shaped relationship between BMI and mortality [4,5]. These findings raise the concern that a low BMI may indicate a risk of mortality, particularly in the elderly [6,7].

Vertebroplasty is commonly performed on patients with osteoporotic vertebral fractures [8,9]. Most patients who undergo a vertebroplasty are from an ageing population [8–10]. Although some postoperative outcomes have been investigated in patients who underwent a vertebroplasty [11,12], the risk factors associated with long-term mortality in this population are not yet clear. In a large population-based cohort study [13], a higher risk of musculoskeletal disease mortality was observed in people with a BMI < 24 (95% CI 24 to 25) kg/m^2, the cut-off point considered the upper limit of normal [14]. Factors associated with short-term (30-day) mortality after vertebroplasty in ageing people have been investigated in several studies [15,16]. Nevertheless, the effect of BMI on the risk of long-term mortality in this population remains unknown. In this study, we aimed to investigate the association of BMI with postoperative long-term mortality in patients who had undergone a vertebroplasty.

2. Materials and Methods

We retrospectively enrolled patients with a vertebral compression fracture of the thoracic or lumbar spine who underwent a vertebroplasty in the Department of Orthopedics at our hospital between May 2013 and June 2020. Patients diagnosed with pathologic fractures and those with no information on the assessment of bone mineral density were excluded. This study was conducted in accordance with the Declaration of Helsinki. The study protocol was approved (approval number CE22167A) by the Institutional Review Board of Taichung Veterans General Hospital, Taichung, Taiwan.

Relevant information, including preoperative BMI, history of smoking, diabetes, hypertension, chronic kidney disease, osteoporosis, and level of vertebral fracture, was recorded from the electronic medical records. The survival status of the study population was confirmed by the end of March 2021 according to data obtained from the Ministry of Health and Welfare, ROC. Thereafter, de-identified data were used for analyses. We divided the study sample into two groups according to their BMI ($\geq$25 kg/m^2 vs. <25 kg/m^2) in order to examine the effect of being overweight/obese (vs. normal weight) on the risk of all-cause mortality.

Statistical Analysis

All statistical analyses were conducted using the Statistical Package for the Social Sciences (IBM SPSS version 22.0; International Business Machines Corp., Armonk, NY, USA). Between-group differences in categorical and continuous variables were examined using the chi-square test and independent t-test, respectively. Kaplan–Meier survival curves were plotted for the groups of overweight/obese (BMI $\geq$ 25 kg/m^2) and normal weight (BMI < 25 kg/m^2). Cox proportional hazard models were conducted to examine the effects of being overweight/obese (vs. normal weight) and BMI (as a continuous variable) on all-cause mortality with adjustments for age, sex, history of smoking, diabetes, hypertension, chronic kidney disease, and osteoporosis. The assumption of a Cox proportional hazard model was tested with scaled Schoenfeld residuals, which confirmed no violation of the assumption. The cubic spline of baseline BMI versus risk of all-cause mortality by a Cox proportional hazards model was performed as a sensitivity test. To validate our findings in the study sample, we examined the associations of preoperative BMI with all-cause mortality in another cohort of patients (validation cohort). Similar to the study sample, these patients underwent a vertebroplasty for a vertebral compression fracture of the thoracic or lumbar spine during the same period. Nevertheless, we did not have information on comorbidities (diabetes, hypertension, chronic kidney disease, and osteoporosis) in this cohort. Statistical significance was determined with a two-sided p value of less than 0.05.

3. Results

A total of 164 patients were analyzed (mean age 75.8 $\pm$ 9.3 years, male 25.6%, mean BMI 24.0 $\pm$ 4.1 kg/m^2), and the median follow-up duration was 785 days. Table 1 shows the baseline characteristics of the study population according to their BMI. Patients who were overweight/obese (BMI $\geq$ 25 kg/m^2, mean 28.2 $\pm$ 2.8 kg/m^2) were younger, more likely to have diabetes, and less likely to have osteoporosis, compared with those who had a normal weight (BMI < 25 kg/m², mean 21.5 ± 2.5 kg/m²). There were no significant between-group differences in the other variables at baseline.

Table 1. Baseline characteristics of the study sample according to body mass index.

Variables	<25 kg/m²	≥25 kg/m²	p Value
N	103	61	
Age, years	77.2 ± 9.4	73.5 ± 8.6	0.013
Male sex, n (%)	30 (29.1)	12 (19.7)	0.180
Body mass index, kg/m²	21.5 ± 2.5	28.2 ± 2.8	<0.001
<18.5 kg/m², n (%)	14 (13.6)	—	—
Smoking, n (%)	10 (9.7)	2 (3.3)	0.126
Diabetes, n (%)	15 (14.6)	18 (29.5)	0.021
Hypertension, n (%)	52 (50.5)	35 (57.4)	0.393
Chronic kidney disease, n (%)	36 (35.0)	20 (32.8)	0.778
Osteoporosis, n (%)	83 (80.6)	38 (62.3)	0.010
Medication for osteoporosis, n (%) [a]	68 (66.0)	36 (59.0)	0.368
Level of vertebral fracture, n (%)			0.847
T-spine	44 (42.7)	27 (44.3)	
L-spine	59 (57.3)	34 (55.7)	

Values are mean ± SD or n (%). [a] Bisphosphonate, receptor activator of nuclear factor kappa-B inhibitor, or parathyroid hormone.

Figure 1 shows the Kaplan–Meier survival curves in patients who were overweight/obese and those who had a normal weight. A total of 27 (16.5%) deaths were identified, and the median survival time was 785 days (interquartile range 595, 1189). We observed that the survival rate was higher in patients who were overweight/obese than it was in those with a normal weight (log rank p = 0.021). We examined the associations of baseline characteristics with all-cause mortality in Table 2. In univariate analysis, age, BMI (≥25 vs. <25 kg/m², HR 0.336, 95% CI 0.127 to 0.890, p = 0.028), smoking, and chronic kidney disease were significantly associated with all-cause mortality. The associations remained significant in BMI (≥25 vs. <25 kg/m², HR 0.297, 95% CI 0.101 to 0.878, p = 0.028), smoking, and chronic kidney disease after multivariate adjustment.

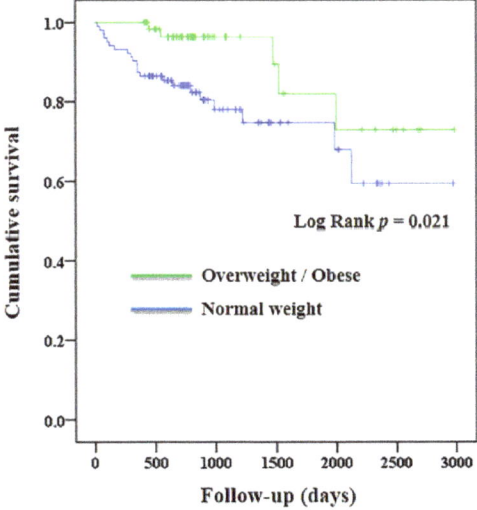

Figure 1. Survival curves of the study patients who were overweight/obese (body mass index ≥ 25 kg/m²) and normal weight (body mass index < 25 kg/m²).

Table 2. Associations of baseline characteristics with all-cause mortality of the study sample.

	Univariate Analysis		Multivariate Analysis [a]	
	HR (95% CI)	p	HR (95% CI)	p
Age, year	1.052 (1.003, 1.104)	0.037	1.028 (0.979, 1.079)	0.265
Sex (male vs. female)	1.018 (0.430, 2.409)	0.968	0.297 (0.088, 1.008)	0.052
BMI ($\geq$25 vs. <25 kg/m^2)	0.336 (0.127, 0.890)	0.028	0.297 (0.101, 0.878)	0.028
Smoking (yes vs. no)	2.844 (1.075, 7.524)	0.035	9.012 (2.166, 37.495)	0.003
Diabetes (yes vs. no)	1.453 (0.614, 3.439)	0.396	1.518 (0.578, 3.986)	0.397
Hypertension (yes vs. no)	2.016 (0.881, 4.617)	0.097	2.216 (0.903, 5.441)	0.082
CKD (yes vs. no)	2.601 (1.211, 5.587)	0.014	3.137 (1.375, 7.157)	0.007
Osteoporosis (yes vs. no)	2.368 (0.815, 6.879)	0.113	1.326 (0.420, 4.188)	0.631

BMI, body mass index. CKD, chronic kidney disease. [a] Adjusted for age, sex, BMI, smoking, diabetes, hypertension, CKD, and osteoporosis.

The findings were consistent when BMI was examined as a continuous variable. An increase in BMI was independently associated with a lower risk of all-cause mortality (adjusted HR 0.874, 95% CI 0.773 to 0.988, p = 0.031, Table 3). Figure 2 shows the cubic spline of BMI versus risk of all-cause mortality in the study sample. The point of BMI below which the risk of mortality started to increase was approximately 22 kg/m^2.

Table 3. Effect of body mass index (as a continuous variable) on all-cause mortality.

	Hazard Ratio (95% CI)	p
Body mass index (kg/m^2)		
Model 1	0.889 (0.808, 0.977)	0.015
Model 2	0.896 (0.810, 0.990)	0.031
Model 3	0.874 (0.773, 0.988)	0.031

Model 1, unadjusted. Model 2, adjusted for age and sex. Model 3, adjusted for variables in Model 2 plus smoking, diabetes, hypertension, chronic kidney disease, and osteoporosis.

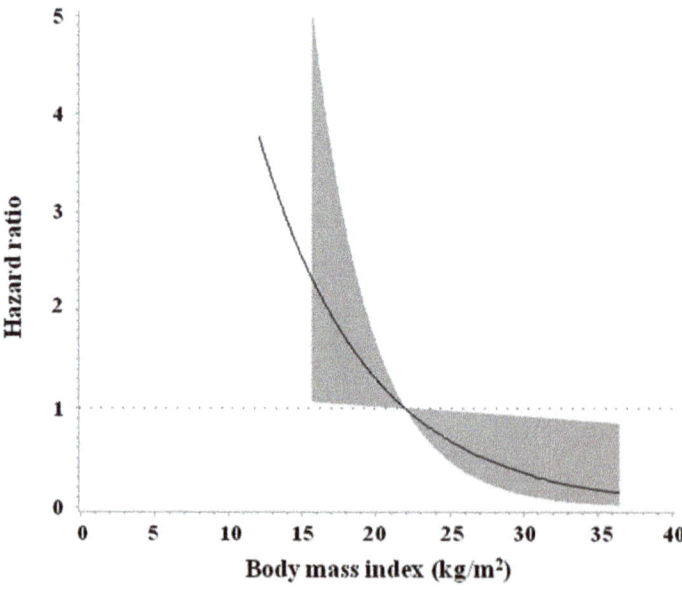

Figure 2. Cubic spline of body mass index versus risk of all-cause mortality in the study sample.

We examined our findings in the validation cohort (n = 266, mean age 76.0 ± 9.4 years, male 22.9%, mean BMI 24.6 ± 4.0 kg/m^2). A total of 101 (38.0%) deaths were identified in this cohort by the end of March 2022, and the median survival time was 1531 days (interquartile range 970, 2358). A preoperative BMI ≥ 25 kg/m^2 (vs. <25 kg/m^2) was associated with a lower risk of all-cause mortality (HR 0.570, 95% CI 0.377 to 0.861, p = 0.008, Table 4). This association remained significant after adjustment for age and sex (HR 0.588, 95% CI 0.387 to 0.891, p = 0.012). The findings were consistent when BMI was examined as a continuous variable (adjusted HR 0.945, 95% CI 0.895 to 0.998, p = 0.041).

Table 4. Effect of body mass index on all-cause mortality in the validation cohort.

	Hazard Ratio (95% CI)	p
Body mass index ≥25 vs. <25 kg/m^2		
Model 1	0.570 (0.377, 0.861)	0.008
Model 2	0.588 (0.387, 0.891)	0.012
Body mass index (kg/m^2)		
Model 1	0.941 (0.893, 0.992)	0.025
Model 2	0.945 (0.895, 0.998)	0.041

Model 1, unadjusted. Model 2, adjusted for age and sex.

4. Discussion

In this study, we demonstrated that being overweight/obese (vs. normal weight) was associated with a lower risk of all-cause mortality (HR 0.297, 95% CI 0.101 to 0.878, p = 0.028) in patients with a compression fracture of the thoracic or lumbar spine who had undergone a vertebroplasty during a median follow-up period of more than 2 years (785 days). Our findings were consistent when BMI was examined as a continuous variable (HR 0.874, 95% CI 0.773 to 0.988, p = 0.031). The point of BMI below which the risk of mortality began to increase was approximately 22 kg/m^2 in this ageing population (mean age 75.8 ± 9.3 years). Our findings suggest that low-BMI (probably <22 kg/m^2) ageing people who had undergone a vertebroplasty for a vertebral compression fracture may be at a higher risk for all-cause mortality.

The "obesity paradox" has been observed in patients with various medical conditions. A lower BMI was associated with a higher risk of mortality in patients with coronary artery disease [17,18] and chronic heart failure [19,20]. Similar findings were noted in patients with cancers [21,22]. Moreover, observation of the "obesity paradox" was more prominent in the elderly [23–25]. The aforementioned results are consistent in surgical patients [26,27]. In a large surgical cohort [27], the perioperative mortality rate was higher in patients with a BMI <25 kg/m^2 compared with those who had a BMI ≥ 25 kg/m^2. In line with previous reports and our findings, patients who were overweight/obese were associated with a lower risk of mortality after orthopedic surgery [28], particularly in the elderly [29,30]. People who underwent a vertebroplasty for vertebral fractures were commonly older than 65 years of age [8–10,31,32]. However, the effect of BMI on the risk of postoperative mortality in this population is not yet clear. Our findings suggest that patients who had undergone a vertebroplasty for a vertebral compression fracture with a BMI less than 25 kg/m^2 (or 22 kg/m^2) were at a higher risk of long-term mortality.

The mechanisms that account for the "obesity paradox" are not yet well understood. Patients who are underweight (BMI < 18.5 kg/m^2) may be of a poor nutritional status. However, even if we had excluded the patients with a BMI <18.5 kg/m^2 (n = 14) from the analyses, a lower risk of mortality was still noted in those with a BMI ≥ 25 kg/m^2 (adjusted HR 0.311, 95% CI 0.102 to 0.951, p = 0.041 vs. BMI 18.5 ≤ 25 kg/m^2). Some researchers have hypothesized that surgical patients who are overweight/obese may have a better preoperative nutritional status than those who are at a normal weight [33,34]. Additionally, there is likely to be an increase in both physiological stress and metabolic demands after surgical intervention, causing those patients with a low BMI to possibly be unable to appropriately adapt to these conditions [35], thus resulting in unfavorable outcomes. This scenario is more likely to be observed in an ageing population [36]. A low BMI in the elderly has been associated with malnutrition and sarcopenia [37,38], both of which have been associated with poor outcomes and mortality in older adults with fractures [39,40]. These findings may help explain the inverse relationship between BMI and mortality in our patients. Given that the effect of BMI on postoperative long-term mortality in patients who have undergone a vertebroplasty for a vertebral fracture has not yet been made clear, our results raise the concern that a low BMI results in adverse patient outcomes in this ageing surgical population.

Our study does have some limitations. First, this was a retrospective study with a relatively small number of study patients. The causal relationship between a low BMI and mortality risk could not be confirmed. Second, we did not have any information on the control status and medication use of some chronic diseases (e.g., blood pressure and diabetes control). Third, we did not investigate the cause-specific mortality in this relatively small study population. These factors should all be taken into account when interpreting our results. Despite these limitations, our findings underline the importance of preoperative BMI on postoperative outcomes in elderly surgical patients. This issue certainly deserves further investigations.

5. Conclusions

In summary, an increase in BMI was associated with a lower risk of all-cause mortality in patients who had undergone a vertebroplasty for a vertebral compression fracture. As these patients are usually older than 65 years of age, a low BMI (e.g., <22 kg/m^2) should be considered a risk factor for postoperative long-term mortality.

Author Contributions: Conceptualization, W.-C.W., J.-S.W. and C.-H.L.; Data curation, Y.-C.W., Y.-H.L., Y.-T.L., K.-H.C., C.-C.P. and C.-H.L.; Formal analysis, W.-C.W. and J.-S.W.; Funding acquisition, J.-S.W.; Investigation, Y.-C.W., Y.-H.L., Y.-T.L., K.-H.C., C.-C.P. and C.-H.L.; Methodology, J.-S.W.; Resources, C.-H.L.; Writing—original draft, W.-C.W. and J.-S.W.; Writing—review and editing, Y.-C.W., Y.-H.L., Y.-T.L., K.-H.C., C.-C.P. and C.-H.L. All authors have read and agreed to the published version of the manuscript.

Funding: This study was supported by research grants from Taichung Veterans General Hospital, Taichung, Taiwan (TCVGH-1103504C and TCVGH-1113502C). The funder was not involved in the study design, data collection, analysis, interpretation of the results, or preparation of the article.

Institutional Review Board Statement: The study was conducted according to the guidelines of the Declaration of Helsinki, and approved by the Institutional Review Board of Taichung Veterans General Hospital, Taichung, Taiwan (approval number CE22167A and date of approval 18 April 2022).

Informed Consent Statement: Patient consent was waived due to the retrospective study design and de-identified data were used for analyses.

Data Availability Statement: The data presented in this study are available on request from the corresponding author. The data are not publicly available due to privacy/ethical restrictions.

Conflicts of Interest: The authors declare no conflict of interest.

References

1. NCD Risk Factor Collaboration (NCD-RisC). Trends in adult body-mass index in 200 countries from 1975 to 2014: A pooled analysis of 1698 population-based measurement studies with 19·2 million participants. *Lancet* **2016**, *387*, 1377–1396. [CrossRef]
2. Global BMI Mortality Collaboration; Di Angelantonio, E.; Bhupathiraju, S.N.; Wormser, D.; Gao, P.; Kaptoge, S.; Berrington de Gonzalez, A. Body-mass index and all-cause mortality: Individual-participant-data meta-analysis of 239 prospective studies in four continents. *Lancet* **2016**, *388*, 776–786. [CrossRef]
3. Prospective Studies Collaboration. Body-mass index and cause-specific mortality in 900,000 adults: Collaborative analyses of 57 prospective studies. *Lancet* **2009**, *373*, 1083–1096. [CrossRef]
4. Berrington de Gonzalez, A.; Hartge, P.; Cerhan, J.R.; Flint, A.J.; Hannan, L.; MacInnis, R.J.; Thun, M.J. Body-mass index and mortality among 1.46 million white adults. *N. Engl. J. Med.* **2010**, *363*, 2211–2219. [CrossRef]

5. Aune, D.; Sen, A.; Prasad, M.; Norat, T.; Janszky, I.; Tonstad, S.; Vatten, L.J. BMI and all cause mortality: Systematic review and non-linear dose-response meta-analysis of 230 cohort studies with 3.74 million deaths among 30.3 million participants. *BMJ* **2016**, *353*, i2156. [CrossRef]
6. Yerrakalva, D.; Mullis, R.; Mant, J. The associations of "fatness", "fitness", and physical activity with all-cause mortality in older adults, a systematic review. *Obesity* **2015**, *23*, 1944–1956. [CrossRef]
7. Javed, A.A.; Aljied, R.; Allison, D.J.; Anderson, L.N.; Ma, J.; Raina, P. Body mass index and all-cause mortality in older adults, A scoping review of observational studies. *Obes. Rev.* **2020**, *21*, e13035. [CrossRef]
8. Buchbinder, R.; Osborne, R.H.; Ebeling, P.R.; Wark, J.D.; Mitchell, P.; Wriedt, C.; Murphy, B. A randomized trial of vertebroplasty for painful osteoporotic vertebral fractures. *N. Engl. J. Med.* **2009**, *361*, 557–568. [CrossRef]
9. Kallmes, D.F.; Comstock, B.A.; Heagerty, P.J.; Turner, J.A.; Wilson, D.J.; Diamond, T.H.; Jarvik, J.G. A randomized trial of vertebroplasty for osteoporotic spinal fractures. *N. Engl. J. Med.* **2009**, *361*, 569–579. [CrossRef]
10. Staples, M.P.; Kallmes, D.F.; Comstock, B.A.; Jarvik, J.G.; Osborne, R.H.; Heagerty, P.J.; Buchbinder, R. Effectiveness of vertebroplasty using individual patient data from two randomised placebo controlled trials: Meta-analysis. *BMJ* **2011**, *343*, d3952. [CrossRef]
11. Ren, H.L.; Jiang, J.M.; Chen, J.T.; Wang, J.X. Risk factors of new symptomatic vertebral compression fractures in osteoporotic patients undergone percutaneous vertebroplasty. *Eur. Spine J.* **2015**, *24*, 750–758. [CrossRef] [PubMed]
12. Lee, B.G.; Choi, J.H.; Kim, D.Y.; Choi, W.R.; Lee, S.G.; Kang, C.N. Risk factors for newly developed osteoporotic vertebral compression fractures following treatment for osteoporotic vertebral compression fractures. *Spine J.* **2019**, *19*, 301–305. [CrossRef] [PubMed]
13. Bhaskaran, K.; Dos-Santos-Silva, I.; Leon, D.A.; Douglas, I.J.; Smeeth, L. Association of BMI with overall and cause-specific mortality: A population-based cohort study of 3·6 million adults in the UK. *Lancet Diabetes Endocrinol.* **2018**, *6*, 944–953. [CrossRef]
14. Flegal, K.M.; Kit, B.K.; Orpana, H.; Graubard, B.I. Association of all-cause mortality with overweight and obesity using standard body mass index categories: A systematic review and meta-analysis. *JAMA* **2013**, *309*, 71–82. [CrossRef] [PubMed]
15. Toy, J.O.; Basques, B.A.; Grauer, J.N. Morbidity, mortality, and readmission after vertebral augmentation: Analysis of 850 patients from the American College of Surgeons National Surgical Quality Improvement Program database. *Spine* **2014**, *39*, 1943–1949. [CrossRef] [PubMed]
16. Kim, H.J.; Zuckerman, S.L.; Cerpa, M.; Yeom, J.S.; Lehman, R.A., Jr.; Lenke, L.G. Incidence and Risk Factors for Complications and Mortality After Vertebroplasty or Kyphoplasty in the Osteoporotic Vertebral Compression Fracture-Analysis of 1,932 Cases From the American College of Surgeons National Surgical Quality Improvement. *Glob. Spine J.* **2022**, *12*, 1125–1134. [CrossRef] [PubMed]
17. Krumholz, H.M.; Chen, J.; Chen, Y.T.; Wang, Y.; Radford, M.J. Predicting one-year mortality among elderly survivors of hospitalization for an acute myocardial infarction: Results from the Cooperative Cardiovascular Project. *J. Am. Coll. Cardiol.* **2001**, *38*, 453–459. [CrossRef]
18. Romero-Corral, A.; Montori, V.M.; Somers, V.K.; Korinek, J.; Thomas, R.J.; Allison, T.G.; Mookadam, F.; Lopez-Jimenez, F. Association of bodyweight with total mortality and with cardiovascular events in coronary artery disease: A systematic review of cohort studies. *Lancet* **2006**, *368*, 666–678. [CrossRef]
19. Kenchaiah, S.; Pocock, S.J.; Wang, D.; Finn, P.V.; Zornoff, L.A.; Skali, H.; Solomon, S.D. CHARM Investigators. Body mass index and prognosis in patients with chronic heart failure: Insights from the Candesartan in Heart failure, Assessment of Reduction in Mortality and morbidity (CHARM) program. *Circulation* **2007**, *116*, 627–636. [CrossRef]
20. Sharma, A.; Lavie, C.J.; Borer, J.S.; Vallakati, A.; Goel, S.; Lopez-Jimenez, F.; Arbab-Zadeh, A.; Mukherjee, D.; Lazar, J.M. Meta-analysis of the relation of body mass index to all-cause and cardiovascular mortality and hospitalization in patients with chronic heart failure. *Am. J. Cardiol.* **2015**, *115*, 1428–1434. [CrossRef]
21. Reichle, K.; Peter, R.S.; Concin, H.; Nagel, G. Associations of pre-diagnostic body mass index with overall and cancer-specific mortality in a large Austrian cohort. *Cancer Causes Control* **2015**, *26*, 1643–1652. [PubMed]
22. Schlesinger, S.; Siegert, S.; Koch, M.; Walter, J.; Heits, N.; Hinz, S.; Jacobs, G.; Hampe, J.; Schafmayer, C.; Nöthlings, U. Postdiagnosis body mass index and risk of mortality in colorectal cancer survivors: A prospective study and meta-analysis. *Cancer Causes Control* **2014**, *25*, 1407–1418. [PubMed]
23. Casas-Vara, A.; Santolaria, F.; Fernández-Bereciartúa, A.; González-Reimers, E.; García-Ochoa, A.; Martínez-Riera, A. The obesity paradox in elderly patients with heart failure: Analysis of nutritional status. *Nutrition* **2012**, *28*, 616–622. [PubMed]
24. Sakuyama, A.; Saitoh, M.; Hori, K.; Adachi, Y.; Iwai, K.; Nagayama, M. Associations of body mass index and hospital-acquired disability with post-discharge mortality in older patients with acute heart failure. *J. Geriatr. Cardiol.* **2022**, *19*, 209–217.
25. Martinez-Tapia, C.; Diot, T.; Oubaya, N.; Paillaud, E.; Poisson, J.; Gisselbrecht, M.; Morisset, L.; Caillet, P.; Baudin, A.; Pamoukdjian, F.; et al. The obesity paradox for mid- and long-term mortality in older cancer patients: A prospective multicenter cohort study. *Am. J. Clin. Nutr.* **2020**, *113*, 129–141.
26. El Moheb, M.; Jia, Z.; Qin, H.; El Hechi, M.W.; Nordestgaard, A.T.; Lee, J.M.; Han, K.; Kaafarani, H.M. The Obesity Paradox in Elderly Patients Undergoing Emergency Surgery, A Nationwide Analysis. *J. Surg. Res.* **2021**, *265*, 195–203.
27. Sood, A.; Abdollah, F.; Sammon, J.D.; Majumder, K.; Schmid, M.; Peabody, J.O.; Preston, M.A.; Kibel, A.S.; Menon, M.; Trinh, Q.D. The Effect of Body Mass Index on Perioperative Outcomes After Major Surgery, Results from the National Surgical Quality Improvement Program (ACS-NSQIP) 2005–2011. *World J. Surg.* **2015**, *39*, 2376–2385.

28. Hennrikus, M.; Hennrikus, W.P.; Lehman, E.; Skolka, M.; Hennrikus, E. The obesity paradox and orthopedic surgery. *Medicine* **2021**, *100*, e26936.
29. Yang, T.I.; Chen, Y.H.; Chiang, M.H.; Kuo, Y.J.; Chen, Y.P. Inverse relation of body weight with short-term and long-term mortality following hip fracture surgery: A meta-analysis. *J. Orthop. Surg. Res.* **2022**, *17*, 249.
30. Modig, K.; Erdefelt, A.; Mellner, C.; Cederholm, T.; Talbäck, M.; Hedström, M. "Obesity Paradox" Holds True for Patients with Hip Fracture, A Registry-Based Cohort Study. *J. Bone Jt. Surg. Am.* **2019**, *101*, 888–895.
31. Rho, Y.J.; Choe, W.J.; Chun, Y.I. Risk factors predicting the new symptomatic vertebral compression fractures after percutaneous vertebroplasty or kyphoplasty. *Eur. Spine J.* **2012**, *21*, 905–911. [PubMed]
32. Buchbinder, R.; Johnston, R.V.; Rischin, K.J.; Homik, J.; Jones, C.A.; Golmohammadi, K.; Kallmes, D.F. Percutaneous vertebroplasty for osteoporotic vertebral compression fracture. *Cochrane Database Syst. Rev.* **2018**, *4*, CD006349. [PubMed]
33. Eminovic, S.; Vincze, G.; Eglseer, D.; Riedl, R.; Sadoghi, P.; Leithner, A.; Bernhardt, G.A. Malnutrition as predictor of poor outcome after total hip arthroplasty. *Int. Orthop.* **2021**, *45*, 51–56. [PubMed]
34. Raad, M.; Amin, R.; Puvanesarajah, V.; Musharbash, F.; Rao, S.; Best, M.J.; Amanatullah, D.F. The CARDE-B Scoring System Predicts 30-Day Mortality After Revision Total Joint Arthroplasty. *J. Bone Jt. Surg. Am.* **2021**, *103*, 424–431.
35. Valentijn, T.M.; Galal, W.; Tjeertes, E.K.; Hoeks, S.E.; Verhagen, H.J.; Stolker, R.J. The obesity paradox in the surgical population. *Surgeon* **2013**, *11*, 169–176. [PubMed]
36. Schneider, S.M.; Al-Jaouni, R.; Pivot, X.; Braulio, V.B.; Rampal, P.; Hebuterne, X. Lack of adaptation to severe malnutrition in elderly patients. *Clin. Nutr.* **2002**, *21*, 499–504. [CrossRef]
37. Coin, A.; Sergi, G.; Beninca, P.; Lupoli, L.; Cinti, G.; Ferrara, L.; Benedetti, G.; Tomasi, G.; Pisent, C.; Enzi, G. Bone mineral density and body composition in underweight and normal elderly subjects. *Osteoporos. Int.* **2000**, *11*, 1043–1050.
38. Tonial, P.C.; Colussi, E.L.; Alves, A.L.S.; Stürmer, J.; Bettinelli, L.A. Prevalence of sarcopenia in elderly users of the primary health care system. *Nutr. Hosp.* **2020**, *34*, 450–455.
39. Meesters, D.M.; Wijnands, K.A.P.; Brink, P.R.G.; Poeze, M. Malnutrition and Fracture Healing: Are Specific Deficiencies in Amino Acids Important in Nonunion Development? *Nutrients* **2018**, *10*, 1597.
40. Chiang, M.H.; Kuo, Y.J.; Chen, Y.P. The Association between Sarcopenia and Postoperative Outcomes among Older Adults with Hip Fracture, a Systematic Review. *J. Appl. Gerontol.* **2021**, *40*, 1903–1913.

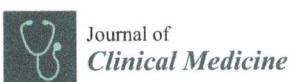

Article

A Prospective Randomized Study Comparing Functional Outcome in Distal Fibula Fractures between Conventional AO Semitubular Plating and Minimal Invasive Intramedullary "Photodynamic Bone Stabilisation"

Michael Zyskowski *, Markus Wurm, Frederik Greve, Philipp Zehnder, Patrick Pflüger, Michael Müller, Peter Biberthaler and Chlodwig Kirchhoff *

Department of Trauma Surgery, Klinikum Rechts der Isar, Technical University of Munich, Ismaninger Str. 22, 81675 Munich, Germany
* Correspondence: michael.zyskowski@mri.tum.de (M.Z.); chlodwig.kirchhoff@mri.tum.de (C.K.)

Abstract: (1) Background: As age in western populations is rising, so too are fractures, e.g., of the distal fibula. The aim of this study was to find out whether a novel, minimally invasive intramedullary osteosynthesis technique for the treatment of distal fibula fractures in elderly patients results in not only a reduction of postoperative complications, but also a shorter hospitalization time, an improved clinical outcome, and preserved autonomy in geriatric trauma patients. (2) Methods: In this prospective study, the results following surgical treatment for distal fibula fractures in geriatric patients after using DePuy Synthes® one-third semitubular plate (Group I) or a minimally invasive intramedullary photodynamic Bone StabilizationSystem (IlluminOss®) (Group II) were compared at 6 weeks, 12 weeks, 6 months, and 1 year after initial treatment. (3) Results: Significant improvement regarding clinical outcome was shown in Group II 6 and 12 weeks after surgery. (4) Conclusions: Our study results demonstrate that the use of this new intramedullary stabilization system in combination with an immediate postoperative weight bearing seems to be a safe and stable treatment option for ankle fractures in geriatric patients, especially in the early stages of recovery.

Keywords: ankle fracture; elderly; fibular; fragility fracture; intramedullary stabilsation; IlluminOss®; osteosynthesis

Citation: Zyskowski, M.; Wurm, M.; Greve, F.; Zehnder, P.; Pflüger, P.; Müller, M.; Biberthaler, P.; Kirchhoff, C. A Prospective Randomized Study Comparing Functional Outcome in Distal Fibula Fractures between Conventional AO Semitubular Plating and Minimal Invasive Intramedullary "Photodynamic Bone Stabilisation". *J. Clin. Med.* **2022**, *11*, 7178. https://doi.org/10.3390/jcm11237178

Academic Editor: Gianluca Testa

Received: 7 November 2022
Accepted: 30 November 2022
Published: 2 December 2022

Publisher's Note: MDPI stays neutral with regard to jurisdictional claims in published maps and institutional affiliations.

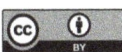

Copyright: © 2022 by the authors. Licensee MDPI, Basel, Switzerland. This article is an open access article distributed under the terms and conditions of the Creative Commons Attribution (CC BY) license (https://creativecommons.org/licenses/by/4.0/).

1. Introduction

Ankle fractures (FX), common injuries constituting about 9% of all FX [1] of the human skeleton, are considered the third most common FX in geriatric patients [2,3]. In recent years, an increasing number of elderly patients have suffered from ankle FX [4,5]. The majority of these elderly patients already suffered from numerous comorbidities at the time of the accident [6]. The focus of fracture treatment in the elderly population is to achieve as much freedom as possible, in combination with maintaining quality of life comparable to the pre-accidental level. Nevertheless, operative treatment is associated with typical complications, such as mal- or nonunion, and especially skin problems ranging from delayed wound healing to severe skin defects [7–12].

Open reduction and internal fixation (ORIF) has become the standard of care for displaced ankle FX in adults [13,14]. Several techniques for internal ankle fixation are commonly used, ranging from simple lag screw fixation to plate osteosynthesis with non-locking to locking screw systems up to biodegradable systems [15–20]. In this context, several studies in the common literature focus on intramedullary (IM) fixation of the distal fibula FX, fracture stabilization, and the appearance of soft tissue-related complications in the older population [21–27].

In addition to fracture healing and the complications related to the surgery itself, postoperative therapy is a prognostic factor for the patient's satisfaction, functional outcome, and return to normal daily activities [28–31]. For older patients suffering from an ankle fracture, returning to their normal daily life is important in terms of their quality of life and freedom [32–34]. In older patients with preexisting comorbidities, surgical treatment must not only respect the soft tissue conditions, but should also have the goal of a shortened pre- and post-operative therapy time window, shortened hospital stay, faster time of recovery, and achievement of full resilience as quickly as possible [6,35]. Therefore, the main goal of any post-operative therapy is to reduce time of recovery to a minimum and to achieve full physical capacity as early as possible. In the past, a few clinical trials have shown that early weight bearing and functional treatment avoiding a plaster cast may shorten the immobilization period, but it also may provoke a loss of reduction, depending on morphology and initial stability of the FX, as well as patients' age and comorbidities [28,32,36–39]. A few clinical trials have demonstrated that IM ankle FX fixation might be a good method to preserve the soft tissue, but it could lead to fibula shortening and loosening of the implant [21,22,26,27,40,41].

Thus far, surgical treatment of FX with IM nailing has already shown promising results in the treatment of various complex fractures of the femur [42], tibial shaft [43], and clavicle [44]; hence, IM nailing has become a standard implant. To the best of our knowledge, there still exists no prospective randomized trial assessing the treatment of distal fibula FX using these modern implants.

In this context, surgical treatment of ankle fractures using IM fixation systems were controversially discussed because of their biomechanical performance and implant costs [45,46].

The aim of this study was to analyze whether open reduction internal fixation (ORIF) of distal fibula FX, using a standard semitubular plate or closed reduction and IM fixation using a new minimally invasive intramedullary Photodynamic Bone Stabilization System (IlluminOss®), allows for a better outcome for immediate postoperative weight bearing and the reduction of complications in older patients with a wide range of comorbidities.

2. Materials and Methods

2.1. Patients

Institutional Review Board approval was obtained prior to this study (IRB approval No: 103/15, Ethical Committee of Technical University Munich, Registration in the German Clinical Trails Register trail number DRKS00025496). This was a prospective randomized single center study with two parallel groups. The study was conducted under consideration of the CONSORT statement (Figure 1). All patients over 65 years suffering from a distal fibula FX according to AO classification (AO 44 B1.1, B1.2, B1.3) with consecutive indication for surgery and a Charlson Comorbidity Index (CCI) greater than one who presented at our academic level-one trauma center between 06/2015 and 06/2018 were prospectively enrolled [47,48]. The CCI predicts the 10-year survival in patients with multiple comorbidities and takes into consideration 19 comorbid diseases, including cardiovascular disorders, diabetes mellitus, liver and lung diseases, cerebrovascular incident and transient ischemic attacks, dementia, COPD, and connective tissue diseases [47]. Written informed consent of the patients was obtained. A randomization plan (Randlist®, DatInf GmbH, Tübingen, Germany) was used to divide patients regarding treatment using either the DePuy Synthes® one-third semitubular plate (DePuy Synthes®, Umkirch, Germany) (Group I) or the IlluminOss® Photodynamic Bone Stabilization System (IlluminOss Medical, Inc., East Providence, RI, USA) (Group II).

Exclusion criteria were mental disorders, patients under comprehensive legal support, and pathological or open FX [40].

2.2. Surgical Technique and Postoperative Therapy

All patients were operated on by expert trauma surgeons, experienced in lower extremity surgery. After assessment by the anesthetists, general anesthesia was performed in all cases. A single prophylactic dose of 1.5 mg cephalosporin was administered preoperatively.

The patients were placed in a supine position on a radiolucent table with a pillow under the ipsilateral gluteal region and the injured ankle.

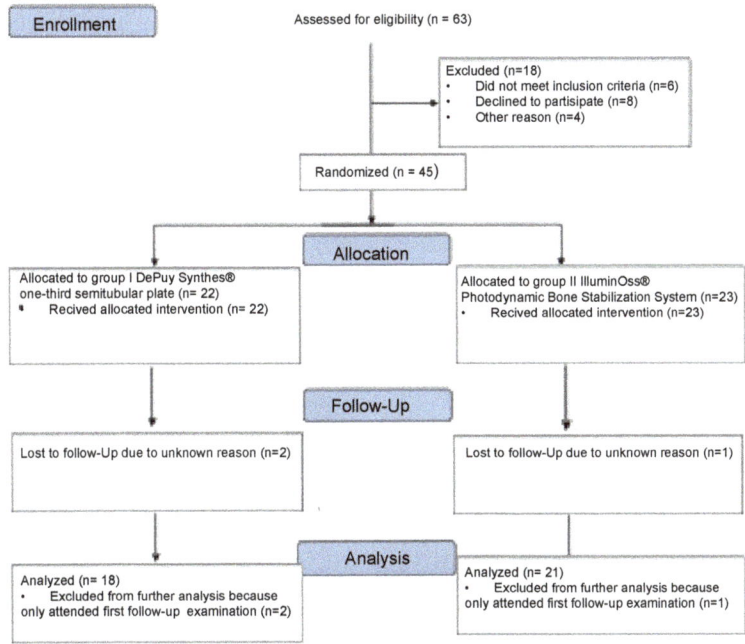

Figure 1. CONSORT (Consolidated Standards of Reporting Trials) flow diagram.

In group I, all surgeries were performed under tourniquet control (250 mmHg) using a standard lateral approach to the distal fibula according to AO recommendations. ORIF was performed according to AO guidelines using a 3.5 mm lag screw and semi-tubular neutralization plate, as well as 3.5 mm cortical screws [41]. The syndesmotic stability was verified with the lateral hook test [49].

Group II required preoperative preparations. The IlluminOss® Photodynamic Bone Stabilization System needs hardening by visible light (436 nm). The length of the light fiber cable is predetermined to 183 cm. Therefore, the light box is placed outside of the sterile surgical field on the fractured side, but as close as under sterile surgery conditions possible to assure the connection between the light cable and light box.

Primarily the closed reduction of the fracture was performed using image intensifier control in two planes. Then, the tip of the fibula was incised using a straight awl under fluoroscopy control. After the correct position was achieved, the entry portal was enlarged. Then, the straight awl was removed, followed by the insertion of a 4 mm cannulated awl (Figure 2A,B) allowing for the insertion of a ball tip guidewire bridging the FX into the medullary canal. Consecutively, the cannulated awl was removed. The ball tip guidewire assured that the now inserted cannulated burrs for reaming the medullary canal stayed in the designated position to be able to clear the fracture site. Reaming was performed in 0.5 mm steps to clean the channel with a minimum diameter of 6 mm up to a maximum diameter of 8.0 mm (Figure 3A,B). To avoid additional fractures of the fibula shaft, additional reamers with a diameter more than 8.00 mm should not be inserted. Furthermore, the surgeon should perform a fluoroscopy while reaming and have experience in intramedullary osteosynthesis. Then, the cannulated burr was removed while the guidewire remained in situ. Consecutively, a dilator and sheath were placed in the fibula under fluoroscopy control. When reaching the correct position, the guidewire and the dilator were removed. During the preceding surgical steps, the OR nurse assembled the implant by removing air from the balloon and transferring the monomer into a syringe. The prepared implant was handed to the surgeon and, finally, the monomer was inserted into the fibula via the already placed sheath (Figure 4A–C). When the right position was confirmed, the sheath was slowly separated and removed. Then the balloon was infused with the monomer (Figure 5). The last two steps were assured under fluoroscopy guidance. When the light cable was handed to the surgeon, the timer was put onto the front of the light box. The specific light emission time was adapted to the length of the chosen implant. The visible light corroborates the monomer (Figure 6); this process should not be disrupted or stopped. After the input hardening time, the light stopped automatically. Then, the catheter connected to the balloon was removed using a slap hammer. As the catheter was removed, the syndesmotic stability was test with the dorsiflexion-external rotation stress test under fluoroscopic control [50]. The last surgical steps include a final fluoroscopic control in two planes, wound closure, and dressing. Postoperatively, physical therapy was initiated. Preoperative ASA Physical Status Classification System was collected from the anesthesia documentation [51].

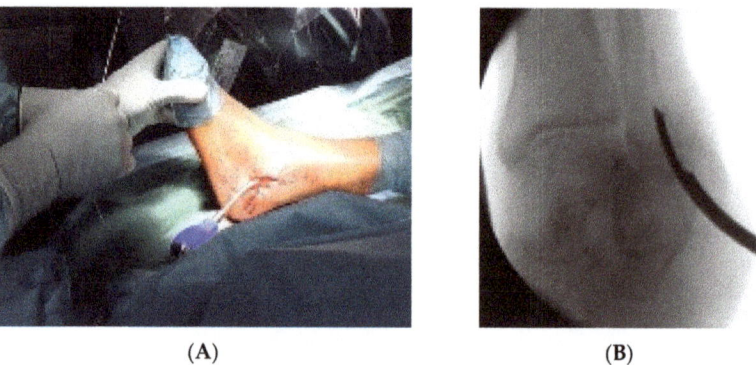

Figure 2. (**A**) demonstrates the insertion of the 4 mm cannulated awl with the corresponding intraoperative fluoroscopic control (**B**).

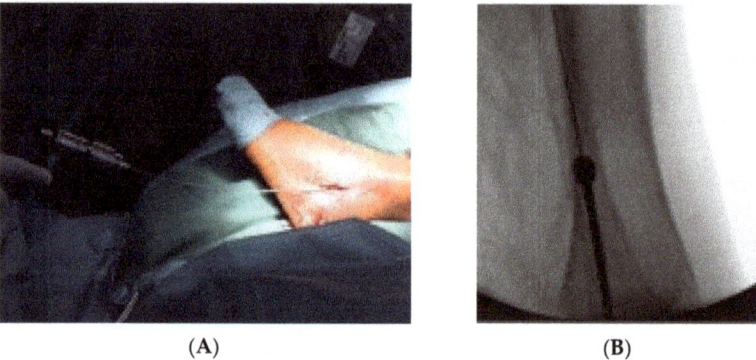

Figure 3. In (**A**) the 1 mm stepwise reaming with a minimum diameter of 4.5 mm is shown with the corresponding intraoperative fluoroscopic image of the reaming procedure (**B**).

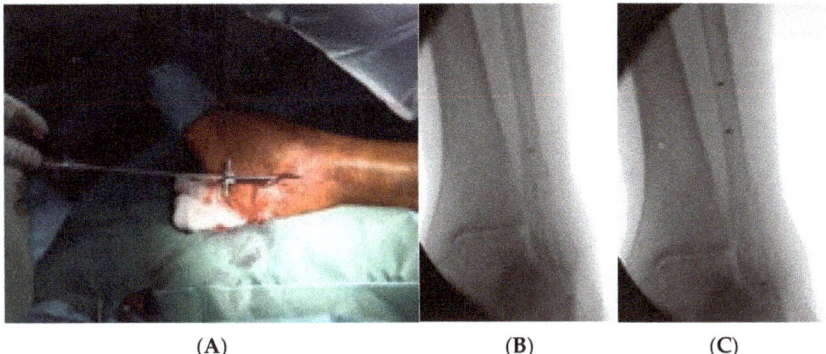

Figure 4. This figure demonstrates the insertion of the implant into the fibula via the already placed sheath (**A**), the fluoroscopic control of the insertion (**B**) and confirmation of the final position via fluoroscopic control and radiopaque markers on the implant (**C**).

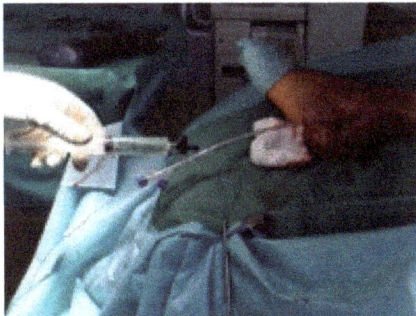

Figure 5. This figure shows the infusion of the balloon with the monomer.

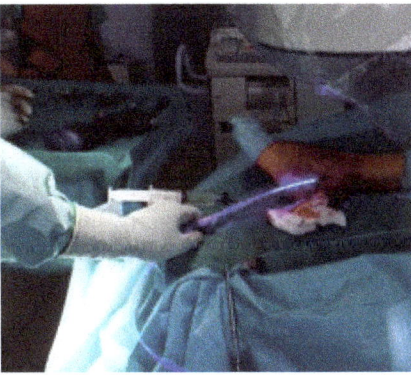

Figure 6. Here, the curing of the monomer by the visible light of 436 nm is shown.

Group I patients were treated following the rehabilitation protocols (Table 1) of our trauma department, which allowed partial weight bearing restricted to 20 kg for 6 weeks, using crouches or a medical walking boot, and pain-adapted motion out of the walking boot without limitations, according to the recommendations of the German Society for Orthopedics and Trauma (DGOU) [44]. After the initial 6 weeks, these patients were allowed to increase the load of weight bearing with the goal to achieve full weight bearing within 10 weeks after surgery.

Table 1. Rehabilitation protocols for both study groups.

Rehabilitation Protocol	Week 1–6 after Surgery	Week 7–12 after Surgery
DePuy Synthes® One-Third Semitubular Plate	partial weight bearing 20 kg	increase weight bearing load
	Walking boot	train away the walking boot
	crouches	crouches till full weight bearing
	pain-adapted motion without limitation	pain-adapted motion without limitation
	Week 1–3 after Surgery	Week 4–12 after Surgery
IlluminOss® Photodynamic Bone Stabilization System	full weight bearing	full weight bearing
	Walking boot	train away the walking boot and switch to an ankle brace
	no crouches	no crouches
	pain-adapted motion without limitation	pain-adapted motion without limitation

In Groupe II, full weight bearing was allowed right after surgery using a medical walking boot without the use of crouches and pain-adapted motion out of the walking boot without limitations. After 3 weeks, the patients were allowed to train the medical walking boot away, with the possibility to switch from the walking boot to an ankle brace.

2.3. Follow-Up Evaluation

The first follow-up exam was set up 6 weeks postoperatively. Additional follow-ups were terminated after 3, 6, and 12 months. The follow-up examinations were performed by independent investigators not involved in patients' initial surgical treatment (PZ, FG, MW) at the outpatient clinic of our level-one university trauma center.

For assessment of pain, the visual analogue scale (VAS) [52], ranging from 0 "no pain" to 10 "worst imaginable pain", was used. ROM and ligament stability were registered during standardized clinical follow-up examination. Moreover, sensomotoric disorders and postoperative complications were recorded. Minor complications were defined as those possibly treatable conservatively (e.g., superficial wound infections, delayed union etc.), whereas major complications needed operative revision (e.g., secondary loss of reduction, non-union, severe wound infections, etc.).

For the assessment of lower extremity and ankle function, the Olerud and Molander ankle score (OMAS) [53,54] and the Karlsson and Peterson Scoring System for Ankle function (KPSS) [55] were comprised and stated the primary outcome markers.

X-rays were taken postoperatively, as well as at the follow-up examinations, and evaluated with special respect to signs of bony healing and secondary loss of reduction.

2.4. Statistics and Sample Size Calculation

Statistical analyses were performed using the statistical software SigmaStat (version 3.5; Systat Software, San Jose, CA, USA). The scores at certain time points were compared with an independent t test after a normality check was passed and equal variances were detected. Normal distributed data with unequal variances would have been compared using the Welch's t test. Arbitrarily, data were tested with the Mann–Whitney U test. The significance level was set at $p = 0.05$.

Power analysis was performed prior to this study using G*Power for Mac. The Wilcoxon signed-rank test was used to compare the means of pre- and postoperative values. The significance threshold was set at a p value of <0.05.

We derived these figures from preliminary studies with OMAS in ankle fractures [56]. At a significance level of 0.05 and using the Welch's t test for independent samples, 20 persons per experimental group are needed to achieve a power of 80%.

3. Results

3.1. Epidemiological Data

At first, 45 patients were enrolled in this study. The mean age was 77 years (range 65–93 years). Of the ankles fractured, 24 were right (53%) and 21 left (47%). Three patients were lost to follow-up for unknown reasons, whereas 3 patients were only able to attend the first follow-up examination due to further health-related causes. The remaining 39 of 45 patients (86%) available for all follow-up examinations presented with a mean age of 77 years (range 65–92 years) and a CCI of 2 (range 1–3 points) at the time of injury, with no statistical differences between both groups. Eighteen patients were assigned to group I (46%) and 21 patients (54%) to group II.

The most common injury type was ankle sprain resulting from supination and external rotation trauma according to the Lauge Hansen classification [57,58]. All accidents happened during spare time and were of low velocity character (100%).

Regarding gender distribution, 16 male (41%) compared to 23 female patients (59%) were included. The interval between trauma and surgery accounted for an average of 8 days (2–20 days). Group I had an interval time of 9 days (5–20 days) and Group II an interval time of 4 days (2–9 days), which reached statistical significance when compared ($p = 0.01$, see Table 2). Correspondingly, the mean length of stay in hospital accounted for an average of 6.2 days (range 2–21 days): for Group I, 9 days (range 4–21 days) and for Group II, 5.3 days (range 2–8 days), which showed a significant difference ($p = 0.05$, Table 2).

Table 2. Patient demographics and injury characteristics of both groups are shown. Data are provided as ⌀ mean and +/− standard deviation.

Characteristics	DePuy Synthes® One-Third Semitubular Plate	IlluminOss® Photodynamic Bone Stabilization System
Mean age (years)	⌀76 ± 8	⌀80 ± 8
Sex (male: female)	8:10	7:14
Side (right:left)	10:8	10:11
Mean BMI	⌀26	⌀24
Mean CCI	⌀2 ± 1	⌀2 ± 1
ASA Scoring		
ASA I	2	3
ASA II	13	12
ASA III	3	6
Surgery time (minutes)	⌀45 ± 5	⌀36 ± 4

Regarding the side of the fracture, 20 right (51.3%) compared to 19 left (48.7%) ankles were fractured. In Group I, 10 right (55.6%) and 8 left (44.4%) ankles were treated versus treatment of 10 right (47.6%) and 11 left (52.4%) ankles in Group II. Regarding the fracture morphology, no difference in distribution considering the AO classification (AO 44 B1.1, B1.2, B1.3) in the treated patients could be shown for both groups. In Group I, 15 patients (83.3%) showed an AO 44 B1.1 type fracture, 2 patients (11.1%) an AO 44 B1.2, and 1 patient (5.6%) an AO 44 B1.3. A similar fracture morphology distribution was detected in Group II, were 17 patients (81.0%) with an AO 44 B1.1, 2 with an AO 44.B1.2 (9.5%), and 2 with an AO 44 B1.3 (9.5%) were treated. The body mass index (BMI) for both groups was similar, with a BMI of 26 in Group I and a BMI of 24 in Group II (see Table 2). The ASA-Score showed no significant differences between the both groups. In addition, regarding the surgical time, in general anesthesia, no significant differences could be shown, with a slight advantage for Group II (see Table 2).

3.2. Clinical Outcome

Only Group I patients ($n = 4$, 22%) presented with minor complications, such as swelling and redness of the wound in two cases (11%) and one deep vein thrombosis (5.5%). In one patient, bronchial pneumonia resulted from a prolonged hospital stay due to difficult postoperative mobilization (5.5%) treated with intravenous antibiotics for one week. Group

I showed a significantly higher incidence of minor complications compared to Group II, which did not have any minor complications ($p = 0.01$, see Table 3).

Table 3. Overview of the complications for both patient groups, Group I treated with DePuy Synthes one-third semitubular® plate and Group II treated with IlluminOss® Photodynamic Bone Stabilization System.

Minor Complication	DePuy Synthes® One-Third Semitubular Plate	IlluminOss® Photodynamic Bone Stabilization System	p-Values
Swelling/redness	2 (11%)		
deep vein thrombosis	1 (5.5%)		
respiratory infection	1 (5.5%)		
			$p = 0.01$
Major Complication			
deep wound infection	1 (5.5%)		
Loss of reposition		1 (4.7%)	
			$p = 0.47$

In both study groups, one major complication was observed. In detail, one Group I patient (5.5%) suffered from a deep wound infection resulting in material loosening followed by operative debridement, material removal, and intravenous antibiotics for ten days. One Group II patient (4.7%) showed a loss of reduction such that the operative procedure was changed to the semitubular plate treatment ($p = 0.47$, see Table 3).

During the first clinical follow-up examination, all patients were asked if they had been able to follow the rehabilitation protocol. All patients, regardless of group assignment, stated that they followed the recommended rehabilitation protocol.

The Olerud and Molander ankle score (OMAS) showed in the first two clinical follow-ups after 6 and 12 weeks significantly better results in Group II compared to Group I ($p = 0.01$, see Table 4). Similar results for the first two clinical follow-ups were recognized in Group II for the Karlsson and Peterson Scoring System for Ankle function (KPSS), confirming the good OMAS results ($p = 0.01$ and 0.02, see Table 4). In the later follow-up exams after 6 and 12 months, no further statistical difference between both groups was found (OMAS $p = 0.06$ and 0.07, KPSS $p = 0.06$ and 0.06, see Table 4). Regarding the VAS, only at the first clinical follow up was a statistical difference detected ($p = 0.01, 0.09, 0.24$ and 0.15, see Table 4). Regarding range of motion (ROM), statistically high significant differences could be identified in our clinical follow-up exams between both groups for extension (dorsiflexion) and flexion ($p = 0.01$, see Table 5).

3.3. Radiological Follow Up

At the final follow-up (12 months postop), 39 patients—18 treated with the DePuy Synthes® semitubular plate and 21 patients using the IlluminOss® Photodynamic Bone Stabilization System—demonstrated complete osseous healing on radiographs without any signs of complications (see Figures 7 and 8). No case of non-union was identified. The one Group I patient who suffered from a deep wound infection and loosening of the implant needed a conversion to a conservative cast treatment. His fracture healed without non-union 15 months after the initial surgery. For the single Group II patient who showed a loss of reduction, fracture healing without non-union was achieved within 14 months after conversion to a semitubular plate fixation treatment.

Table 4. Functional Ankle Scoring was assessed using VAS, OMAS, and KPSS for both treatment/patient groups separately at 6 and 12 weeks as well as 6 and 12 months postoperatively. Results are given as ∅ mean and +/− standard deviation. Group I was treated by DePuy Synthes one third semitubular, Group II with the IlluminOss® Photodynamic Bone Stabilization System.

Treatment Group	Scores	6 Weeks	12 Weeks	6 Months	12 Months
	VAS				
Group I		4 ±.1	2.94 ± 0.89	2.41 ± 1.00	1.94 ± 0.65
Group II		3.19 ± 0.9	2.52 ± 0.92	2.2 ± 0.76	1.70 ± 0.73
	p value	0.01	0.09	0.24	0.15
	OMAS				
Group I		∅44.3 ± 18	∅55.9 ± 16	∅63.8 ± 15	∅70.3 ± 8
Group II		∅63.7 ± 12	∅67.5 ± 14	∅71.2 ± 10	∅76.2 ± 10
	p value	0.01	0.01	0.06	0.07
	KPSS				
Group I		∅40.61 ± 10	∅52.30 ± 11	∅66.52 ± 12	∅69.98 ± 13
Group II		∅57.04 ± 10	∅61.17 ± 9	∅72.3 ± 11	∅76.63 ± 9
	p value	0.01	0.02	0.06	0.06

Table 5. Range of Motion at each single follow-up exam. Results are given as ∅ mean and +/− standard deviation. Group I was treated by DePuy Synthes one third semitubular, Group II with the IlluminOss® Photodynamic Bone Stabilization System.

ROM	6 Weeks	12 Weeks	6 Months	12 Months
Group I				
Extension(dorsiflexion)	∅4 ± 2	∅10 ± 3	∅14 ± 2	∅18 ± 2
Flexion	∅20 ± 4	∅23 ± 4	∅32 ± 4	∅35 ± 3
Group II				
Extension(dorsiflexion)	∅10 ± 2	∅15 ± 4	∅18 ± 4	∅18 ± 2
Flexion	∅25 ± 4	∅32 ± 3	∅34 ± 4	∅36 ± 2
p value				
Extension(dorsiflexion)	0.01	0.01	0.03	0.47
Flexion	0.01	0.01	0.07	0.19

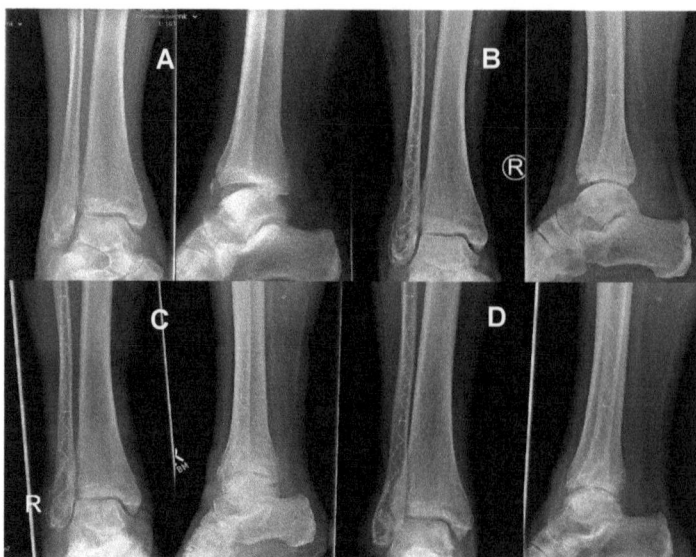

Figure 7. Radiograph of a 77-year-old female patient with an AO type 44 B1.1 ((**A**) a preoperative) fracture treated with the IlluminOss® Photodynamic Bone Stabilization System. Postoperative results after 6 (**B**) and 12 weeks (**C**) as well as after 14 months (**D**) showed excellent fracture healing.

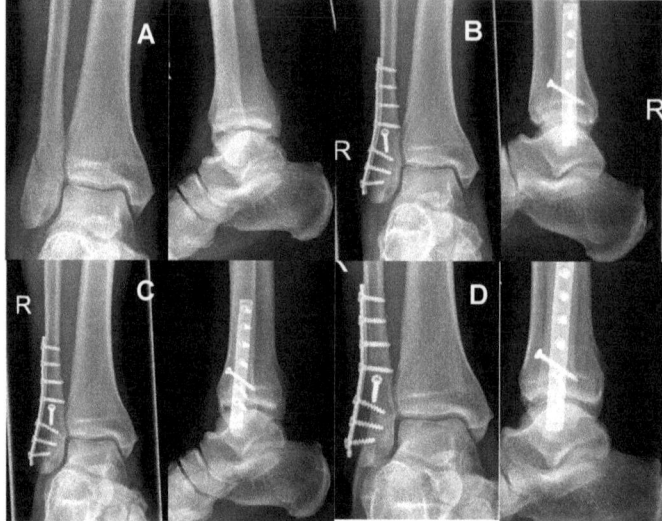

Figure 8. (**A**) shows the preoperative radiograph of a 72-year-old male patient with an AO type 44B1.1 fracture. The patient was treated with the DePuy Synthes® one-third semi tubular plate system. Figure (**B**) presents the postoperative results after 6 and Figure (**C**) after 12 weeks. In addition, the 14 months postoperative control (**D**) shows good fracture healing without any secondary complications.

4. Discussion

To the best of our knowledge, this is the first randomized controlled study to compare semitubular plates with the presented new intramedullary stabilization system in distal fibula fracture treatment with an immediate postoperative weight bearing regime in the intramedullary stabilization patient group. With increasing age, the probability of fracture occurrence rises, and also the number of ankle fractures (9% of all human skeleton fractures [1]) increases; thus, ankle fractures are considered the third most common FX in geriatric patients [2,3]. Usually, many of these elderly patients with ankle FX already suffer from numerous comorbidities at the time of the accident [6]. In this context, treatment of ankle fractures in the elderly population should result in achieving as much freedom as possible, in combination with quality of life comparable to before the accident. Nevertheless, operative treatment is usually associated with typical complications, such as mal- or nonunion, and especially skin problems ranging from delayed wound healing to severe skin defects [7–12]. Commonly known open reduction and internal fixation (ORIF) using various techniques is the standard of care for displaced ankle FX in adults [15–17]. Generally speaking, a recent advance in the treatment of fractures of different bones was the introduction of intramedullary nails [43,44]. Thus far, the use of intramedullary nailing systems in distal fibula fractures has been investigated under the aspects of FX stabilization, soft tissue management, and complication rates [25–27]. The majority of these studies were of retrospective character. The presented prospective randomized study focused on the comparison of treating ankle fractures of patients at an age over 65 years either using a rather established semitubular plate AO-system or an intramedullary Photodynamic Bone Stabilization System (IlluminOss®). Our results show that the IlluminOss® system allows for a progressive postoperative rehabilitation protocol performing full weight bearing immediately after surgery, leading to reliable results along with a good functional outcome.

In the general literature, complication rates of up to 25% have been reported for ankle fractures, especially in geriatric patients [10,13]. These complications include wound healing problems, redness, hyperthermia, superficial and deep infections, deep leg vein thrombosis, and loosening of the material resulting in a loss of reposition. Previous studies in elderly patients with preexisting comorbidities demonstrated that intramedullary nailing systems in distal fibula FX have a significantly lower incidence of soft tissue complications and lead to adequate FX stability compared to conventional plate osteosynthesis [26,28–30]. White et al. described in their prospective randomized study on 100 patients ($n = 50$ ORIF, $n = 50$ IM nailing) no superficial wound infections in the IM group compared to eight (16%) superficial wound infections in the ORIF group [22]. Similar results for wound infections following IM nailing were described by Cofiman et al. [27]. In their study, only 1 deep infection occurred in the 34 patients available for follow-up after IM nailing [27]. Both studies consider small incisions as beneficial for soft tissue healing [22,27]. In the actual study, the rate of postoperative complications was lower in the Photodynamic Bone Stabilization System group (Group II). Similar to White et al. and Cofiman et al., no single minor complication (superficial wound infection, delayed union etc.) was detected in this treatment Group II. In contrast, in Group I treated with the DePuy Synthes® one-third semitubular plate with a rather greater incision, four minor complications (22%) occurred. In terms of major complications, such as secondary loss of reduction, non-union, major wound infections, etc., only one major complication was detected in both groups without reaching significance (Group I 5.5%, Group II 4.7%. See Table 3).

Considering the consistently low complication rates in the above mentioned studies (White et al., Cofiman et al. [22,27]) as well as in the presented study for the patients treated with the IM IlluminOss® Photodynamic Bone Stabilization System, we are convinced that the significantly reduced size of the surgical incision wound plays a decisive role in the reduction of wound healing disorders, especially in older patients with significant comorbidities. Moreover, our data suggest that the small surgical incision allows for an overlook of the posttraumatic soft-tissue swelling and is not considered as a contraindication to a potentially earlier surgery, along with earlier mobilization and an earlier discharge from the hospital.

Early weight bearing and postoperative mobilization are very controversially discussed in the literature. In this context, patient-related factors, such as age, comorbidities, and fracture morphology, have a strong impact on the postoperative treatment [14,33,45,48,59].

Smeeing et al. showed in a normal-aged patient population (18–65 y) without comorbidities suffering from Lauge-Hansen supination external rotation type 2–4 ankle fractures treated with ORIF that a postoperative unlimited weight-bearing and mobilization regimen improved short-term functional outcome after six weeks, shortened the absence from work, and improved the time to return to sports compared to the patients who only followed a limited weight-bearing or unprotected non-weight-bearing therapy regimen. The mean OMAS (61.2 ± 19.0) after six weeks was up to 10 to 15 points higher compared to the two other groups [35].

In this context, we were able to prove in the actual study that treatment of distal fibula fractures with IM stabilization using the innovative IlluminOss® Photodynamic Bone Stabilization System allowing for an immediate weight bearing in elder patients with a wide range of comorbidities leads to similar good functional results six weeks postoperatively, as described by Smeeing in patients under 65 (see Table 4). Therefore, the actual data present a significant better outcome at the first two follow-up exams (6 and 12 weeks postoperatively) compared to the ORIF group who followed a restricted postoperative rehabilitation protocol including partial weight bearing (see Table 1).

We believe this new IM implant used in the presented study allows for a safe and stable fracture fixation, and it is the key to the early full weight bearing and good clinical outcome in the enrolled elderly patients with significant comorbidities.

Regarding the hospital length of stay, a significant difference between the two groups was identified in favor of Group II ($p = 0.05$, see Table 6). This result confirmed the significant differences between patients from Group I and Group II in terms of range of motion and the assessed outcome scores (see Table 4). In addition, patients in Group II had a significantly shorter preoperative delay caused by posttraumatic swelling of the ankle compared to patients in Group I ($p = 0.01$, see Table 6).

Table 6. Interval between trauma and surgery as well as mean length of hospital stay for both groups.

Interval between Trauma and Surgery	Days
general	∅8 days
DePuy Synthes® one-third semitubular plate	∅9 days
IlluminOss® Photodynamic Bone Stabilization System	∅4 days
	$p = 0.01$
Length of Hospital Stay	**Days**
general	∅6 days
DePuy Synthes® one-third semitubular plate	∅9 days
IlluminOss® Photodynamic Bone Stabilization System	∅5 days
	$p = 0.05$

The outcome scores assessed in the presented study are self-assessment questionnaires that reflect the subjective physical well-being and clinical outcome of the individual patients [60]. All used outcome scores have a graduation divided into five scales, ranging from poor to fair over good to excellent. Especially in the early follow-up exams after 6 and 12 weeks of the postoperative treatment, functional ankle scoring results showed a very significant difference (OMAS $p = 0.01$, KPSS $p = 0.01$ and 0.02 see Table 4) for the used scores in favor of Group II (see Table 4). No statistical differences regarding the used outcome scores were detected in the follow up examination after 6 and 12 months (OMAS $p = 0.06/0.07$, KPSS $p = 0.06/0.06$, see Table 4).

The distinct lack of comparability due to different applied postoperative treatment regimens is considered a basic limitation. While Group I patients (semitubular plate) were treated with partial weight bearing for 6 weeks, Group II patients (IlluminOss® Photodynamic Bone Stabilization System) started full weight bearing right after surgery. However, recommendations for patients treated with the new intramedullary implant are still missing the guidelines of the DGOU, as well as of the AO, for patients treated with semitubular plates involving partial weight bearing [59]. The allowance of full weight bearing led to an improved clinical outcome in patients treated with the intramedullary Photodynamic Bone Stabilization System. The presented results seem to be reliable and safe, and they should be considered an important contribution of our research.

Due to the small number of patients, the influence of implant removal was not analyzed. However, the presented follow-up rate of 86.5%, the wide assessment of functional parameters, and the prospective randomized character of the study certainly present the strengths of the presented work.

Studies with higher sample sizes are necessary in the future to demonstrate the benefits and possible disadvantages of these novel implant systems in the treatment of ankle fractures. Although we were able to show in our clinical prospective study for the first time a comparison of outcomes in geriatric patients for both implant groups, this study has its limitations. The fact that in our population, no fracture-related or implant-related infection occurred in the Photodynamic Bone Stabilization System, thus there was no necessity for implant removal in this group, does not mean that this complication is impossible. The used blue light might have antibacterial effects that must be investigated in future studies. Nevertheless, there is still the question to answer of how to remove this implant. An implant removal kit is provided on the market by the manufacturer, but still only a few cases of implant removal are known. Further investigations of possible complications in the usage of this novel implant have to be done in the future.

Although the current literature shows a trend towards the use of locking plate systems in distal fibula FX, and especially in osteoporotic FX, we showed that the use of this new intramedullary system provides a benefit for the geriatric population regarding postoperative clinical outcome, as well as shorter time period to full recovery and full weight bearing, plus very gentle soft tissue management due to the small incision site as compared to the locking plate treatment [49,61,62]. For this study, the use of locking one-third semitubular plates instead of the applied non-locking one-third semitubular plates could have been beneficial for patients randomized in Group I. Thus far, it could be shown that the use of locking plates allows an early weight bearing in younger patients suffering from a distal fibula fracture [20,35]. Nevertheless, the extended surgical approach and operative soft tissue stress can pose a disadvantage in geriatric patients and lead to soft tissue problems as compared to minimally invasive surgical methods; hence, minimally invasive surgical treatment should experience a renaissance [63–65]. Overall, all geriatric patients will benefit individually from a faster recovery, but also the cost of medical care could be reduced in general due to shorter hospital stays. Nevertheless, this study focused on the patient's outcome; therefore, an additional economic analysis could provide supplementary information regarding cost effectiveness. In addition, an analysis of the assumed reduction of health-related costs is advisable.

In general, adding two more groups to the study—e.g., (a) conservative treatment and (b) current intramedullary fibular nail—would add an interesting additional aspect regarding the treatment of distal fibula fractures in geriatric patients, as well as provide broader coverage of all aspects in the treatment of such fractures.

5. Conclusions

The presented results demonstrate that the Photodynamic Bone Stabilization System for treating distal fibula fractures in elderly patients with significant comorbidities leads to good clinical results. In fact, the immediate postoperative weight bearing showed that the FX stabilization with this new intramedullary system is a safe method for treating these fragile FXs. However, in comparing the treatment of distal fibula fractures using semitubular plates with the innovative IM system, the first two follow-up exams after 6 and 12 weeks raised our confidence that this new implant system provides a safe and stable treatment option. In addition, the patients treated with this new implant will benefit from the possibility of immediate postoperative full weight-bearing and, therefore, from a faster return to their normal daily life and freedom.

In summary, the successful treatment of distal fibula fractures in elderly patients is essentially dependent on sufficient wound healing and high primary stability to allow for immediate postoperative full weight bearing and initial functional rehabilitation.

Author Contributions: C.K. and M.Z. were substantially involved in the conception and design of the study. M.Z., P.Z. and M.W. carried out patients evaluation and drafted the manuscript. F.G., M.M. and P.P. assisted in the literature research and performed the statistical analysis. P.B. and C.K. participated in the design of the study, helped to draft the manuscript, and noted critical revisions of the manuscript for important intellectual content. All authors have read and agreed to the published version of the manuscript.

Funding: This research received no external funding.

Institutional Review Board Statement: The study was approved by the local ethics committee (Ethics Committee of the medical faculty, Klinikum rechts der Isar, Technical University of Munich, Germany; study number: 86/19S). Registration in the German Clinical Trails Register trail number DRKS00025496. Written informed consent to participate was obtained from all participants.

Informed Consent Statement: Written informed consent for publication was obtained from all participants.

Data Availability Statement: Availability of data and materials. To request the raw data: the first author of the manuscript can be contacted: Michael Zyskowski, Department of Trauma Surgery, Klinikum rechts der Isar, Technical University of Munich, Ismaninger Strasse 22, 81675 Munich, Germany, Tel.: 0049-89-4140-2126, e-mail: michael.zyskowski@mri.tum.de.

Acknowledgments: We thank Fritz Seidl, M.A., Interpreting and Translating, for professional language editing. We thank our emergency department team, including the nursing team, for the support.

Conflicts of Interest: The authors declare that there are no financial or personal conflict of interest that could have influenced this work.

Abbreviations

DGOU: German Society for Orthopedics and Trauma, FAOS: Foot and Ankle Outcome Score, Fx: Fracture, IM: intramedullary, KPSS: Karlsson and Peterson Scoring System for Ankle function, OMAS: Olerud-Molander Ankle Score, ORIF: Open reduction internal fixation.

References

1. Court-Brown, C.M.; Caesar, B. Epidemiology of adult fractures: A review. *Injury* **2006**, *37*, 691–697. [CrossRef]
2. Grutter, R.; Cordey, J.; Wahl, D.; Koller, B.; Regazzoni, P. A biomechanical enigma: Why are tibial fractures not more frequent in the elderly? *Injury* **2000**, *31* (Suppl. S3), C72–C77. [CrossRef]
3. Crevoisier, X.; Baalbaki, R.; Dos Santos, T.; Assal, M. Ankle fractures in the elderly patient. *Rev. Med. Suisse* **2014**, *10*, 2420–2423.
4. Koval, K.J.; Lurie, J.; Zhou, W.; Sparks, M.B.; Cantu, R.V.; Sporer, S.M.; Weinstein, J. Ankle fractures in the elderly: What you get depends on where you live and who you see. *J. Orthop. Trauma* **2005**, *19*, 635–639. [CrossRef]
5. Kannus, P.; Palvanen, M.; Niemi, S.; Parkkari, J.; Jrvinen, M. Increasing number and incidence of low-trauma ankle fractures in elderly people: Finnish statistics during 1970–2000 and projections for the future. *Bone* **2002**, *31*, 430–433. [CrossRef]
6. Karlamangla, A.; Tinetti, M.; Guralnik, J.; Studenski, S.; Wetle, T.; Reuben, D. Comorbidity in older adults: Nosology of impairment, diseases, and conditions. *J. Gerontol. Ser. A* **2007**, *62*, 296–300. [CrossRef]
7. Leyes, M.; Torres, R.; Guillén, P. Complications of open reduction and internal fixation of ankle fractures. *Foot Ankle Clin.* **2003**, *8*, 131–147. [CrossRef]
8. Tsukada, S.; Otsuji, M.; Shiozaki, A.; Yamamoto, A.; Komatsu, S.; Yoshimura, H.; Ikeda, H.; Hoshino, A. Locking versus non-locking neutralization plates for treatment of lateral malleolar fractures: A randomized controlled trial. *Int. Orthop.* **2013**, *37*, 2451–2456. [CrossRef]
9. Yeo, E.D.; Kim, H.J.; Cho, W.I.; Lee, Y.K. A Specialized Fibular Locking Plate for Lateral Malleolar Fractures. *J. Foot Ankle Surg.* **2015**, *54*, 1067–1071. [CrossRef]
10. Jain, S.; Haughton, B.A.; Brew, C. Intramedullary fixation of distal fibular fractures: A systematic review of clinical and functional outcomes. *J. Orthop. Traumatol.* **2014**, *15*, 245–254. [CrossRef]
11. Dabash, S.; Eisenstein, E.D.; Potter, E.; Kusnezov, N.; Thabet, A.M.; Abdelgawad, A.A. Unstable Ankle Fracture Fixation Using Locked Fibular Intramedullary Nail in High-Risk Patients. *J. Foot Ankle Surg.* **2019**, *58*, 357–362. [CrossRef]

12. Swart, E.; Bezhani, H.; Greisberg, J.; Vosseller, J.T. How long should patients be kept non-weight bearing after ankle fracture fixation? A survey of OTA and AOFAS members. *Injury* **2015**, *46*, 1127–1130. [CrossRef]
13. Kristensen, K.D. Ankle Fractures: Supination-Eversion Fractures of Stage IV: Primary and Late Results of Operative and Non—Operative Treatment AU—Yde, Johannes. *Acta Orthop. Scand.* **1980**, *51*, 981–990.
14. Makwana, N.K.; Bhowal, B.; Harper, W.M.; Hui, A.W. Conservative versus operative treatment for displaced ankle fractures in patients over 55 years of age. *J. Bone Jt. Surgery. Br.* **2001**, *83*, 525–529. [CrossRef]
15. Eckel, T.T.; Glisson, R.R.; Anand, P.; Parekh, S.G. Biomechanical Comparison of 4 Different Lateral Plate Constructs for Distal Fibula Fractures. *Foot Ankle Int.* **2013**, *34*, 1588–1595. [CrossRef]
16. Kim, T.; Ayturk, U.M.; Haskell, A.; Miclau, T.; Puttlitz, C.M. Fixation of Osteoporotic Distal Fibula Fractures: A Biomechanical Comparison of Locking Versus Conventional Plates. *J. Foot Ankle Surg.* **2007**, *46*, 2–6. [CrossRef]
17. Klos, K.; Sauer, S.; Hoffmeier, K.; Gras, F.; Fröber, R.; Hofmann, G.O.; Mückley, T. Biomechanical Evaluation of Plate Osteosynthesis of Distal Fibula Fractures with Biodegradable Devices. *Foot Ankle Int.* **2009**, *30*, 243–251. [CrossRef]
18. McKenna, P.B.; O'Shea, K.; Burke, T. Less is more: Lag screw only fixation of lateral malleolar fractures. *Int. Orthop.* **2006**, *31*, 497–502. [CrossRef]
19. Sain, A.; Garg, S.; Sharma, V.; Meena, U.K.; Bansal, H. Osteoporotic Distal Fibula Fractures in the Elderly: How to Fix Them. *Cureus* **2020**, *12*, e6552. [CrossRef]
20. Zyskowski, M.; Wurm, M.; Greve, F.; Pesch, S.; von Matthey, F.; Pflüger, P.; Crönlein, M.; Biberthaler, P.; Kirchhoff, C. Is early full weight bearing safe following locking plate ORIF of distal fibula fractures? *BMC Musculoskelet. Disord.* **2021**, *22*, 159. [CrossRef]
21. Rehman, H.; McMillan, T.; Rehman, S.; Clement, A.; Finlayson, D. Intrmedullary versus extramedullary fixation of lateral malleolus fractures. *Int. J. Surg.* **2015**, *22*, 54–61. [CrossRef]
22. White, T.O.; Bugler, K.E.; Appleton, P.; Will, E.; McQueen, M.M.; Court-Brown, C.M. A prospective randomised controlled trial of the fibular nail versus standard open reduction and internal fixation for fixation of ankle fractures in elderly patients. *Bone Jt. J.* **2016**, *98*, 1248–1252. [CrossRef]
23. Fleming, J.J. Intramedullary Nailing of Fibular Fractures. *Clin. Podiatr. Med. Surg.* **2018**, *35*, 259–270. [CrossRef]
24. Ebraheim, N.A.; Maten, J.W.V.; Delaney, J.R.; White, E.; Hanna, M.; Liu, J. Cannulated Intramedullary Screw Fixation of Distal Fibular Fractures. *Foot Ankle Spéc.* **2018**, *12*, 264–271. [CrossRef]
25. Challagundla, S.R.; Shewale, S.; Cree, C.; Hawkins, A. Intramedullary fixation of lateral malleolus using Fibula Rod System in ankle fractures in the elderly. *Foot Ankle Surg.* **2018**, *24*, 423–426. [CrossRef]
26. Tas, D.B.; Smeeing, D.P.; Emmink, B.L.; Govaert, G.A.; Hietbrink, F.; Leenen, L.P.; Houwert, R.M. Intramedullary Fixation Versus Plate Fixation of Distal Fibular Fractures: A Systematic Review and Meta-Analysis of Randomized Controlled Trials and Observational Studies. *J. Foot Ankle Surg.* **2019**, *58*, 119–126. [CrossRef]
27. Coifman, O.; Bariteau, J.T.; Shazar, N.; Tenenbaum, S.A. Lateral malleolus closed reduction and internal fixation with intramedullary fibular rod using minimal invasive approach for the treatment of ankle fractures. *Foot Ankle Surg.* **2019**, *25*, 79–83. [CrossRef]
28. Amaha, K.; Arimoto, T.; Saito, M.; Tasaki, A.; Tsuji, S. Shorter recovery can be achieved from using walking boot after operative treatment of an ankle fracture. *Asia-Pac. J. Sport. Med. Arthrosc. Rehabil. Technol.* **2016**, *7*, 10–14. [CrossRef]
29. Di Stasio, A.J., 2nd; Jaggears, F.R.; DePasquale, L.V.; Frassica, F.J.; Turen, C.H. Protected early motion versus cast immobilization in postoperative management of ankle fractures. *Contemp. Orthop.* **1994**, *29*, 273–277.
30. Bonness, E.K.; Siebler, J.C.; Reed, L.K.; Lyden, E.R.; Mormino, M.A. Immediate Weight-Bearing Protocol for the Determination of Ankle Stability in Patients with Isolated Distal Fibular Fractures. *J. Orthop. Trauma* **2018**, *32*, 534–537. [CrossRef]
31. Curtis, E.M.; van der Velde, R.; Moon, R.J.; van den Bergh, J.P.; Geusens, P.; de Vries, F.; van Staa, T.P.; Cooper, C.; Harvey, N.C.W. Epidemiology of fractures in the United Kingdom 1988-2012: Variation with age, sex, geography, ethnicity and socioeconomic status. *Bone* **2016**, *87*, 19–26. [CrossRef]
32. Van Laarhoven, C.J.; Meeuwis, J.D.; der Werken, C.V. Postoperative treatment of internally fixed ankle fractures: A prospective randomised study. *J. Bone Jt. Surg. Br. Vol.* **1996**, *78*, 395–399. [CrossRef]
33. Kortekangas, T.; Haapasalo, H.; Flinkkilä, T.; Ohtonen, P.; Nortunen, S.; Laine, H.-J.; Järvinen, T.; Pakarinen, H. Three week versus six week immobilisation for stable Weber B type ankle fractures: Randomised, multicentre, non-inferiority clinical trial. *BMJ* **2019**, *364*, k5432. [CrossRef] [PubMed]
34. Appleton, P.; McQueen, M.; Court-Brown, C. The Fibula Nail for Treatment of Ankle Fractures in Elderly and High Risk Patients. *Tech. Foot Ankle Surg.* **2006**, *5*, 204–208. [CrossRef]
35. Smeeing, D.P.J.; Houwert, R.M.; Briet, J.P.; Groenwold, R.H.H.; Lansink, K.W.W.; Leenen, L.P.H.; van der Zwaal, P.; Hoogendoorn, J.M.; van Heijl, M.; Verleisdonk, E.J.; et al. Weight-bearing or non-weight-bearing after surgical treatment of ankle fractures: A multicenter randomized controlled trial. *Eur. J. Trauma Emerg. Surg.* **2018**, *46*, 121–130. [CrossRef]
36. Gauthé, R.; Desseaux, A.; Rony, L.; Tarissi, N.; Dujardin, F. Ankle fractures in the elderly: Treatment and results in 477 patients. *Orthop. Traumatol. Surg. Res.* **2016**, *102*, S241–S244. [CrossRef]
37. Wukich, D.K.; Joseph, A.; Ryan, M.; Ramirez, C.; Irrgang, J.J. Outcomes of Ankle Fractures in Patients with Uncomplicated versus Complicated Diabetes. *Foot Ankle Int.* **2011**, *32*, 120–130. [CrossRef]
38. Ahl, T.; Dalen, N.; Selvik, G. Mobilization after operation of ankle fractures Good results of early motion and weight bearing. *Acta Orthop. Scand.* **1988**, *59*, 302–306. [CrossRef]

39. Simanski, C.J.; Maegele, M.G.; Lefering, R.; Lehnen, D.M.; Kawel, N.; Riess, P.; Nedim, Y.; Thomas, T.; Bertil, B. Functional treatment and early weightbearing after an ankle fracture: A prospective study. *J. Orthop. Trauma* **2006**, *20*, 108–114. [CrossRef]
40. Zyskowski, M.; Crönlein, M.; Heidt, E.; Biberthaler, P.; Kirchhoff, C. Osteosynthesis of distal fibular fractures with IlluminOss: Video article. *Unfallchirurg* **2017**, *120*, 6–11. [CrossRef]
41. Weber, B.G.; Colton, C. Malleolar Fractures. In *Manual of Internal Fixation: Techniques Recommended by the AO-ASIF Group*; Springer: Berlin/Heidelberg, Germany, 1991; pp. 595–612.
42. Benirschke, S.K.; Melder, I.; Henley, M.B.; Routt, M.L.; Smith, D.G.; Chapman, J.R.; Swiontkowski, M.F. Closed interlocking nailing of femoral shaft fractures: Assessment of technical complications and functional outcomes by comparison of a prospective database with retrospective review. *J. Orthop. Trauma* **1993**, *7*, 118–122. [CrossRef] [PubMed]
43. Hooper, G.J.; Keddell, R.G.; Penny, I.D. Conservative management or closed nailing for tibial shaft fractures. A randomised prospective trial. *J. Bone Jt. Surg.* **1991**, *73*, 83–85. [CrossRef] [PubMed]
44. Yuan, H.; Wang, R.; Zheng, J.; Yang, Y. Intramedullary Nailing and Minimally Invasive Percutaneous Plate Osteosynthesis in Treatment of Displaced Clavicular Mid-shaft Fractures: A Prospective Study. *Z. Orthopädie Und Unf.* **2019**, *158*, 604–610. [CrossRef] [PubMed]
45. Peeperkorn, S.; Nijs, S.; Hoekstra, H. Why Fibular Nailing Can Be an Efficient Treatment Strategy for AO Type 44-B Ankle Fractures in the Elderly. *J. Foot Ankle Surg.* **2018**, *57*, 961–966. [CrossRef] [PubMed]
46. Switaj, P.J.; Fuchs, D.; Alshouli, M.; Patwardhan, A.G.; Voronov, L.I.; Muriuki, M.; Havey, R.M.; Kadakia, A.R. A biomechanical comparison study of a modern fibular nail and distal fibular locking plate in AO/OTA 44C2 ankle fractures. *J. Orthop. Surg. Res.* **2016**, *11*, 100. [CrossRef]
47. Charlson, M.E.; Pompei, P.; Ales, K.L.; MacKenzie, C.R. A new method of classifying prognostic comorbidity in longitudinal studies: Development and validation. *J. Chronic Dis.* **1987**, *40*, 373–383. [CrossRef]
48. Malleolar Segment. *J. Orthop. Trauma* **2018**, *32*, 67.
49. Bhimani, R.; Lubberts, B.; Hagemeijer, N.; Zhao, J.Z.; Saengsin, J.; Sato, G.; Waryasz, G.R.; DiGiovanni, C.W.; Guss, D. The Lateral Hook Test: What is the Amount of Force that Should Be Applied to Evaluate Syndesmotic Instability Using Arthroscopy? *Foot Ankle Orthop.* **2022**, *7*, 2473011421S00117. [CrossRef]
50. Sman, A.D.; Hiller, C.E.; Rae, K.; Linklater, J.; Black, D.; Nicholson, L.; Burns, J.; Refshauge, K. Diagnostic accuracy of clinical tests for ankle syndesmosis injury. *Br. J. Sport. Med.* **2013**, *49*, 323–329. [CrossRef]
51. Hocevar, L.A.; Fitzgerald, B.M. American Society of Anesthesiologists Staging. In *StatPearls*; StatPearls Publishing LLC.: Treasure Island, FL, USA, 2019.
52. Hayes, M.J.P.B. Experimental developement of the graphics rating method. *Physiol. Bull.* **1921**, *18*, 98–99.
53. Olerud, C.; Molander, H. A scoring scale for symptom evaluation after ankle fracture. *Arch. Orthop. Trauma Surg.* **1984**, *103*, 190–194. [CrossRef] [PubMed]
54. Karlsson, J.; Peterson, L. Evaluation of ankle joint function: The use of a scoring scale. *Foot* **1991**, *1*, 15–19. [CrossRef]
55. Lauge, N. Fractures of the ankle: Analytic Historic Survey as the Basis of New Experimental, Roentgenologic and Clinical Investigations. *Arch. Surg.* **1948**, *56*, 259–317. [CrossRef]
56. Schepers, T.; Van Lieshout, E.; De Vries, M.; Van der Elst, M. Increased rates of wound complications with locking plates in distal fibular fractures. *Injury* **2011**, *42*, 1125–1129. [CrossRef] [PubMed]
57. Yde, J. The Lauge Hansen Classification of Malleolar Fractures. *Acta Orthop. Scand.* **1980**, *51*, 181–192. [CrossRef]
58. Dogra, A.; Rangan, A. Early mobilisation versus immobilisation of surgically treated ankle fractures. Prospective randomised control trial. *Injury* **1999**, *30*, 417–419. [CrossRef]
59. Autoren, H.; Belzl, U.; Ernst, S.; Heining, U.; Hirsch, T.; Riedel, J.; Schmidt, M.; Settner, S. Deutsche Gesellschaft für Orthopädie und Unfallchirurgie (DGOU). Available online: https://dgou.de/fileadmin/dgou/dgou/Dokumente/News/News/2020/2020_Nachbehandlungsempfehlungen.pdf (accessed on 1 February 2022).
60. Müller, M.; Greve, F.; Rittstieg, P.; Beirer, M.; Biberthaler, P. Documentation of self-reported patient outcomes in trauma surgery: Clinical benefits of patient reported outcome measures. *Unfallchirurg* **2020**, *123*, 354–359. [CrossRef]
61. Giordano, V.; Boni, G.; Godoy-Santos, A.L.; Pires, R.E.; Fukuyama, J.M.; Koch, H.A.; Giannoudis, P.V. Nailing the fibula: Alternative or standard treatment for lateral malleolar fracture fixation? A broken paradigm. *Eur. J. Trauma Emerg. Surg.* **2020**, *47*, 1911–1920. [CrossRef]
62. Milstrey, A.; Baumbach, S.F.; Pfleiderer, A.; Evers, J.; Boecker, W.; Raschke, M.J.; Polzer, H.; Ochman, S. Trends of incidence and treatment strategies for operatively treated distal fibula fractures from 2005 to 2019: A nationwide register analysis. *Arch. Orthop. Trauma. Surg.* **2021**, *142*, 3771–3777. [CrossRef]
63. Asloum, Y.; Bedin, B.; Roger, T.; Charissoux, J.-L.; Arnaud, J.-P.; Mabit, C. Internal fixation of the fibula in ankle fractures. A prospective, randomized and comparative study: Plating versus nailing. *Orthop. Traumatol. Surg. Res.* **2014**, *100*, S255–S259. [CrossRef]
64. Shih, C.-A.; Jou, I.-M.; Lee, P.-Y.; Lu, C.-L.; Su, W.-R.; Yeh, M.-L.; Wu, P.-T. Treating AO/OTA 44B lateral malleolar fracture in patients over 50 years of age: Periarticular locking plate versus non-locking plate. *J. Orthop. Surg. Res.* **2020**, *15*, 1–9. [CrossRef] [PubMed]
65. Dingemans, S.A.; Lodeizen, O.A.; Goslings, J.C.; Schepers, T. Reinforced fixation of distal fibula fractures in elderly patients; A meta-analysis of biomechanical studies. *Clin. Biomech.* **2016**, *36*, 14–20. [CrossRef] [PubMed]

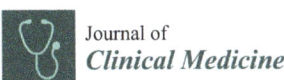

Article

Changes in Sleep Problems in Patients Who Underwent Surgical Treatment for Degenerative Spinal Disease with a Concurrent Sleep Disorder: A Nationwide Cohort Study in 3183 Patients during a Two-Year Perioperative Period

Jihye Kim [1], Jang Hyun Kim [2] and Tae-Hwan Kim [2,*]

[1] Division of Infection, Department of Pediatrics, Kangdong Sacred Heart Hospital, Hallym University College of Medicine, 150 Seongan-ro, Gangdong-gu, Seoul 05355, Republic of Korea
[2] Spine Center, Department of Orthopedics, Hallym University Sacred Heart Hospital, Hallym University College of Medicine, 22 Gwanpyeong-ro, 170beon-gil, Dongan-gu, Anyang 14068, Republic of Korea
* Correspondence: paragon0823@gmail.com; Tel.: +82-31-380-6000; Fax: +82-31-380-6008

Abstract: Sleep disturbance is prevalent in patients with degenerative spinal disease, and recent studies have reported that surgical treatment is more effective for improving sleep quality than conservative treatment. We aimed to investigate the perioperative changes of sleep problems in patients who underwent surgical treatment for degenerative spinal disease with a concurrent sleep disorder, and presented them according to various clinical profiles possibly associated with sleep disturbance. In addition, we identified factors associated with poor sleep improvement after surgery. This study used data from the Korea Health Insurance Review and Assessment Service database from 2016 to 2018. We included 3183 patients aged ≥19 years who underwent surgery for degenerative spinal disease and had a concurrent sleep disorder. Perioperative changes in the two target outcomes, including the use of sleep medication and hospital visits owing to sleep disorders, were precisely investigated according to factors known to be associated with sleep disturbance, including demographics, comorbidities, and spinal regions. Logistic regression analysis was performed to identify factors associated with poor improvement in terms of sleep medication after surgery. All estimates were validated using bootstrap sampling. During the 1-year preoperative period, the use of sleep medications and hospital visits owing to sleep disorder increased continuously. However, they abruptly decreased shortly after surgical treatment, and throughout the 1-year postoperative period, they remained lower than those in the late preoperative period. At the 1-year follow-up, 75.6% (2407 of 3183) of our cohort showed improvement in sleep medication after surgery. Multivariable analysis identified only two variables as significant factors associated with non-improvement in sleep medication after surgery: depressive disorder (odds ratio (OR) = 1.25 [1.06–1.48]; $p = 0.008$), and migraine (OR = 1.42 [1.04–1.94]; $p = 0.028$). We could not investigate the actual sleep quality and resultant quality of life; however, our results justify the necessity for further high-quality studies that include such information and would arouse clinicians' attention to the importance of sleep disturbance in patients with degenerative spinal disease.

Keywords: change; sleep disturbance; sleep medication; sleep improvement; surgery; degenerative spinal disease; sleep disorder

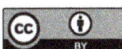

1. Introduction

Despite the importance of sleep for physiologic function [1–4], falling asleep is not easy for modern people, and sleep disturbance is prevalent in the general population [5–7]. The importance of sleep has been particularly emphasized for older patients with chronic medical conditions because they frequently experience sleep disturbance which significantly influences their disease outcome and life expectancy [4,8–12]. Therefore, sleep is an important topic for clinicians. Sleep has not been a subject of interest for researchers and clinicians caring for patients with spinal disease. However, studies have begun to address the fact that sleep disturbance is also highly prevalent in these patient populations [13–17], suggesting various mechanisms for their sleep disturbance [13,14].

Recently, two single-center prospective studies reported changes in patients' sleep quality after surgery for degenerative spinal disease and compared these results with those experienced by patients after conservative treatment [18,19]. They concluded that surgical treatment for degenerative spinal disease improves sleep quality more effectively than conservative treatment, especially after a long-term follow-up. Degenerative spinal disease is a common medical problem globally [20], and 11 to 74% of these diseases are accompanied by sleep disturbance [13–15,17–19,21]. Therefore, the results of the two prospective studies are promising for numerous patients with degenerative spinal disease and chronic sleep disorder.

However, the limitations of these two studies should be addressed. First, these comparative studies were single-center studies with small sample sizes. The studies focused on a narrow range of patients with specific types of degenerative spinal disease in a specific spinal region, such as lumbar stenosis or cervical myelopathy. Therefore, they could not comprehensively analyze various types of degenerative spinal disease, which include the entire spinal region. In addition, because the primary purpose of the two studies was to compare sleep improvement between the conservative and surgical groups, they did not require a large number of patients who underwent surgical treatment. Therefore, the number of surgical cohorts was small (<50 patients), and multivariable analysis to identify factors associated with adverse sleep outcomes after surgery could not be performed because of the limited sample size. Second, patients' sleep disturbance was identified using only single-time questionnaire-based surveys, which could result in the overestimation of sleep problems [18,19]. Therefore, there was a higher chance of including patients with temporary or minor sleep problems.

We planned a nationwide, population-based cohort study using a claims database. This study had two research purposes. First, we investigated changes in sleep problems in patients who underwent surgical treatment for degenerative spinal disease and had a concurrent sleep disorder. The use of sleep medication and hospital visits owing to sleep disorders were chosen as target outcomes in our study. This is because the claims database guarantees the reliability and accuracy of these two pieces of information as important objective measures of sleep disturbance [22,23]. In addition, perioperative changes in the two target outcomes were thoroughly presented according to the various clinical profiles possibly associated with sleep disturbance, including demographics, comorbidities, and spinal regions. Second, we identified the factors associated with poor sleep improvement after surgery for degenerative spinal disease.

2. Materials and Methods

2.1. Database

The data were obtained from the Health Insurance Review and Assessment Service (HIRA) database which contains data from all the hospitals and community clinics in Korea. In the database, the seventh revision of the Korean Classification of Diseases and tenth revision of the International Classification of Diseases (ICD-10) were used to identify diseases. The anatomical therapeutic chemical (ATC) codes and HIRA general name codes were used to identify the drugs used. In addition, this study was approved by the Institutional Review Board of our hospital (IRB No. 2020-03-009-001).

2.2. Study Patients

Patients aged >19 years who underwent surgical treatment (index surgery) for degenerative spinal disease from 1 January 2016 to 31 December 2018, were included (Figure 1). We identified degenerative spinal diseases using the following ICD-10 codes: spinal stenosis (M48.0), spondylolisthesis (M43.1), spondylolysis (M43.0), other spondylosis (M47.1

and M47.2), and cervical disc disorder (M50). Information regarding spinal surgery and its regions were identified using the corresponding electronic data interchange codes (Supplementary Materials Table S1). Subsequently, we excluded patients with spinal infection, spinal fractures, or malignancy within 2 years before the index surgery (Figure 1). The ICD-10 codes for exclusion are presented in Supplementary Materials Table S2.

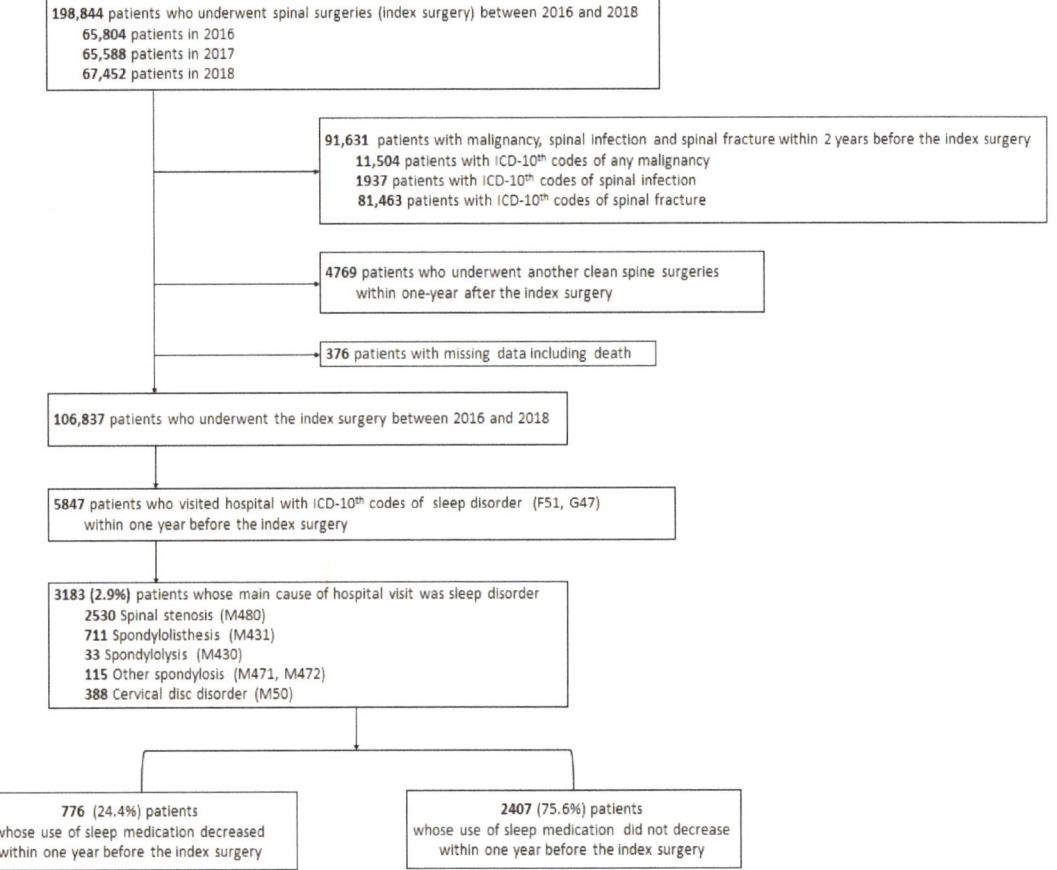

Figure 1. Patient enrollment.

Sleep disorder of the cohort patients was initially identified using the following ICD-10 codes: nonorganic sleep disorders (F51) and sleep disorders (G47). To identify patients with a concurrent sleep disorder, we only included patients who visited the hospital with the two ICD-10th codes as the primary diagnosis of the visits within 1 year before the index surgery.

2.3. Two Target Outcomes Associated with Sleep Disturbance: Use of Sleep Medication and Hospital Visits Owing to Sleep Disorders

Our main target outcome of interest was the use of sleep medication during the perioperative period. Sleep medication was defined as currently available drugs for insomnia approved by the Korean Food and Drug Administration [24]. They included flurazepam, triazolam, flunitrazepam, brotizolam, zolpidem, eszopiclone, doxepin, doxylamine, and diphenhydramine. Among them, antihistamines such as doxylamine and diphenhydramine were excluded. The sleep medication codes are presented in Supplementary Materials Table S3. Based on this definition, we investigated both the types of the sleep medication and their prescribed duration during the perioperative period. In addition, we investigated the number of hospital visits with a sleep disorder as the primary diagnosis during the perioperative period.

2.4. Definition of the Eight Quarters of Perioperative Periods

To observe the changes in the two target outcomes, we defined the perioperative period as the period between 1 year before and after the index surgery. Subsequently, we divided each preoperative and postoperative period into four intervals (quarters), each lasting 90 days (Figure 2). The 1-year preoperative period was divided into the following four quarters: (1) within 90 days before the index surgery (preoperative 4th quarter); (2) between the 91st and 180th day before the index surgery (preoperative 3rd quarter); (3) between the 181st and 270th day before the index surgery (preoperative 2nd quarter); and (4) between the 271st and 360th day before the index surgery (preoperative 1st quarter). The 1-year postoperative period was also divided into the following four quarters: (1) within 90 days after the index surgery (postoperative 1st quarter); (2) between the 91st and 180th day after the index surgery (postoperative 2nd quarter); (3) between the 181st and 270th day after the index surgery (postoperative 3rd quarter); and (4) between the 271st and 360th day before the index surgery (postoperative 4th quarter).

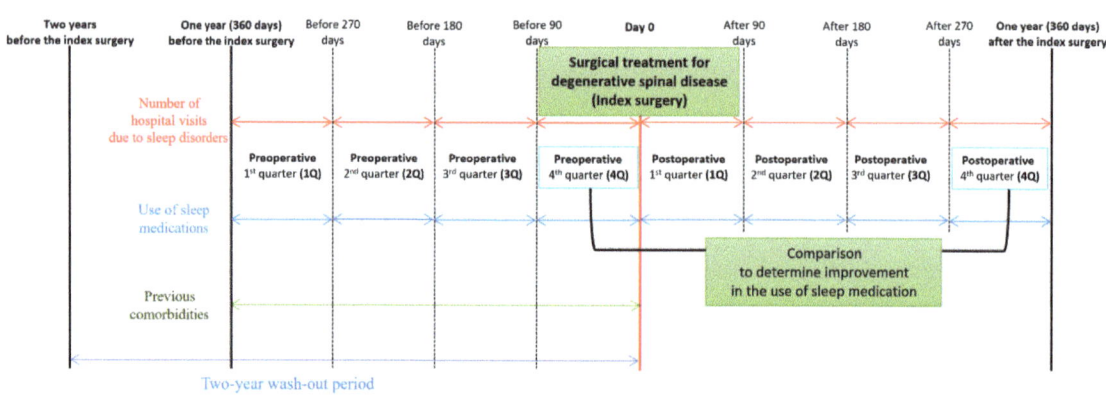

Figure 2. Study designs and definitions of the eight perioperative periods.

2.5. Evaluation of Perioperative Changes in the Two Target Outcomes

We investigated the use of sleep medication and hospital visits owing to sleep disorders during the perioperative period. The two target outcomes were thoroughly investigated and presented according to four groups of factors known to be associated with sleep disturbance in patients with degenerative spinal disease [21]: demographics; general medical comorbidities; neuropsychiatric disorders; and concurrent osteoarthritis of the extremities.

Information on the four groups of factors was retrieved using the previously described method [21]. Demographic data at the time of index surgery, including age, sex, region of residence, and hospital type, were initially retrieved. General medical comorbidities and neuropsychiatric disorders diagnosed within 1 year before the index surgery were investigated using the corresponding ICD-10 codes (Supplementary Materials Table S4), and the Charlson comorbidity index (CCI) score was calculated using an optimized method for the database using ICD-10 codes [25–28]. Diagnosis of depression was confirmed by the use of antidepressants (ATC code: N06A, Supplementary Materials Table S5). Osteoarthritis in the extremities was identified using the validated method for our database: [29] (1) ICD-10 codes for osteoarthritis (M15 to M19), and (2) corresponding X-rays of the extremities. The x-ray codes are presented in Supplementary Materials Table S6.

2.6. Statistical Analysis

During eight quarters of the perioperative period, changes in the use of sleep medication and number of hospital visits owing to sleep disorder were precisely presented according to the four groups of factors known to be associated with sleep disturbance in patients with degenerative spinal disease [21].

Expecting an overall postoperative decrease (improvement) in the use of sleep medication, [18,19] we tried to analyze factors associated with poor sleep improvement regarding the use of sleep medication. To assess the changes in sleep medication at 1-year follow-up after surgery, we compared the prescribed duration of the sleep medication between the preoperative and postoperative 4th quarters (Figure 2) and identified patients who showed no improvement in the duration of sleep medication between the two periods. Subsequently, we calculated the proportions of patients (%) who showed no postoperative improvement in the duration of sleep medication according to the four groups of factors associated with sleep disorder. The statistical difference of the proportions was presented with a standardized mean difference (SMD) known as Cohen's *d*. Logistic regression analysis was performed to identify independent factors associated with patients who showed no postoperative improvement in the use of sleep medication. Adjustments were made for variables identified as significant in the univariable analysis (SMD > 0.1).

The statistical model was internally validated using the bootstrap method. All estimates in the multivariable model were presented with relative bias estimated on 1000 bootstrapped samples. Relative bias was defined as the difference between the mean bootstrapped regression coefficient estimates and the mean parameter estimates of the multivariable model divided by the mean parameter estimates of the multivariable model. In addition, the variance inflation factor was used to evaluate multicollinearity between covariates. Data extraction and statistical analysis were performed using the SAS Enterprise Guide 6.1 (SAS Institute, Cary, NC, USA).

3. Results

Among the 198,844 patients who underwent spinal surgeries (index surgery) for degenerative spinal diseases from 2016 to 2018, we excluded patients who had malignancy (n = 11,504), spinal infection (n = 1937), spinal fracture (n = 81,463) within 2 years before the index surgery, and those with missing data (n = 376, Figure 1). Among the remaining 106,837 patients, 3148 (2.9%) who visited the hospital because of sleep disorders were included in our study. Baseline information regarding the cohort patients is presented in Table 1. Their mean age was 66.7 years, and 59% (n = 1875) were women.

3.1. Overall Perioperative Changes in the Two Target Outcomes

In the entire cohort, both the use of sleep medication and hospital visits owing to sleep disorders increased continuously throughout the preoperative period (Figure 3). The rate of this increase also increased continuously during the preoperative period, which was highest immediately before the index surgery, in the preoperative 4th quarter. However, shortly after the index surgery, the use of sleep medication and hospital visits owing to sleep disorders decreased abruptly. The rate of this decrease was highest in the postoperative 1st quarter. There were fluctuations in the subsequent postoperative period; however, the postoperative use of sleep medication and hospital visits were persistently lower than those in the preoperative 4th quarter. At the 1-year follow-up, 24.4% (776 of 3183) of patients in the cohort showed improvement in the prescribed duration of sleep medication (Table 1).

The two most commonly used sleep medications were zolpidem and triazolam (Figure 4). The proportions of these two drugs increased continuously during the preoperative period and decreased during the subsequent postoperative period. Except for these two drugs, there were no remarkable changes in the use of other drugs.

3.2. Perioperative Changes in the Two Target Outcomes: According to the Demographics and Spinal Regions

Hospital visits owing to sleep disorders decreased after surgery regardless of age group and sex; however, the postoperative decrease in the use of sleep medication was more pronounced in the female and older age groups (Figure 5).

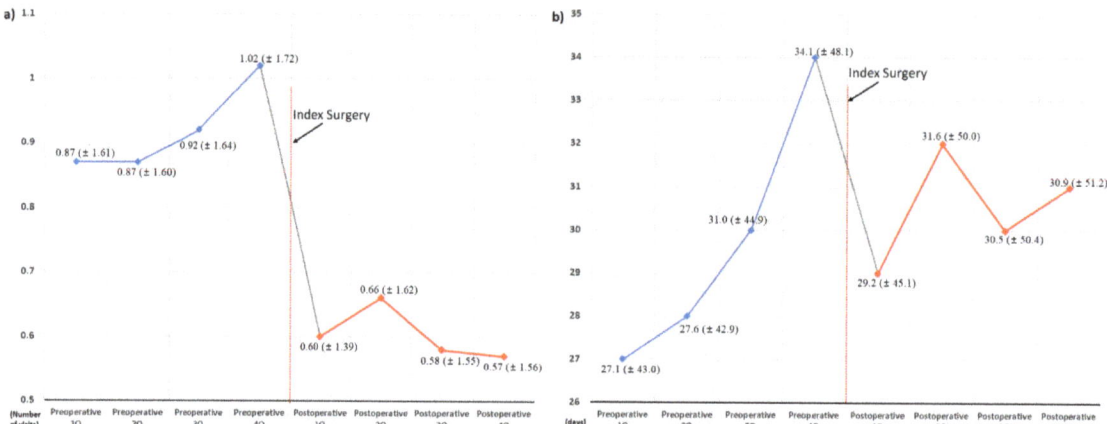

Figure 3. Overall perioperative changes in the use of sleep medication and hospital visits owing to sleep disorder: (**a**) changes in the number of hospital visits, and (**b**) changes in the prescribed duration of sleep medication.

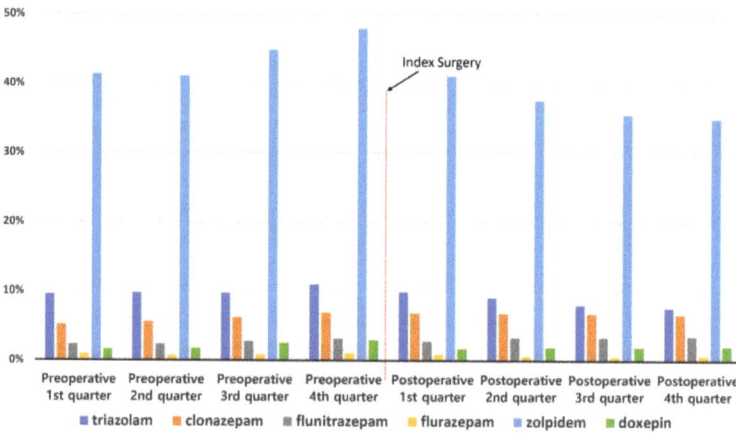

Figure 4. Types of sleep medication used during the perioperative period.

Perioperative changes in the use of sleep medication and hospital visits owing to sleep disorders are presented according to the spinal regions in Figure 6. The patterns of perioperative changes in the cervical and lumbar regions were similar to those in the entire cohort. In contrast, the preoperative pattern in the use of sleep medication and hospital visits owing to sleep disorders in patients with thoracic lesions differed from the overall pattern shown in Figure 3. The use of medication and hospital visits in patients with thoracic lesions decreased continuously, even during the preoperative period, although the most abrupt decrease occurred after surgery.

Table 1. Baseline characteristics of the cohort patients.

Variables	Categories	All	Patients without Postoperative Improvement in Sleep Medication	Patients with Postoperative Improvement in Sleep Medication	Proportions of Patients without Improvement	Standardized Mean Difference
Number of patients		3183	776	2407	24.4%	
Age	Mean ± SD	66.7 ± 10.7	67.2 ± 10.5	66.5 ± 10.8		0.065
	20–49	213 (7)	50 (6)	163 (7)	23.5%	
	50–69	1525 (48)	366 (47)	1159 (48)	24.0%	
	70+	1445 (45)	360 (46)	1085 (45)	24.9%	
Sex	Men	1308 (41)	307 (40)	1001 (42)	23.5%	0.046
	Women	1875 (59)	469 (60)	1406 (58)	25.0%	
Region	Urban	2714 (85)	660 (85)	2054 (85)	24.3%	0.012
	Rural	469 (15)	116 (15)	353 (15)	24.7%	
Hospital	Tertiary	640 (20)	153 (20)	487 (20)	23.9%	0.062
	General	660 (21)	172 (22)	488 (20)	26.1%	
	Others	1883 (59)	451 (58)	1432 (59)	24.0%	
Spinal regions	Cervical	461 (14)	96 (12)	365 (15)	20.8%	0.134
	Thoracic	35 (1)	7 (1)	28 (1)	20.0%	
	Lumbar	2687 (84)	673 (87)	2014 (84)	25.0%	
Charlson comorbidity index score	Mean ± SD	1.61 ± 1.46	1.75 ± 1.52	1.56 ± 1.44		0.136
	0–2	2427 (76)	572 (74)	1855 (77)	23.6%	
	3–5	696 (22)	185 (24)	511 (21)	26.6%	
	≥6	60 (2)	19 (2)	41 (2)	31.7%	

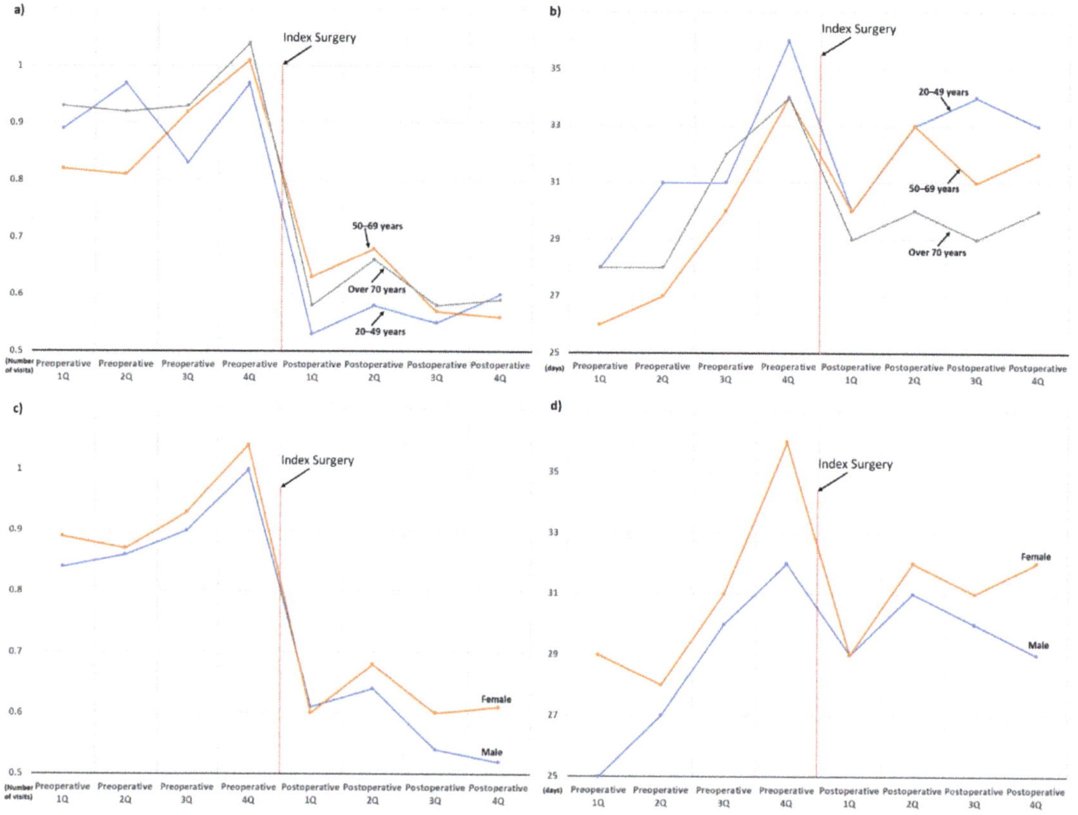

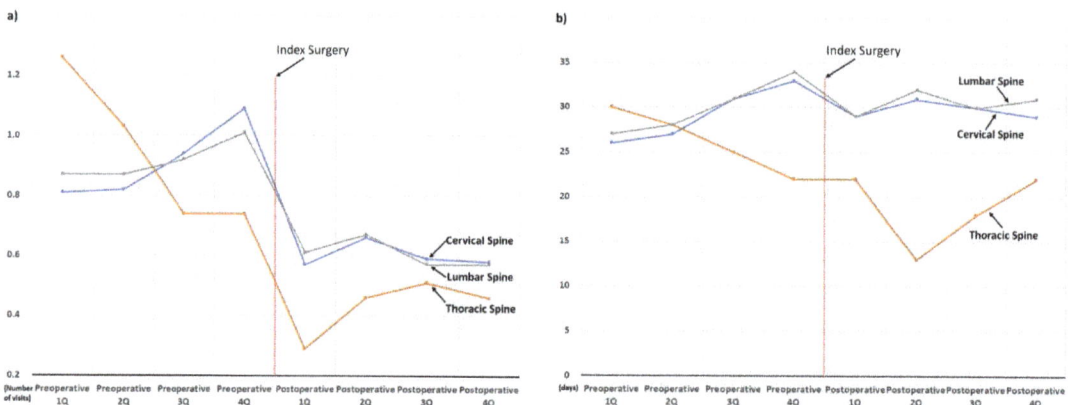

Figure 5. Perioperative changes in the use of sleep medication and hospital visits owing to sleep disorder according to the demographics: (**a**) changes in the number of hospital visits according to the age groups; (**b**) changes in the prescribed duration of sleep medication according to the age groups; (**c**) changes in the number of hospital visits according to sex groups; and (**d**) changes in the prescribed duration of sleep medication according to sex groups.

Figure 6. Perioperative changes in the use of sleep medication and hospital visits owing to sleep disorder according to the spinal regions: (**a**) changes in the number of hospital visits, and (**b**) changes in the prescribed duration of sleep medication.

3.3. Perioperative Changes in the Two Target Outcomes: According to the Comorbidities

Information about the comorbidities of the cohort patients is presented in Table 2. We also presented the changes in the use of sleep medication and hospital visits owing to sleep disorders according to the CCI scores (Figure 7), neuropsychiatric diseases (Figure 8), and concurrent osteoarthritis of the extremities (Figure 9).

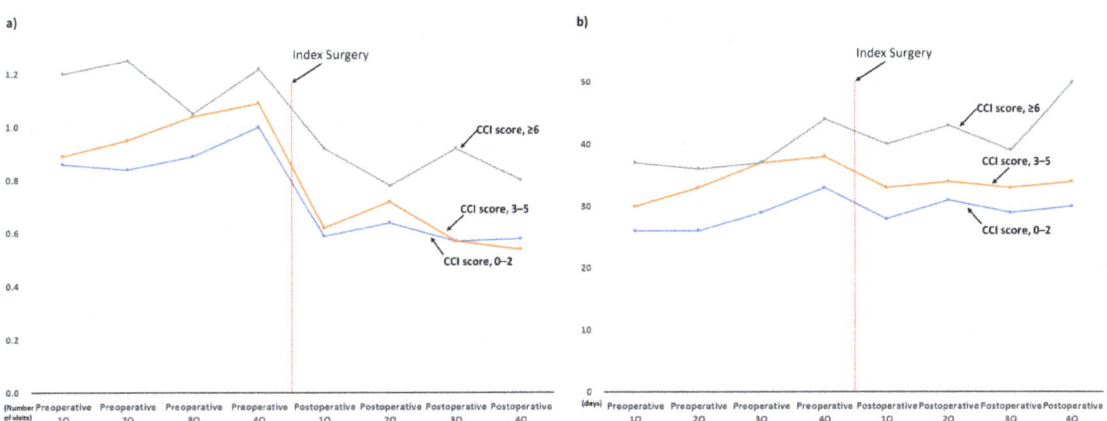

Figure 7. Perioperative changes in the use of sleep medication and hospital visits owing to sleep disorder according to the Charlson comorbidity index (CCI) score: (**a**) changes in the number of hospital visits, and (**b**) changes in the prescribed duration of sleep medication.

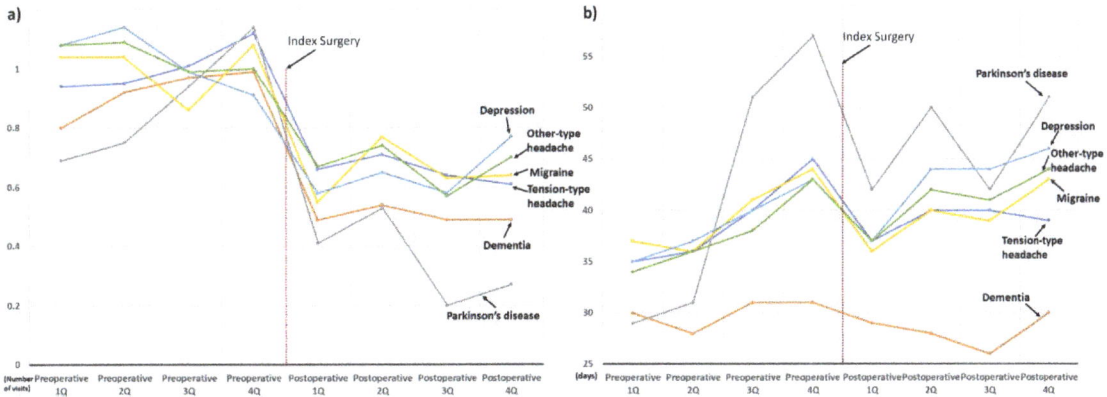

Figure 8. Perioperative changes in the use of sleep medication and hospital visits owing to sleep disorder according to the neuropsychiatric disorders: (**a**) changes in the number of hospital visits, and (**b**) changes in the prescribed duration of sleep medication.

Regardless of the type of comorbidity, the use of sleep medication and hospital visits owing to sleep disorders decreased abruptly in the postoperative 1st quarter, shortly after surgery. Subsequent postoperative use of sleep medication showed a rebound increase in the postoperative 2nd quarter; however, the use of sleep medication in the postoperative 4th quarter was lower than that in the preoperative 4th quarter in most patient subgroups (Figures 7–9). On the other hand, in three patient subgroups, including those with CCI score ≥ 6 (Figure 7b), depression, and other-type headaches (Figure 8b), the mean use of sleep medication in the postoperative 4th quarter exceeded that in the preoperative 4th quarter.

Table 2. Comorbidities of the cohort patient.

Variables	Categories	All	Patients without Postoperative Improvement in Sleep Medication	Patients with Postoperative Improvement in Sleep Medication	Proportions of Patients without Improvement	Standardized Mean Difference
General comorbidities	Myocardial infarction	40 (1)	7 (1)	33 (1)	17.5%	0.233
	Congestive heart failure	159 (5)	45 (6)	114 (5)	28.3%	0.118
	Cerebrovascular disease	441 (14)	113 (15)	328 (14)	25.6%	0.043
	Peripheral vascular disease	531 (17)	140 (18)	391 (16)	26.4%	0.070
	Chronic pulmonary disease	1059 (33)	285 (37)	774 (32)	26.9%	0.112
	Rheumatologic disease	161 (5)	42 (5)	119 (5)	26.1%	0.053
	Peptic ulcer disease	745 (23)	205 (26)	540 (22)	27.5%	0.119
	Liver disease					
	Mild	273 (9)	70 (9)	203 (8)	25.6%	0.041
	Moderate to severe	5 (0)	1 (0)	4 (0)	20.0%	0.140
	Diabetes					
	Uncomplicated	828 (26)	206 (27)	622 (26)	24.9%	0.020
	Complicated	245 (8)	70 (9)	175 (7)	28.6%	0.129
	Hemiplegia or paraplegia	26 (1)	1 (0)	25 (1)	3.8%	1.156
	Renal disease	105 (3)	34 (4)	71 (3)	32.4%	0.226
	End-stage renal disease	16 (1)	6 (1)	10 (0)	37.5%	0.344
	Osteoporosis	609 (19)	144 (19)	465 (19)	23.6%	0.027
Concurrent neuropsychiatric disorders	Depressive disorder	1560 (49)	423 (55)	1137 (47)	27.1%	0.161
	Dementia	106 (3)	29 (4)	77 (3)	27.4%	0.089
	Parkinson disease	51 (2)	13 (2)	38 (2)	25.5%	0.033
	Migraine	202 (6)	67 (9)	135 (6)	33.2%	0.256
	Tension-type headache	180 (6)	59 (8)	121 (5)	32.8%	0.243
	Other-type headache	246 (8)	76 (10)	170 (7)	30.9%	0.197
Concurrent osteoarthritis of extremities	Shoulder	349 (11)	90 (12)	259 (11)	25.8%	0.047
	Elbow	78 (2)	18 (2)	60 (2)	23.1%	0.041
	Wrist	94 (3)	27 (3)	67 (3)	28.7%	0.127
	Hip	299 (9)	80 (10)	219 (9)	26.8%	0.076
	Knee	991 (31)	258 (33)	733 (30)	26.0%	0.071
	Ankle	189 (6)	53 (7)	136 (6)	28.0%	0.111

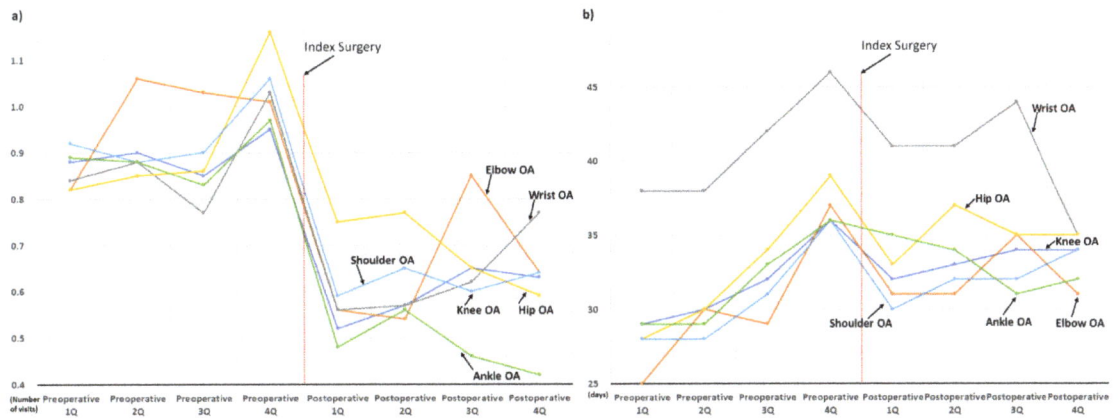

Figure 9. Perioperative changes in the use of sleep medication and hospital visits owing to sleep disorder according to the osteoarthritis of the extremities: (**a**) changes in the number of hospital visits, and (**b**) changes in the prescribed duration of sleep medication.

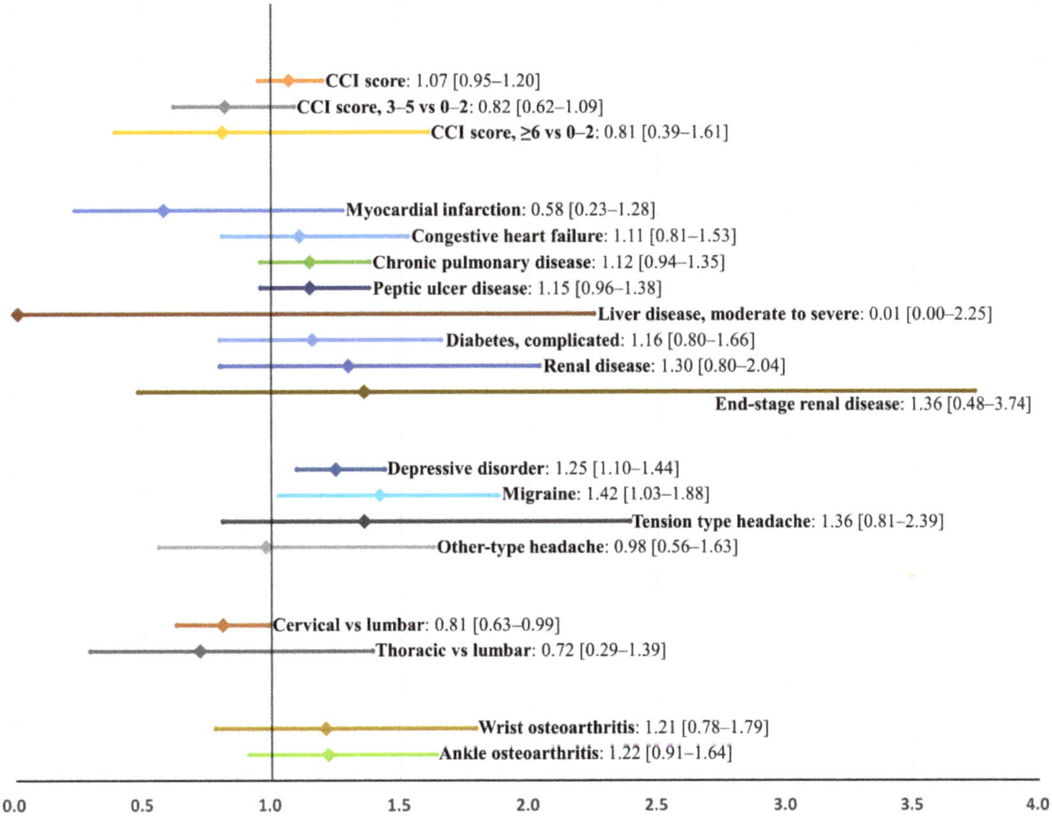

Figure 10. Factors associated with non-improvement in sleep medication after surgery: a multivariable analysis. Bootstrap-adjusted odds ratios and their 95% confidence intervals are presented.

Table 3. Factors associated with poor improvement in the sleep medication after surgery: internal validation using bootstrap sampling.

Variables	Categories	Univariable		Model 2 (Fully Adjusted)		Model 3 (Bootstrap Validation after Fully Adjusted)	
		Odds Ratio (95% Confidence Interval)	p-Value	Adjusted Odds Ratio (95% Confidence Interval)	p-Value	Adjusted Odds Ratio (95% Confidence Interval)	Bias (%)
Charlson comorbidity index score							
	3–5 vs. 0–2	1.09 [1.03–1.15]	0.002	1.07 [0.93–1.22]	0.364	1.07 [0.95–1.20]	−6.7
	≥6 vs. 0–2	1.17 [1.77–2.02]	0.102	0.83 [0.59–1.17]	0.284	0.82 [0.62–1.09]	4.7
		1.50 [0.87–2.61]	0.148	0.81 [0.35–1.89]	0.624	0.81 [0.39–1.61]	2.4
Comorbidities	Myocardial infarction	0.66 [0.29–1.49]	0.312	0.64 [0.28–1.47]	0.291	0.58 [0.23–1.28]	22.5
	Congestive heart failure	1.24 [0.87–1.77]	0.238	1.12 [0.75–1.62]	0.607	1.11 [0.81–1.53]	−10.3
	Chronic pulmonary disease	1.23 [1.03–1.45]	0.019	1.13 [0.92–1.39]	0.259	1.12 [0.94–1.35]	−3.8
	Peptic ulcer disease	1.24 [1.03–1.50]	0.023	1.15 [0.92–1.43]	0.233	1.15 [0.96–1.38]	1.5
	Liver disease, moderate to severe	0.78 [0.09–6.95]	0.820	0.56 [0.06–5.38]	0.615	0.01 [0.00–2.25]	678.3
	Diabetes, complicated	1.27 [0.95–1.69]	0.112	1.16 [0.78–1.72]	0.478	1.16 [0.80–1.66]	−2.3
	Renal disease	1.51 [0.99–2.29]	0.054	1.29 [0.77–2.16]	0.338	1.30 [0.80–2.04]	2.2
	End-stage renal disease	1.87 [0.68–5.16]	0.227	1.37 [0.45–4.16]	0.578	1.36 [0.48–3.74]	−3.4
Comorbidities associated with neuropsychiatric disorders	Depressive disorder	1.34 [1.14–1.57]	<0.001	1.25 [1.06–1.48]	0.008	1.25 [1.10–1.44]	1.4
	Migraine	1.59 [1.17–2.16]	0.003	1.42 [1.04–1.94]	0.028	1.42 [1.03–1.88]	−0.6
	Tension-type headache	1.56 [1.13–2.15]	<0.001	1.28 [0.68–2.44]	0.445	1.36 [0.81–2.39]	23.1
	Other-type headache	1.43 [1.08–1.90]	0.014	1.04 [0.59–1.84]	0.889	0.98 [0.56–1.63]	−139.0
Surgical regions	Cervical vs. lumbar	0.79 [0.62–1.00]	0.052	0.82 [0.64–1.04]	0.100	0.81 [0.63–0.99]	8.9
	Thoracic vs. lumbar	0.75 [0.33–1.72]	0.495	0.77 [0.33–1.78]	0.539	0.72 [0.29–1.39]	26.9
Concurrent osteoarthritis	Wrist	1.26 [0.80–1.98]	0.320	1.21 [0.76–1.92]	0.426	1.21 [0.78–1.79]	0.3
	Ankle	1.22 [0.88–1.70]	0.227	1.22 [0.87–1.71]	0.244	1.22 [0.91–1.64]	1.2

3.4. Factors Associated with Poor Improvement in the Sleep Medication after Surgery: Internal Validation Using Bootstrap Sampling

At the 1-year follow-up after surgery, the duration of the sleep medication decreased (improved) in 75.6% of patients (2407 of 3183, Table 1). In the univariable analysis, various factors showed statistical significance by the standard of SMD > 0.1 (Tables 1 and 2); however, the multivariable analysis identified only two variables as significant factors associated with non-improvement in sleep medication after surgery (Table 3): depressive disorder (odds ratio (OR), 95% confidence interval [CI] = 1.25 [1.06–1.48]; p = 0.008), and migraine (OR = 1.42 [1.04–1.94], p = 0.028). The relative bias of the estimates for most risk factors was low, except for moderate-to-severe liver disease (678.3%) and other-type headaches (−139.0%). Bootstrap-adjusted odds ratios and their 95% CIs for the multivariable model are presented in Table 3 and Figure 10.

4. Discussions

Chronic pain and its intensity are major risk factors for sleep disturbance [30–33]. However, overall pain intensity is not a significant risk factor for sleep disturbance in patients with degenerative spinal disease [13,14]. Instead, the radiologic degree of degeneration is a stronger predictor for sleep disturbance. For example, sleep disturbance in patients with lumbar stenosis was closely associated with the degree of foraminal-type stenosis [14], and sleep disturbance in patients with cervical myelopathy was associated with the degree of central-type stenosis [13]. If severe radiologic degeneration is a major component of sleep disturbance in patients with degenerative spinal disease, sleep disturbance will be prevalent in patients who undergo surgical treatment for degenerative spinal disease [14,18,19,21], and sleep disturbance might have influenced their choice of surgical treatment. In addition, we can reasonably expect that 'decompressive' surgical treatment for degenerative spinal disease will positively influence sleep quality. These hypotheses are clinically important and should be verified because sleep disturbance in patients with a severe degree of degenerative spinal disease is not easily improved by conservative treatment [18,19].

In this regard, we attempted to clearly visualize perioperative changes in sleep medication and hospital visits owing to sleep disorders in patients who underwent surgery for degenerative spinal disease with concurrent sleep disorders. During the preoperative period, the use of sleep medication and hospital visits owing to sleep disorders increased continuously (Figure 3). However, they abruptly decreased shortly after surgical treatment. In addition, throughout the 1-year postoperative period, they remained lower than those in the preoperative 4th quarter. When the use of sleep medication immediately before surgery (in the preoperative 4th quarter) was compared with that of 1 year after surgery (in the postoperative 4th quarter), 75.6% (2407 of 3183) of the patients in our cohort showed improvement in sleep medication after surgery. Multivariable analysis identified that the two neuropsychiatric disorders, depressive disorder and migraine, were associated with poor outcomes in the use of sleep medication after surgery.

One of the major advantages of our study is that we obtained accurate information about the two target outcomes during the 1-year preoperative period in all cohorts. As a claims database based on an obligatory national health insurance system, the HIRA database contains all inpatient and outpatient data for the entire population. In our claims database, information about the two target outcomes, including sleep medication and hospital visits owing to sleep disorders, has been prospectively recorded and reviewed by government officials; thus, it is available for all patients, regardless of the time interval. Investigating sleep problems during the 1-year preoperative period in all the study cohorts is theoretically impossible, even in randomized or prospective studies. This is because researchers would defer surgical treatment for degenerative spinal disease for 1 year without exception to prospectively collect such information during the 1-year preoperative period.

Therefore, one of the most important findings of our study is the changes in the two target outcomes during the year before the index surgery. During the preoperative period, the use of sleep medication and hospital visits owing to sleep disorders increased continuously. The increasing rates continued during the 1-year preoperative period, culminating in the preoperative 4th (last) quarter (Figure 3). However, the accelerated preoperative increase in the use of sleep medication and hospital visits immediately reversed after surgery and abruptly decreased in the postoperative 1st quarter. The decreasing rate at the postoperative 1st quarter was even faster than the increasing rate, which culminated in the preoperative 4th quarter (Figure 3).

In addition, this is the largest study investigating changes in sleep problems after surgical treatment for degenerative spinal disease and has several advantages. First, through a comprehensive analysis based on a sufficient number of patients (n = 3183), perioperative changes in the two target outcomes were clearly presented according to various factors possibly associated with sleep disturbance (Figures 5–9). Second, we included enough patients with evident preoperative sleep disorders. In the two previous studies, sleep disturbance in the cohorts was identified using only single-time questionnaire-based surveys, with a high possibility of including patients with temporary or minor sleep problems despite their prospective study design. [18,19] However, we only included patients who visited the hospital with sleep disorders as the main reason for the hospital visit. In similar patient populations, the prevalence rates of sleep disturbance from large database studies conducted using ICD-10 codes (3.8 to 10.8%) are lower than those from survey-based single- or multi-center studies (42 to 74%) [13–17,21]. Therefore, our 3183 (2.9%) cohort patients, chosen using concordant ICD-10 codes for sleep disorder among 106,837 patients who underwent surgery for degenerative spinal disease, were expected to have more severe sleep disturbance than those chosen from questionnaire-based surveys [18,19] (Figure 1). They are more appropriate for evaluating the influence of spinal surgical treatment on sleep disturbance.

Accordingly, throughout the 1-year preoperative period, the mean duration of sleep medication use was approximately 30 days per quarter (90 days, Figure 3), which indirectly reflects their severe and chronic sleep disturbance. Nevertheless, their severe and chronic dependency on sleep medication and resultant hospital visits strikingly decreased after surgical treatment, regardless of various known risk factors for sleep disturbances (Figures 5–9) [21]. After surgery, 75.6% (2407 of 3183) of the patients in our cohort with preoperative sleep disorders showed improvement in sleep medication. Among numerous independent variables, only two factors, depressive disorder and migraine, were significantly associated with poor outcomes regarding sleep medication in the multivariable analysis (Table 3 and Figure 10).

However, our study has limitations. First, our claims database was not originally designed for research. Therefore, important information possibly related to sleep disturbance, such as the anatomical degree of spinal degeneration or neurologic impairment, was not included. We can propose that most patients who underwent surgical treatment had severe degrees of degeneration; however, such additional information could have influenced our results [13,14]. To reduce the influence of such unknown confounders, we validated our results using bootstrap sampling, and the results were consistent. In addition, we used validated data-retrieving methods for the HIRA database, and thoroughly presented the exact diagnostic and therapeutic codes for all types of diseases and drugs to ensure the reproducibility of our results. Second, the two target outcomes, the use of sleep medication and hospital visits owing to sleep disorders, are not precise measures for sleep quality. Based on our results, we cannot assert that surgical treatment in patients with degenerative spinal disease and concurrent sleep disorders can improve actual sleep quality and the resultant quality of life. This conclusion is beyond the scope of our study. Instead, as a comprehensive preliminary study, our results justify the necessity of further high-quality studies investigating improvements in actual sleep quality after spine surgery in patients with degenerative spinal disease and concurrent sleep disorders.

In conclusion, our population-based study using a nationwide database clearly presented perioperative changes in the use of sleep medication and hospital visits owing to sleep disorders in patients who underwent surgery for degenerative spinal disease with a concurrent sleep disorder. During the 1-year preoperative period, the use of sleep medication and hospital visits owing to sleep disorder increased continuously. However, they abruptly decreased shortly after surgical treatment. In addition, throughout the 1-year postoperative period, they remained lower than those in the preoperative 4th quarter. At the 1-year follow-up, 75.6% (2407 of 3183) of patients in our cohort showed improvement in sleep medication after surgery. Multivariable analysis identified that the two neuropsychiatric disorders, depressive disorder and migraine, were associated with poor outcomes in the use of sleep medications after surgery. We could not investigate the actual sleep quality and resultant quality of life in our cohort; however, our results justify the necessity of further high-quality studies which include such information and would arouse clinicians' attention to the importance of sleep disturbance in patients with degenerative spinal disease.

Supplementary Materials: The following supporting information can be downloaded at: https://www.mdpi.com/article/10.3390/jcm11247402/s1, Table S1: HIRA therapeutic codes for spinal surgery; Table S2: ICD-10 codes for spinal infection, spinal fracture, and malignancy; Table S3: Types of the used sleep medication; Table S4: ICD-10 codes for comorbidities including Charlson comorbidities index items and scores; Table S5: ATC and HIRA codes for the used antidepressant; Table S6: HIRA codes for the x-rays of the extremities.

Author Contributions: Conceptualization, J.K. and T.-H.K.; Formal analysis, J.K. and J.H.K.; Investigation, J.K. and J.H.K.; Methodology, J.K. and J.H.K.; Software, J.K. and J.H.K.; Supervision, T.-H.K.; Validation, J.H.K.; Visualization, J.H.K.; Writing—original draft, J.K.; Writing—review and editing, T.-H.K. All authors have read and agreed to the published version of the manuscript.

Funding: This research received no external funding.

Institutional Review Board Statement: This study was approved by the Institutional Review Board of our hospital (IRB No. 2020-03-009-001).

Informed Consent Statement: Patient consent was waived because of the retrospective study design and anonymity of the HIRA database.

Data Availability Statement: The datasets generated for the current study are not publicly available because of Data Protection Laws and Regulations in Republic of Korea; however, the analyzed results are available from the corresponding authors upon reasonable request.

Conflicts of Interest: The authors declare no conflict of interest.

References

1. Dattilo, M.; Antunes, H.K.; Medeiros, A.; Mônico Neto, M.; Souza, H.S.; Tufik, S.; de Mello, M.T. Sleep and muscle recovery: Endocrinological and molecular basis for a new and promising hypothesis. *Med. Hypotheses* **2011**, *77*, 220–222. [CrossRef]
2. Cirelli, C.; Tononi, G. Is sleep essential? *PLoS Biol.* **2008**, *6*, e216. [CrossRef]
3. Luyster, F.S.; Strollo, P.J., Jr.; Zee, P.C.; Walsh, J.K. Sleep: A health imperative. *Sleep* **2012**, *35*, 727–734. [CrossRef]
4. Cappuccio, F.P.; D'Elia, L.; Strazzullo, P.; Miller, M.A. Sleep duration and all-cause mortality: A systematic review and meta-analysis of prospective studies. *Sleep* **2010**, *33*, 585–592. [CrossRef]
5. Stranges, S.; Tigbe, W.; Gómez-Olivé, F.X.; Thorogood, M.; Kandala, N.B. Sleep problems: An emerging global epidemic? Findings from the INDEPTH WHO-SAGE study among more than 40,000 older adults from 8 countries across Africa and Asia. *Sleep* **2012**, *35*, 1173–1181. [CrossRef]
6. Sutton, D.A.; Moldofsky, H.; Badley, E.M. Insomnia and health problems in Canadians. *Sleep* **2001**, *24*, 665–670. [CrossRef]
7. Hossain, J.L.; Shapiro, C.M. The prevalence, cost implications, and management of sleep disorders: An overview. *Sleep Breath. = Schlaf Atm.* **2002**, *6*, 85–102. [CrossRef]
8. Schubert, C.R.; Cruickshanks, K.J.; Dalton, D.S.; Klein, B.E.; Klein, R.; Nondahl, D.M. Prevalence of sleep problems and quality of life in an older population. *Sleep* **2002**, *25*, 889–893.
9. Mystakidou, K.; Parpa, E.; Tsilika, E.; Pathiaki, M.; Gennatas, K.; Smyrniotis, V.; Vassiliou, I. The relationship of subjective sleep quality, pain, and quality of life in advanced cancer patients. *Sleep* **2007**, *30*, 737–742. [CrossRef]
10. Nagasaka, T.; Washida, N.; Uchiyama, K.; Hama, E.Y.; Kusahana, E.; Nakayama, T.; Yasuda, I.; Morimoto, K.; Itoh, H. Health-Related Quality of Life Sleep Score Predicts Transfer to Hemodialysis among Patients on Peritoneal Dialysis. *Healthcare* **2022**, *10*, 1030. [CrossRef]

11. Broström, A.; Strömberg, A.; Dahlström, U.; Fridlund, B. Sleep difficulties, daytime sleepiness, and health-related quality of life in patients with chronic heart failure. *J. Cardiovasc. Nurs.* **2004**, *19*, 234–242. [CrossRef] [PubMed]
12. Nunes, D.M.; Mota, R.M.; de Pontes Neto, O.L.; Pereira, E.D.; de Bruin, V.M.; de Bruin, P.F. Impaired sleep reduces quality of life in chronic obstructive pulmonary disease. *Lung* **2009**, *187*, 159–163. [CrossRef] [PubMed]
13. Kim, J.; Oh, J.K.; Kim, S.W.; Yee, J.S.; Kim, T.H. Risk factors for sleep disturbance in patients with cervical myelopathy and its clinical significance: A cross-sectional study. *Spine J. Off. J. N. Am. Spine Soc.* **2021**, *21*, 96–104. [CrossRef] [PubMed]
14. Kim, J.; Park, J.; Kim, S.W.; Oh, J.K.; Park, M.S.; Kim, Y.W.; Kim, T.H. Prevalence of sleep disturbance in patients with lumbar spinal stenosis and analysis of the risk factors. *Spine J. Off. J. N. Am. Spine Soc.* **2020**, *20*, 1239–1247. [CrossRef] [PubMed]
15. Kim, H.J.; Hong, S.J.; Park, J.H.; Ki, H. Sleep Disturbance and Its Clinical Implication in Patients with Adult Spinal Deformity: Comparison with Lumbar Spinal Stenosis. *Pain Res. Manag.* **2020**, *2020*, 6294151. [CrossRef] [PubMed]
16. Artner, J.; Cakir, B.; Spiekermann, J.-A.; Kurz, F.; Leucht, F.; Reichel, H.; Lattig, F. Prevalence of sleep deprivation in patients with chronic neck and back pain: A retrospective evaluation of 1016 patients. *J. Pain Res.* **2013**, *6*, 1–6. [CrossRef] [PubMed]
17. Becker, K.N.; Gifford, C.S.; Qaqish, H.; Alexander, C.; Ren, G.; Caras, A.; Miller, W.K.; Schroeder, J.L. A Population-Based Study of Patients with Sleep-Wake Disorders Undergoing Elective Instrumented Spinal Surgery. *World Neurosurg.* **2022**, *160*, e335–e343. [CrossRef]
18. Kim, J.; Kim, G.; Kim, S.W.; Oh, J.K.; Park, M.S.; Kim, Y.W.; Kim, T.H. Changes in sleep disturbance in patients with cervical myelopathy: Comparison between surgical treatment and conservative treatment. *Spine J. Off. J. N. Am. Spine Soc.* **2021**, *21*, 586–597. [CrossRef]
19. Kim, J.; Lee, S.H.; Kim, T.H. Improvement of sleep quality after treatment in patients with lumbar spinal stenosis: A prospective comparative study between conservative versus surgical treatment. *Sci. Rep.* **2020**, *10*, 14135. [CrossRef]
20. Buser, Z.; Ortega, B.; D'Oro, A.; Pannell, W.; Cohen, J.R.; Wang, J.; Golish, R.; Reed, M.; Wang, J.C. Spine Degenerative Conditions and Their Treatments: National Trends in the United States of America. *Glob. Spine J.* **2017**, *8*, 57–67. [CrossRef]
21. Kim, J.; Kang, M.S.; Kim, T.-H. Prevalence of Sleep Disturbance and Its Risk Factors in Patients Who Undergo Surgical Treatment for Degenerative Spinal Disease: A Nationwide Study of 106,837 Patients. *J. Clin. Med.* **2022**, *11*, 5932. [CrossRef]
22. Buysse, D.J.; Reynolds, C.F., 3rd; Monk, T.H.; Berman, S.R.; Kupfer, D.J. The Pittsburgh Sleep Quality Index: A new instrument for psychiatric practice and research. *Psychiatry Res.* **1989**, *28*, 193–213. [CrossRef]
23. Ibáñez, V.; Silva, J.; Cauli, O. A survey on sleep assessment methods. *PeerJ* **2018**, *6*, e4849. [CrossRef]
24. Choi, H.; Youn, S.; Um, Y.H.; Kim, T.W.; Ju, G.; Lee, H.J.; Lee, C.; Lee, S.D.; Bae, K.; Kim, S.J.; et al. Korean Clinical Practice Guideline for the Diagnosis and Treatment of Insomnia in Adults. *Psychiatry Investig.* **2020**, *17*, 1048–1059. [CrossRef]
25. Kim, J.; Ryu, H.; Kim, T.-H. Early Reoperation Rates and Its Risk Factors after Instrumented Spinal Fusion Surgery for Degenerative Spinal Disease: A Nationwide Cohort Study of 65,355 Patients. *J. Clin. Med.* **2022**, *11*, 3338. [CrossRef]
26. Lim, J.S.; Kim, T.-H. Recurrence Rates and Its Associated Factors after Early Spinal Instrumentation for Pyogenic Spondylodiscitis: A Nationwide Cohort Study of 2148 Patients. *J. Clin. Med.* **2022**, *11*, 3356. [CrossRef]
27. Kim, J.; Kim, T.-H. Risk Factors for Postoperative Deep Infection after Instrumented Spinal Fusion Surgeries for Degenerative Spinal Disease: A Nationwide Cohort Study of 194,036 Patients. *J. Clin. Med.* **2022**, *11*, 778. [CrossRef]
28. Frenkel, W.J.; Jongerius, E.J.; van Mandjes Uitert, M.J.; van Munster, B.C.; de Rooij, S.E. Validation of the Charlson Comorbidity Index in acutely hospitalized elderly adults: A prospective cohort study. *J. Am. Geriatr. Soc.* **2014**, *62*, 342–346. [CrossRef]
29. Park, H.-R.; Im, S.; Kim, H.; Jung, S.-Y.; Kim, D.; Jang, E.; Sung, Y.-K.; Cho, S.-K. Validation of algorithms to identify knee osteoarthritis patients in the claims database. *Int. J. Rheum. Dis.* **2019**, *22*, 890–896. [CrossRef]
30. Burgess, H.J.; Burns, J.W.; Buvanendran, A.; Gupta, R.; Chont, M.; Kennedy, M.; Bruehl, S. Associations Between Sleep Disturbance and Chronic Pain Intensity and Function: A Test of Direct and Indirect Pathways. *Clin. J. Pain* **2019**, *35*, 569–576. [CrossRef]
31. Onen, S.H.; Onen, F. Chronic Medical Conditions and Sleep in the Older Adult. *Sleep Med. Clin.* **2018**, *13*, 71–79. [CrossRef] [PubMed]
32. Sasaki, E.; Tsuda, E.; Yamamoto, Y.; Maeda, S.; Inoue, R.; Chiba, D.; Okubo, N.; Takahashi, I.; Nakaji, S.; Ishibashi, Y. Nocturnal knee pain increases with the severity of knee osteoarthritis, disturbing patient sleep quality. *Arthritis Care Res.* **2014**, *66*, 1027–1032. [CrossRef] [PubMed]
33. Khazzam, M.S.; Mulligan, E.P.; Brunette-Christiansen, M.; Shirley, Z. Sleep Quality in Patients with Rotator Cuff Disease. *J. Am. Acad. Orthop. Surg.* **2018**, *26*, 215–222. [CrossRef] [PubMed]

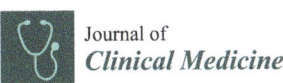

Review

Non-Adherence to Anti-Osteoporosis Medication: Factors Influencing and Strategies to Overcome It. A Narrative Review

Giulia Rita Agata Mangano [1], Marianna Avola [1], Chiara Blatti [2], Alessia Caldaci [2], Marco Sapienza [2], Rita Chiaramonte [1], Michele Vecchio [1], Vito Pavone [2] and Gianluca Testa [2,*]

[1] Department of Biomedical and Biotechnological Sciences, Section of Pharmacology, University Hospital Policlinico-San Marco, University of Catania, 95123 Catania, Italy
[2] Department of General Surgery and Medical Surgical Specialties, Section of Orthopaedics and Traumatology, University Hospital Policlinico-San Marco, University of Catania, 95123 Catania, Italy
* Correspondence: gianpavel@hotmail.com

Abstract: To evaluate the reasons for inadequate adherence to osteoporosis therapy and to describe the strategies for improving adherence to and persistence with regular medications, we conducted a review of the literature. The primary outcome of the study was the determination of the factors adverse to the onset and maintenance of anti-osteoporosis therapies. Secondly, we focused on studies whose efforts led to finding different strategies to improve adherence and persistence. We identified a total of 26 articles. The most recurrent and significant factors identified were aging, polypharmacy, and smoking habits. Different strategies to guide patients in their osteoporosis care have been identified, such as monitoring and follow-up via telephone calls, email, and promotional meetings, and proactive care interventions such as medication monitoring, post-fracture care programs, and decision aids. Changes in the drugs regimen and dispensation are strategies tried to lead to better adherence and persistence, but also improved satisfaction of patients undergoing anti-osteoporosis treatment. Patient involvement is an important factor to increase medication persistence while using a flexible drugs regimen.

Keywords: osteoporosis; adherence medications; elderly; frailty; postmenopausal; fractures; post-fracture care; educational meeting; drug regimen; medication monitoring

1. Introduction

Osteoporosis is one of the main health problems, affecting more than 200 million people worldwide [1] and a major public health issue considering that fragility fractures, one of the most serious complications, result in significant increases in morbidity and mortality, as well as socioeconomic burden [2].

Safe and effective medications are available to reduce the risk of fractures, but numerous patients do not start or do not appropriately follow treatment for osteoporosis, leading to a significant clinical and financial burden [3,4].

The utilization of health services in a general way is determined by the interaction between predisposing factors (e.g., race, age, and health beliefs), enabling factors (e.g., social support and access to health services), and the perceived and actual need for healthcare services [5].

The process by which patients take their medications as prescribed is defined by the term adherence and includes initiation, implementation, and discontinuation. Terms such us compliance and persistence are used in the literature as well [6].

Initiation, implementation, and persistence with osteoporosis medications, especially oral bisphosphonates, but also other medications such us teriparatide, raloxifene, denosumab, and zoledronic acid, are proven to be suboptimal by several studies [7]. For instance, after medical prescription, about 20–30% of patients do not initiate taking oral bisphosphonates, [7] and the persistence rates at 1 year are commonly estimated between 16 and

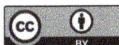

60% [8]. Numerous and multidimensional reasons and factors influence nonadherence, varying for each patient [9].

This trend of poor persistence and adherence to osteoporosis medications lowers the gains in bone mineral density (BMD), which is the protecting factor against fragility fractures [10].

Furthermore, investing the interventions to increase drug adherence could improve health outcomes and the efficiency of the health system [11]. Economic studies have also suggested that improving adherence results in cost-effectiveness benefits [12]. Improving medication adherence could lead to greater benefits than designing a new, more effective drug [6].

Therefore, improving adherence to osteoporosis medications remains a pivotal, but challenging task. Several interventions and programs have therefore been developed to improve osteoporosis medications adherence [3].

The primary outcome of the study was the determination of the factors adverse to the onset and maintenance of anti-osteoporosis therapies. Secondly, we focused on studies whose efforts led to finding different strategies to improve adherence and persistence.

2. Materials and Methods

We performed an extensive literature search in PubMed, Scopus, and Web of Science to identify relevant studies published from January 2012 to January 2022, analyzing the factors influencing osteoporosis medication adherence and interventions to improve it. The following search was used: (Osteoporosis AND (compliance OR adherence)) AND (prevention OR medications for treatment of therapy or follow up or exam or diagnosis). We limited our search to English language publications. A total of 308 studies were found. Upon reviewing the titles, excluding those articles which did not examine the barriers to starting or continuing anti-osteoporosis intervention and did not study the methods to ameliorate it, we identified a total of 26 articles.

3. Results

We identified 8 studies exploring the barriers and factors influencing patients' adherence, 10 studies testing and analyzing methods (healthcare systems, interventions, programs) to improve medication adherence, and 8 more studies which had as a main focus changes in administration methods as a strategy to increase persistence. The characteristics of the studies, samples, outcome measures and/or results are set out in Tables 1–3.

Table 1. Characteristics of studies analyzing factors and barriers influencing adherence and persistence.

Author	Study Design	Sample Size	Outcome Measures	Results/Conclusions
Fahrleitner-Pammer et al., 2017 [13]	Multicenter, prospective, noninterventional study	1500	24 months Denosumab persistance. Medical CRatio and Morisky Medication Adherence Scale (MMAS-8) questionnaire	Falling episodes before enrolling, multiple comobidities, age > 75 years, smoking habit
Garcia-Sempere et al., 2017 [14]	Population-based retrospective cohort	4856	Primary and secondary non-adherence (proportion of days covered (PDC) and persistence) to osteoporosis medications 1 year and 4 years after the first prescription	Age, dementia, polypharmacy, previous diagnosis of osteoporosis, rheumatoid arthritis
Alamri et al., 2015 [15]	Qualitative study	40	Interviews about barriers to implementing osteoporosis and fracture prevention guidelines	Lack of information and educational resources, difficulty obtaining required patient information for fracture risk assessment, inconsistent prescribing of vitamin D and calcium at the time of admission

Table 1. Cont.

Author	Study Design	Sample Size	Outcome Measures	Results/Conclusions
Gonnelli et al., 2016 [16]	Retrospective and prospective study	3206 + 816	4-item Morisky Medication Adherence Scale (MMAS)	History of osteoporotic fractures, frequency of drug administration, condition of being overweight/obese, age, smoking habit
Hall et al., 2017 [17]	Randomized controlled trial	790	Patient information and knowledge of osteoporosis through interview, FRAX	Osteoporosis knowledge, fear of medicine
McAlister et al., 2018 [18]	Randomized controlled trial	129	2 months' adherence (>80% of dose assumed), rate of non-adherence, 24 months' adherence to biphosphonates through self-report and pills report, SF-12, DASH, OptQol	Family members with osteoporosis, physician–patient relation
Parsons et al., 2019 [19]	Exploratory study	12,483	Self-reported adherence questionnaire	Incident fracture, prior medication, age, screening for fracture risk using FRAX
Salter et al., 2014 [20]	Longitudinal qualitative study	30	Interviews about understanding of osteoporosis, responses to screening results, current usage of preventive medicine, motivators and detractors from taking medication, follow-up with healthcare professionals	Severe side effects, confusion, lack of knowledge about the risks of osteoporosis

Table 2. Characteristics of studies analyzing methods and healthcare systems to enhance adherence and persistence.

Author	Study Design	Treatment	Sample Size	Outcome Measures	Results/Conclusions
Tüzün et al., 2013 [21]	Multicenter randomized controlled study	Use of bisphosphonate guide and osteoporosis training booklets. Intervention group received four phone calls and participated in four interactive social/training meetings held in groups of 10 patients.	448 aged 45–75 years with postmenopausal osteoporosis	1. Self-reported persistence and compliance with the treatment. 2. Quality of life of the patients assessed by the 41-item Quality of Life European Foundation for Osteoporosis (QUALEFFO-41) questionnaire.	No significant differences between AT and PT groups in both visit 1 and visit 5.
Akarırmak et al., 2016 [22]	Prospective non-interventional observational cohort registry study	Use of "Training Kit", including four training booklets ("General Information on Osteoporosis", "Osteoporosis and Exercise", "Osteoporosis and Nutrition", "Osteoporosis and Patient Rights") During 12-month follow-up, four telephone calls and four individual face-to-face interactive/educational meetings.	979 mean age 63.2(7.2) with postmenopausal osteoporosis	1. Persistence and compliance. 2. Effect of bisphosphonate treatment on withdrawals from the study due to adverse event.	No significant difference in terms of compliance and persistence (79.4% of the patients).
Solomon et al., 2012 [23]	Randomized pilot study	Telephonic motivational interviewing intervention.	2087 with osteoporosis	1. Medication regimen adherence.	In an intention to treat analysis, median adherence was 49% in the intervention arm and 41% in the control arm.

Table 2. Cont.

Author	Study Design	Treatment	Sample Size	Outcome Measures	Results/Conclusions
Bianchi et al., 2015 [24]	Randomized prospective study	Booklets providing information on osteoporosis and the importance of adherence to treatment. Colored memo stickers for a calendar or diary. Alarm clock. Phone calls.	334 post-menopausal women	1. Adherence to therapy. 2. Persistence with therapy.	247 of 334 patients (74%) started the prescribed therapy.
Kessous et al., 2014 [25]	Prospective randomized l trial	Use of explanatory pamphlet, article concerning OP, and a letter addressed to primary care physician that recommended further diagnostic workup.	99 with distal fractures radius	Referral to their primary care physician and undergoing an OP workup.	Intervention increased the number of patients who turned to their primary care physician from 22.9% to 68.6% and boosted the proportion of patients undergoing a diagnostic examination from 14.3% to 40% ($p < 0.001$).
Stuurman-Bieze et al., 2014 [26]	Prospective intervention study	Medication. Monitoring and Optimization (MeMO) intervention, compared to usual pharmacy care.	937 with osteoporosis	1. Therapy discontinuation and nonadherence. 2. Patients' satisfaction.	32.8% of patients in the usual care group initiating osteoporosis medication were nonadherent or discontinued, compared to 19.0% of patients in the intervention group ($p < 0.001$).
Ganda et al., 2014 [27]	Randomized controlled trial	Secondary-fracture prevention handled by specialists, compared with usual care.	102 men and women with osteoporotic fractures	1. Patient compliance and persistence.	At 24 months' medication persistence the medication possession ratio was similar in both groups (64% versus 61%, respectively; $p = 0.75$).
Merle et al., 2017 [28]	Multicenter, randomized controlled trial	PREVOST population-based patient-centered post-fracture care program, compared to usual care.	436 women aged 50–85 years (fracture of the wrist or humerus)	1. Proportion of women who reported the initiation of an appropriate post-fracture care program. 2. Proportion of bone mineral density scans performed.	At 6 months, 53% of patients in the intervention group began a post-fracture care program versus 33% in the control group.

Table 3. Characteristics of Studies analyzing different drug regimens.

Author	Study Design	Sample Size	Outcome Measures	Results/Conclusions
Oral et al., 2015 [29]	Multicentric, prospective, crossover, randomized, parallel	448 postmenopausal women	Persistence and compliance	Patients on a flexible daily dose of risedronate are more compliant and persistent than patients on fixed regimens.
Finigan et al., 2013 [30]	Single-center, prospective, randomized	75 women	Adherence	Monitoring caps assesses adherence more accurately than tablet counts.
Freementle et al. 2012 [31]	Single-center, randomized, open-label, crossover	250 women	Adherence, compliance, persistence, and satisfaction	Patients were more adherent, compliant, persistent, and satisfied with subcutaneous denosumab injections every 6 months than with once-weekly alendronate tablets.
Kendler et al., 2014 [32]	Multicenter, randomized, open-label, crossover	250 women	BMQ (Beliefs about Medicines Questionnaire)	Participants preferred denosumab to alendronate while on treatment and had more positive perceptions of denosumab than alendronate. These perceptions were associated with better adherence.

Table 3. Cont.

Author	Study Design	Sample Size	Outcome Measures	Results/Conclusions
Muratore et al., 2013 [33]	Randomized, open-label, parallel-group, single centre	87 women	Adherence	Neridronate is associated with higher adherence and a better effect on BMD compared to alendronate and risedronate.
Palacios et al., 2015 [34]	Single-center, retrospective, randomized, open-label	1703	TSQM (Treatment Satisfaction Questionnaire for Medication)	Patients were more satisfied when transitioned to denosumab versus switching to a monthly oral bisphosphonate.
Roh et al., 2018 [35]	Single-center, randomized	439	Adherence	Patients with limited health literacy showed better adherence to quarterly intravenous bisphosphonates compared to weekly oral bisphosphonates, similar to rates among patients with appropriate literacy.
Tamechika et al., 2018 [36]	Multicentric, randomized, prospective, open-label	130	Satisfaction, BMD	Patients were more satisfied with monthly minodronate compared to weekly alendronate or risedronate, it also showed an improvement in BMD.

3.1. Factors and Barriers Influencing Adherence and Persistence

The most frequent factors influencing anti-osteoporosis medication adherence or persistence identified are aging, polypharmacy, and smoking habits. Alamri et al.'s study, [15] in 2015, found that the Clinical Practice Guidelines for the Diagnosis and Management of Osteoporosis in Canada, [37] are underutilized in long-term care (LTC).

The most commonly reported barriers to providing optimal bone health care in LTC were a lack of information and educational resources, difficulty obtaining the required patient information for a fracture risk assessment and the inconsistent prescribing of vitamin D and calcium at the time of admission, as well as the difficulty in including osteoporosis and fracture prevention strategies as topics for quarterly reviews.

In 2017 Fahrleitner-Pammer conducted a study assessing persistence, adherence, and medication coverage ratio (MCR) in postmenopausal women receiving denosumab in routine practice in Germany, Austria, Greece, and Belgium [13]. Lower persistence was associated with elderly age, a history of previous interruptions in therapy, patients' intolerance to other osteoporosis medications, smoking habit, and a history of falls in the year before enrollment. Individuals with multiple comorbidities are likely to have a high medication burden [38] which may be confusing and could result in osteoporosis treatment being considered a low priority. In addition, when attempting to reduce the medication burden, physicians and patients may deprioritize osteoporosis therapy.

In García-Sempere's study, aging was associated with both non-adherence and non-persistence, similar to what has been seen previously [14]. Poor adherence-only was associated with sedative treatment and previous stroke, while being male and having dementia led mostly to impaired persistence. A high medication burden, due to multiple comorbidities, led to lower non-adherence in this study as well.

Aging, comorbidities, and smoking attitude were identified as worsening factors for adherence to osteoporosis therapy, probably because these conditions could express the reduced attention of the patients to their state of health as was explained in the randomized prospective study conducted by Gonnelli et al. in 2016 [16]. Moreover, being overweight was associated with worse compliance too. The authors explained this finding with a likely reduced attention of the patients towards their health condition. They tried to ameliorate compliance through patient information about fracture risk using the DeFRA algorithm [39], but this strategy only marginally improved adherence. Osteoporosis prior to fracture is asymptomatic, and patients are more likely to prioritize other diseases that have a more direct impact on their daily lives.

On the other hand, in the study conducted by Parsons et al., [19] the use of systematic screening for fracture risk using FRAX® in primary care led to the increased use of, and adherence to, anti-osteoporosis medications, compared to usual care.

Hall et al. examined the effects of a patient-activation intervention on osteoporosis pharmacotherapy through osteoporosis knowledge, conducting interviews about the reasons for non-adherence to therapy [17]. The most common reasons for non-adherence were the fear of side effects or contraindications, a dislike of taking medications, and believing that the prescribed medication would not improve their condition.

McAlister et al. analyzed the effect of an educational program, comparing it with usual care from a primary care physician through an RCT, identifying the factors influencing compliance to biphosphonates [18]. The most commonly reported reasons for stopping bisphosphonate therapy were the side effects, mostly gastrointestinal ones. Moreover, this study highlights the importance of established physician–patient relationships and continuity of care in the decision to take long-term preventive therapies. In fact, patients who were managed by their physician, had a better 2-year adherence than patients dealt with by the educational program.

A similar scenario is encountered in the Salter et al. trial [20], in which it is suggested that preventive health measures often pose a challenge in which the general practitioner has to make individual decisions dependent on the beliefs, understanding, needs, and expectations of the patient in front of them, debating every new health issue in the context of the person's whole life, maximizing health gain, and minimizing adverse consequences [40].

3.2. Methods and Healthcare Systems to Enhance Adherence and Persistence

Different strategies to guide patients in their osteoporosis care have been identified, such as monitoring and follow-up via telephone calls, email and education meetings, proactive care interventions, such as medication monitoring, post-fracture care programs, and decision aids.

3.2.1. Telephone Calls, Emails, Educational Meetings

In an RCT, Tuzun et al. randomized patients with postmenopausal osteoporosis undergoing treatment with weekly oral bisphosphonates into two groups, an active training group (AT) and a passive training group (PT). Both groups received a Starter Training Kit including a bisphosphonate guide and osteoporosis training booklets. The AT group was, in addition, trained through a standard training package including telephone calls and interactive educational meetings. The authors evaluated persistency, treatment compliance, adverse events, vertebral and non-vertebral fractures, and quality of life. There were no significant differences between the AT and PT groups, most of the patients always used their drugs regularly according to the recommended days and dosages; the most common reason for not receiving treatment regularly was forgetfulness and most of the patients were highly satisfied with the treatment and wanted to continue [21].

In another Turkish study patients with post-menopausal osteoporosis undergoing treatment with weekly or monthly bisphosphonates were included and randomized into two groups. The training group was provided with a training kit including booklets containing information about osteoporosis and followed up with telephone calls and individual face-to-face interactive/educational meetings focused on disease awareness. The patients in the control group were followed up by physicians without supplying training booklets. The authors did not find significant differences between the training and control groups in terms of compliance and persistence. The patients on the monthly bisphosphonate regimen showed significantly longer persistence in comparison to patients on the weekly regimen [22].

In an RCT, Solomon et al. enrolled patients who had been newly prescribed a medication for osteoporosis and divided them into two groups. Both received information material on osteoporosis by e-mail, while the patients in the intervention group also received motivational interviewing counseling sessions via telephone with health educators discussing osteoporosis medication. They could not find a statistically significant improvement in adherence to an osteoporosis medication regimen using this method [23].

Post-menopausal women, receiving an oral prescription for osteoporosis for the first time were recruited and randomized into three groups in an RCT conducted by Bianchi et al. Group 1 were managed according to standard clinical practice, group 2 received educational booklets providing information on osteoporosis and reminders as well an alarm clock to prompt medication administration, group 3 also received phone calls from physicians and nurses who discussed the topic of osteoporosis with patients. The outcomes were adherence and persistence to therapy. There were no significant differences among the three groups. The authors point out that monthly intake of the drug had a higher adherence than weekly and daily intake [24].

Kessous et al. in an RCT investigated whether a clinical intervention after a distal radial fracture would encourage patients to visit their primary care physician and start an OP therapy. Seventy patients were divided into two groups. Both groups were contacted by telephone 6–8 weeks after the fracture and asked to respond to a questionnaire about their awareness of osteoporosis and fragility fractures. Only the intervention group received an explanatory pamphlet and an article about osteoporosis with a letter to their primary care physician that recommended further diagnostic workup. The outcome was evaluated by a second call for both groups after 6–8 weeks and was considered positive if the patients' referral to their primary care physician had resulted in them undergoing an osteoporosis workup. The intervention increased the number of patients who turned to their primary care physician and boosted the proportion of patients undergoing a diagnostic examination [25].

3.2.2. Medication Monitoring

In a study by Stuurman-Bieze the pharmacy provided structured counseling on aspects regarding administration, efficacy, and possible side-effects. The pharmacists checked whether the patients returned for their next prescriptions. If the patients did not redeem their medication they were contacted if warranted. The results were compared to a reference group receiving the usual pharmacy care. This intervention can decrease patients' non-adherence; 93% of patients were satisfied and mentioned that the pharmacy was the only place where they received explanations regarding osteoporosis [26].

3.2.3. Post-Fracture Care

Ganda et al. evaluated whether a secondary fracture prevention (SFP) program could improve compliance and persistence with oral bisphosphonate therapy. An intervention group was followed by a specialist in the SFP service for the entire duration of the study, while a control group was seen by the SFP service twice and then followed up by their primary care physician. At 24 months the medication persistence and medication possession ratio (MPR) were similar in both groups. Time-based changes in BMD or bone turnover were not associated with persistence and compliance. These results indicate that one of the main functions of an SFP program may be the initiation of therapy rather than continuous patient monitoring [27].

Merle et al. evaluated the impact of a population-based patient-centered post-fracture care program, PREVOST, in an RCT. The intervention group received a phone call where a trained case manager focused on the association between fragility fractures and the high risk of osteoporosis and encouraged the patient to visit their primary care physician to discuss their personal risk of fragility, fracture, and osteoporosis, to schedule a BMD test, and to start a pharmacological treatment for osteoporosis if necessary. An information summary booklet was then mailed to each subject. Reminder phone calls were performed following the telephone discussion. The patients from the control group received the usual care. The primary outcome was the percentage of patients who reported the beginning of appropriate post-fracture care. The secondary outcomes were the percentage of patients who reported that a BMD had been performed, a treatment prescription and/or a calcium–

vitamin D supplementation had been given, and information on osteoporosis had been delivered by the primary care physician. The authors described a significantly improved post-fracture BMD investigation [28].

3.2.4. Decision Aid

LeBlanc et al. enrolled women with a diagnosis of osteopenia or osteoporosis who were not taking medications to treat their condition and compared the patients' estimated risk of fracture using the FRAX calculator with Osteoporosis Choice, an encounter decision aid. The latter included the individualized 10-year risk of having a bone fracture, using the FRAX calculator, with and without the use of bisphosphonate, and the possible harms and other disadvantage of using bisphosphonates. The primary outcomes were the patients' decisional conflict, knowledge, decision whether to start medication, adherence to medication, involvement in decision making by the clinician, fidelity to the intended intervention, acceptability, satisfaction, and quality of life. The secondary outcome was decision quality. The Osteoporosis Choice decision aid was found to be better than usual care with or without the FRAX calculation. More patients started taking a bisphosphonate and filled their prescriptions in the decision aid group arm compared to the FRAX/usual care group. The FRAX calculator alone as a clinical decision support tool during the encounter was no different from usual care across all the measured parameters [41].

In a pilot randomized trial the authors tested the feasibility of a fracture prevention decision aid in an online patient portal. The patients in the intervention group received the decision aid which contained a 10-year fracture risk calculator, a summary of the medication risks and benefits (prescription and nonprescription), and an elicitation of values, while those in the control group were directed to the National Institute on Aging homepage which provided web-based information relevant to aging but not specific to osteoporosis. The first outcomes were decisional conflict and preparation for decision making; the second outcomes were feasibility and planning for a larger trial. The patients in the intervention group reported being more prepared for making decisions about their treatment and having decreased decisional conflict compared to the patients in the control group [42].

3.3. Drug Regimen

Changes in drug regimen and dispensation are strategies attempted to lead not only to better adherence and persistence, but also improved satisfaction of patients undergoing treatment with anti-osteoporosis medication. Various studies explore this issue.

Oral et al. conducted a multicentric study including women with post-menopausal osteoporosis (OP) [29]. They evaluated the level of compliance and persistence over 26 weeks in women receiving risedronate daily, following two different regimens: flexible doses or fixed doses either before breakfast, in-between meals or before bedtime. In both groups the effect on the urinary N-terminal telopeptide of type 1 collagen was evaluated. The study resulted in a higher rate of persistence among patients under the flexible regimen; however, no statistical significance was noted in terms of compliance between the two groups.

Finigan et al. analyzed adherence to raloxifene for 2 years among post-menopausal women [30]. They compared the methods of tablet counts and of electronic monitoring with electronic bottle caps and eventually they examined the degree of bone response to raloxifene. Simple counts of returned tablets may mask irregular patterns of tablet-taking, therefore electronic monitoring is the most accurate way to monitor actual behavior and the resulting adherence levels are consistently lower than those obtained by counting returned tablets.

Freemantle et al. conducted a study that compared adherence, compliance, and persistence in a group of post-menopausal osteoporotic women who were firstly administered once-weekly alendronate tablets for 12 months and then for another 12 months were administered subcutaneous denosumab injections every 6 months; the other group followed the opposite pattern of osteoporosis therapy medication [31]. Denosumab was associated with less non-adherence than alendronate. Postmenopausal osteoporotic women were shown to be more adherent, compliant, and persistent with subcutaneous denosumab injections every 6 months than with once-weekly alendronate tablets. These results are aligned to the degree of satisfaction: women preferred injectable denosumab over oral alendronate. The BMD variation was analyzed, and further improvements were described when subjects received alendronate first followed by denosumab, with BMD after the opposite pattern remaining stable.

In addition, Kendler et al. conducted a study of a group of post-menopausal osteoporotic women who during the first year were administered 70 mg of alendronate daily, and during the second year were given a subcutaneous denosumab injection every 6 months [32]. At baseline, 6, 12, 18, and 24 months, patients answered a questionnaire about the necessity of treatment and their concerns regarding osteoporosis therapy. The BMQ (Beliefs about Medicines Questionnaire) results showed that the subjects included in the study reported a greater preference for denosumab to alendronate in both treatment periods.

Muratore et al. conducted a 3-year randomized study with post-menopausal women affected by rheumatic arthritis and glucocorticoid induced osteopenia (T score $\geq$ 2.5) [33]. A total of 87 patients receiving methylprednisolone therapy were randomized into three treatment pattern groups for 1 year: 30 on neridronate, 27 on alendronate, and 30 on risedronate. They compared the adherence to intramuscular neridronate versus oral alendronate or risedronate therapy. The results from the study showed a higher adherence to intramuscular neridronate administered monthly than oral alendronate or risedronate administered weekly. Neridronate was shown to have similar efficacy to alendronate or risedronate in terms of BMD.

Palacios et al. considered the TSQM (Treatment Satisfaction Questionnaire for Medication) for the first time for the evaluation of osteoporosis treatment satisfaction [34]. They enrolled in the study post-menopausal osteoporotic women that had already been undergoing osteoporotic therapy for at least 1 month prior to screening with daily or weekly oral alendronate for transition to risedronate, and any oral bisphosphonate for transition to ibandronate. The patients were randomized to be administered subcutaneous denosumab every 6 months, or oral ibandronate or risedronate monthly for 12 months. The study showed that women with post-menopausal osteoporosis were more satisfied after transitioning to subcutaneous denosumab every 6 months compared with transitioning to risedronate or ibandronate every month.

Roh et al. conducted a study of women with distal radius fractures and limited health literacy [35]. These patients were randomized into two groups: one underwent intravenous ibandronate injections every 3 months for 1 year and the other group were administered weekly alendronate orally for 1 year. They reported a higher adherence in the subjects receiving intravenous ibandronate injections treatment than those receiving alendronate per os every 3 months, justified both by the pattern of administration and by the gastrointestinal adverse events.

Tamechika et al. conducted a study with patients affected by glucocorticoids induced osteoporosis, treated with weekly alendronate or risedronate [36]. These patients were randomized into two groups: one group continued their original bisphosphonate treatment weekly, the other group switched to monthly minodronate. Satisfaction therapy and BMD at the lumbar spine level were evaluated. Even though drug compliance in both groups was excellent and not statistically significant, switching to monthly minodronate considerably improved patient satisfaction as well as decreasing TRACP-5b (a bone resorption marker) and increasing BMD; however, serum BAP level (a bone formation marker) showed no significant difference between the two groups.

4. Discussion

In the literature it is well established that osteoporosis treatment considerably decreases the risk of non-vertebral and vertebral fractures. The management of osteoporosis is arduous since patients with osteoporosis can be totally asymptomatic until they have a fracture, contrarily to other chronic pathologies such as diabetes or heart failure. Due to poor adherence to osteoporosis treatment, patients develop poor clinical conditions. Therefore, the need to improve this situation is one of the most important issues in the treatment of osteoporosis. Improving adherence to osteoporosis medications is a challenging task. The reasons for nonadherence to osteoporosis treatment are several and multifaceted and differ for each patient [9].

It is clear that the current usual practice regarding the assessment of osteoporosis after a fragility fracture is insufficient. There are no appropriate guidelines regarding the correct follow-up and treatment of patients with fragility fractures; furthermore, a fragility fracture patient is seen by numerous doctors who may lack the required lines of communication with one another. Usually patients with a femoral neck fracture tend to experience a long hospital placement and for this reason they are more likely to receive an explanation concerning the association between their fracture and osteoporosis.

Various interventions and programs have been designed to improve osteoporosis medications adherence. Most of the studies evaluating adherence to and persistence in osteoporosis treatment are based on patient education, using different methods. The use of telephone calls, emails, and alarm clocks as a reminder to take medication as prescribed compared with the usual care pathways seems not to improve adherence and persistence [21–25].

Explanatory pamphlets, articles, and training booklets regarding the correlation between fragility fractures and osteoporosis can increase awareness and consequently the percentage of patients who start a diagnostic examination pattern for osteoporosis, as well as increasing the number of patients who turned to their primary care physician. In the studies evaluated there was a significant difference in patient participation and involvement. If the patient was advised about and involved in the therapeutic prescription decision regarding their drug regimen, there was an improvement in continuation; conversely there was no improvement in adherence when the patient was not involved [26]. Well-informed patients seem to take their medication regularly [21]. Patient involvement is an important factor to increase medication persistence while using a flexible dosing regimen. Coherent with the concept that reducing the complexity and frequency of dosing regimens improves adherence to and persistence with bisphosphonates in patients with osteoporosis, several authors point out that a monthly intake of osteoporosis medications has a higher adherence and persistence in comparison to patients on weekly and daily regimens [22,24]. Switching from a weekly to a monthly bisphosphonate regimen seems to offer a helpful strategy for improving long-term fracture prevention [22]. It seems that changing the drug regimen is only helpful for patients already using osteoporosis drugs and not for new medication treatments [43].

Other interventions to increase adherence and persistence include Medication Monitoring and Optimization, where pharmacies provided structured counseling on aspects regarding the administration, efficacy, and possible side-effects of medications, in order to reduce the fear of therapy and encourage take-up, showing that this decision aid or better-than-usual care decreases decisional conflict and increases patient knowledge and involvement in deciding to start therapy [41,42]. Decision aid communicates not only the risk of fracture but also quantifies the potential risk reduction with bisphosphonate therapy. Decision aid also brings various essential patient topics (i.e., side effects, cost) to the forefront and serves as an invitation for the patient and clinician to address these [41]. Patient portal-based decision aid was also effective at decreasing decisional conflict, preparing patients to make a decision on how to prevent fractures, and increasing patients' self-reported decision making [42].

Secondary fracture prevention programs should identify patients and initiate treatment rather than facilitate continuous patient management. These programs not only overcome the aversion to initiating the appropriate management of patients with incident osteoporotic fractures, but also result in high compliance and persistence with treatment over time [27]. Some authors have suggested that the initiation of bisphosphonate therapy soon after an incident fracture may improve compliance and persistence because the acute fracture event provides a window of opportunity to instigate positive behavioral change [44].

Moreover, understanding patients' perceptions and preferences for treatment may be an effective method for improving adherence to the appropriate osteoporosis therapy selected [32]. Medications with longer intervals between doses and a reduced risk of gastrointestinal issues, such as neridronate, minodronate, or denosumab compared with a weekly intake of bisphosphonate, are proven to increase patients' satisfaction and therefore compliance [33,34].

5. Conclusions

This review tried to explore the limitations, barriers, and factors influencing anti-osteoporosis medication adherence, finding that generally patient education, monitoring, changes in drug regimens combined with patient support, and patient education through interdisciplinary collaboration has been shown to have positive effects on adherence to and persistence with treatment. Greater treatment satisfaction may lead to better treatment adherence and, ultimately, improvements in treatment effectiveness.

Author Contributions: Conceptualization, M.A.; methodology, G.R.A.M.; software, A.C.; validation, G.T.; formal analysis, C.B.; investigation, M.S.; resources, R.C.; data curation, G.R.A.M. and M.A.; writing—original draft preparation, G.R.A.M.; writing—review and editing, M.A.; visualization, V.P.; supervision, G.T.; project administration, M.V. All authors have read and agreed to the published version of the manuscript.

Funding: This research received no external funding.

Institutional Review Board Statement: Not applicable.

Informed Consent Statement: Not applicable.

Data Availability Statement: Non applicable.

Acknowledgments: Not applicable.

Conflicts of Interest: The authors declare no conflict of interest.

References

1. Dhanwal, D.K.; Dennison, E.M.; Harvey, N.C.; Cooper, C. Epidemiology of hip fracture: Worldwide geographic variation. *Indian J. Orthop.* **2011**, *45*, 15–22. [CrossRef] [PubMed]
2. Iolascon, G.; Moretti, A.; Toro, G.; Gimigliano, F.; Liguori, S.; Paoletta, M. Pharmacological Therapy of Osteoporosis: What's New? *Clin. Interv. Aging* **2020**, *15*, 485–491. [CrossRef] [PubMed]
3. Hiligsmann, M.; Cornelissen, D.; Vrijens, B.; Abrahamsen, B.; Al-Daghri, N.; Biver, E.; Brandi, M.; Bruyère, O.; Burlet, N.; Cooper, C.; et al. Determinants, consequences and potential solutions to poor adherence to anti-osteoporosis treatment: Results of an expert group meeting organized by the European Society for Clinical and Economic Aspects of Osteoporosis, Osteoarthritis and Musculoskeletal Diseases (ESCEO) and the International Osteoporosis Foundation (IOF). *Osteoporos. Int.* **2019**, *30*, 2155–2165. [CrossRef] [PubMed]
4. Jaleel, A.; Saag, K.G.; Danila, M.I. Improving drug adherence in osteoporosis: An update on more recent studies. *Ther. Adv. Musculoskelet. Dis.* **2018**, *10*, 141–149. [CrossRef]
5. Vrijens, B.; De Geest, S.; Hughes, D.; Przemyslaw, K.; Demonceau, J.; Ruppar, T.; Dobbels, F.; Fargher, E.; Morrison, V.; Lewek, P.; et al. A new taxonomy for describing and defining adherence to medications. *Br. J. Clin. Pharmacol.* **2012**, *73*, 691–705. [CrossRef]
6. De Geest, S.; Sabaté, E. Adherence to Long-Term Therapies: Evidence for Action. *Eur. J. Cardiovasc. Nurs.* **2003**, *2*, 323. [CrossRef]
7. Reynolds, K.; Muntner, P.; Cheetham, T.C.; Harrison, T.N.; Morisky, D.E.; Silverman, S.; Gold, D.T.; Vansomphone, S.S.; Wei, R.; O'Malley, C.D. Primary non-adherence to bisphosphonates in an integrated healthcare setting. *Osteoporos. Int.* **2013**, *24*, 2509–2517. [CrossRef]
8. Rabenda, V.; Hiligsmann, M.; Reginster, J.-Y. Poor adherence to oral bisphosphonate treatment and its consequences: A review of the evidence. *Expert Opin. Pharmacother.* **2009**, *10*, 2303–2315. [CrossRef]
9. Yeam, C.T.; Chia, S.; Tan, H.C.C.; Kwan, Y.H.; Fong, W.; Seng, J.J.B. A systematic review of factors affecting medication adherence among patients with osteoporosis. *Osteoporos. Int.* **2018**, *29*, 2623–2637. [CrossRef]
10. Siris, E.S.; Selby, P.L.; Saag, K.G.; Borgström, F.; Herings, R.M.; Silverman, S.L. Impact of Osteoporosis Treatment Adherence on Fracture Rates in North America and Europe. *Am. J. Med.* **2009**, *122*, S3–S13. [CrossRef]

11. Sabaté, E. *Adherence to Long-Term Therapies: Evidence for Action*; World Health Organization: Geneva, Switzerland, 2003.
12. Hiligsmann, M.; McGowan, B.; Bennett, K.; Barry, M.; Reginster, J.-Y. The Clinical and Economic Burden of Poor Adherence and Persistence with Osteoporosis Medications in Ireland. *Value Health* **2012**, *15*, 604–612. [CrossRef] [PubMed]
13. Fahrleitner-Pammer, A.; Papaioannou, N.; Gielen, E.; Tepie, M.F.; Toffis, C.; Frieling, I.; Geusens, P.; Makras, P.; Boschitsch, E.; Callens, J.; et al. Factors associated with high 24-month persistence with denosumab: Results of a real-world, non-interventional study of women with postmenopausal osteoporosis in Germany, Austria, Greece, and Belgium. *Arch. Osteoporos.* **2017**, *12*, 58. [CrossRef] [PubMed]
14. García-Sempere, A.; Hurtado, I.; Sanfélix-Genovés, J.; Rodríguez-Bernal, C.L.; Gil Orozco, R.; Peiró, S.; Sanfélix-Gimeno, G. Primary and secondary non-adherence to osteoporotic medications after hip fracture in Spain. The PREV2FO population-based retrospective cohort study. *Sci. Rep.* **2017**, *7*, 11784. [CrossRef] [PubMed]
15. Alamri, S.H.; Kennedy, C.C.; Marr, S.K.; Lohfeld, L.; Skidmore, C.J.; Papaioannou, A. Strategies to overcome barriers to implementing osteoporosis and fracture prevention guidelines in long-term care: A qualitative analysis of action plans suggested by front line staff in Ontario, Canada. *BMC Geriatr.* **2015**, *15*, 94. [CrossRef] [PubMed]
16. Gonnelli, S.; Caffarelli, C.; Rossi, S.; Di Munno, O.; Malavolta, N.; Isaia, G.; Muratore, M.; D'Avola, G.; Gatto, S.; Minisola, G.; et al. How the knowledge of fracture risk might influence adherence to oral therapy of osteoporosis in Italy: The ADEOST study. *Aging Clin. Exp. Res.* **2016**, *28*, 459–468. [CrossRef]
17. Hall, S.F.; Edmonds, S.W.; Lou, Y.; Cram, P.; Roblin, D.W.; Saag, K.G.; Wright, N.C.; Jones, M.P.; Wolinsky, F.D. Patient-reported reasons for nonadherence to recommended osteoporosis pharmacotherapy. *J. Am. Pharm. Assoc.* **2017**, *57*, 503–509. [CrossRef]
18. McAlister, F.A.; Ye, C.; Beaupre, L.A.; Rowe, B.H.; Johnson, J.A.; Bellerose, D.; Hassan, I.; Majumdar, S.R. Adherence to osteoporosis therapy after an upper extremity fracture: A pre-specified substudy of the C-STOP randomized controlled trial. *Osteoporos. Int.* **2018**, *30*, 127–134. [CrossRef]
19. Parsons, C.M.; Harvey, N.; Shepstone, L.; Kanis, J.; Lenaghan, E.; Clarke, S.; Fordham, R.; Gittoes, N.; Harvey, I.; Holland, R.; et al. Systematic screening using FRAX® leads to increased use of, and adherence to, anti-osteoporosis medications: An analysis of the UK SCOOP trial. *Osteoporos. Int.* **2019**, *31*, 67–75. [CrossRef]
20. Salter, C.; McDaid, L.; Bhattacharya, D.; Holland, R.; Marshall, T.; Howe, A. Abandoned Acid? Understanding Adherence to Bisphosphonate Medications for the Prevention of Osteoporosis among Older Women: A Qualitative Longitudinal Study. *PLoS ONE* **2014**, *9*, e83552. [CrossRef]
21. Tüzün, Ş.; Akyüz, G.; Eskiyurt, N.; Memiş, A.; Kuran, B.; Içağasıoğlu, A.; Sarpel, T.; Özdemir, F.; Özgirgin, N.; Günaydın, R.; et al. Impact of the Training on the Compliance and Persistence of Weekly Bisphosphonate Treatment in Postmenopausal Osteoporosis: A Randomized Controlled Study. *Int. J. Med. Sci.* **2013**, *10*, 1880–1887. [CrossRef]
22. Akarırmak, Ü.; Koçyiğit, H.; Eskiyurt, N.; Esmaeilzadeh, S.; Kuru, Ö.; Yalçinkaya, E.Y.; Peker, Ö.; Ekim, A.A.; Özgirgin, N.; Çalış, M.; et al. Influence of patient training on persistence, compliance, and tolerability of different dosing frequency regimens of bisphosphonate therapy: An observational study in Turkish patients with postmenopausal osteoporosis. *Acta Orthop. Traumatol. Turc.* **2016**, *50*, 415–423. [CrossRef] [PubMed]
23. Solomon, D.H.; Iversen, M.D.; Avorn, J.; Gleeson, T.; Brookhart, M.A.; Patrick, A.R.; Rekedal, L.; Shrank, W.H.; Lii, J.; Losina, E.; et al. Osteoporosis Telephonic Intervention to Improve Medication Regimen Adherence. *Arch. Intern. Med.* **2012**, *172*, 477–483. [CrossRef] [PubMed]
24. Bianchi, M.L.; Duca, P.; Vai, S.; Guglielmi, G.; Viti, R.; Battista, C.; Scillitani, A.; Muscarella, S.; Luisetto, G.; Camozzi, V.; et al. Improving adherence to and persistence with oral therapy of osteoporosis. *Osteoporos. Int.* **2015**, *26*, 1629–1638. [CrossRef] [PubMed]
25. Kessous, R.; Weintraub, A.Y.; Mattan, Y.; Dresner-Pollak, R.; Brezis, M.; Liebergall, M.; Kandel, L. Improving compliance to osteoporosis workup and treatment in postmenopausal patients after a distal radius fracture. *Taiwan. J. Obstet. Gynecol.* **2014**, *53*, 206–209. [CrossRef]
26. Stuurman-Bieze, A.G.G.; Hiddink, E.G.; Van Boven, J.F.M.; Vegter, S. Proactive pharmaceutical care interventions decrease patients' nonadherence to osteoporosis medication. *Osteoporos. Int.* **2014**, *25*, 1807–1812. [CrossRef]
27. Ganda, K.; Schaffer, A.; Pearson, S.; Seibel, M.J. Compliance and persistence to oral bisphosphonate therapy following initiation within a secondary fracture prevention program: A randomised controlled trial of specialist vs. non-specialist management. *Osteoporos. Int.* **2014**, *25*, 1345–1355. [CrossRef]
28. Merle, B.; Chapurlat, R.; Vignot, E.; Thomas, T.; Haesebaert, J.; Schott, A.-M. Post-fracture care: Do we need to educate patients rather than doctors? The PREVOST randomized controlled trial. *Osteoporos. Int.* **2017**, *28*, 1549–1558. [CrossRef]
29. Oral, A.; Lorenc, R.; FLINT-ACT Study. Compliance, persistence, and preference outcomes of postmenopausal osteoporotic women receiving a flexible or fixed regimen of daily risedronate: A multicenter, prospective, parallel group study. *Acta Orthop. Traumatol. Turc.* **2015**, *49*, 67–74. [CrossRef]
30. Finigan, J.; Naylor, K.; Paggiosi, M.A.; Peel, N.F.; Eastell, R. Adherence to raloxifene therapy: Assessment methods and relationship with efficacy. *Osteoporos. Int.* **2013**, *24*, 2879–2886. [CrossRef]
31. Freemantle, N.; on behalf of the DAPS Investigators; Satram-Hoang, S.; Tang, E.-T.; Kaur, P.; Macarios, D.; Siddhanti, S.; Borenstein, J.; Kendler, D.L. Final results of the DAPS (Denosumab Adherence Preference Satisfaction) study: A 24-month, randomized, crossover comparison with alendronate in postmenopausal women. *Osteoporos. Int.* **2011**, *23*, 317–326. [CrossRef]

32. Kendler, D.L.; Macarios, D.; Lillestol, M.J.; Moffett, A.; Satram, S.; Huang, J.; Kaur, P.; Tang, E.-T.; Wagman, R.B.; Horne, R. Influence of patient perceptions and preferences for osteoporosis medication on adherence behavior in the Denosumab Adherence Preference Satisfaction study. *Menopause* **2014**, *21*, 25–32. [CrossRef] [PubMed]
33. Muratore, M.; Quarta, E.; Quarta, L. Intramuscular neridronate in patients with rheumatoid arthritis using corticosteroids: Evaluation of treatment adherence in a randomized, open-label comparison with other bisphosphonates. *Acta Biomed.* **2013**, *84*, 23–29. [PubMed]
34. Palacios, S.; Agodoa, I.; Bonnick, S.; Bergh, J.P.V.D.; Ferreira, I.; Ho, P.-R.; Brown, J.P. Treatment Satisfaction in Postmenopausal Women Suboptimally Adherent to Bisphosphonates Who Transitioned to Denosumab Compared With Risedronate or Ibandronate. *J. Clin. Endocrinol. Metab.* **2015**, *100*, E487–E492. [CrossRef] [PubMed]
35. Roh, Y.H.; Noh, J.H.; Gong, H.S.; Baek, G.H. Comparative adherence to weekly oral and quarterly intravenous bisphosphonates among patients with limited heath literacy who sustained distal radius fractures. *J. Bone Miner. Metab.* **2017**, *36*, 589–595. [CrossRef] [PubMed]
36. Tamechika, S.-Y.; Sasaki, K.; Hayami, Y.; Ohmura, S.-I.; Maeda, S.; Iwagaitsu, S.; Naniwa, T. Patient satisfaction and efficacy of switching from weekly bisphosphonates to monthly minodronate for treatment and prevention of glucocorticoid-induced osteoporosis in Japanese patients with systemic rheumatic diseases: A randomized, clinical trial. *Arch. Osteoporos.* **2018**, *13*, 67. [CrossRef]
37. Papaioannou, A.; Morin, S.; Cheung, A.M.; Atkinson, S.; Brown, J.P.; Feldman, S.; Hanley, D.A.; Hodsman, A.; Jamal, S.A.; Kaiser, S.M.; et al. 2010 clinical practice guidelines for the diagnosis and management of osteoporosis in Canada: Summary. *Can. Med. Assoc. J.* **2010**, *182*, 1864–1873. [CrossRef]
38. Briesacher, B.A.; Andrade, S.E.; Fouayzi, H.; Chan, K.A. Comparison of Drug Adherence Rates Among Patients with Seven Different Medical Conditions. *Pharmacother. J. Hum. Pharmacol. Drug Ther.* **2008**, *28*, 437–443. [CrossRef]
39. Adami, S.; Bertoldo, F.; Gatti, D.; Minisola, G.; Rossini, M.; Sinigaglia, L.; Varenna, M. FRI0302 Analysis of the Defra Algorithm for Definition of Risk Fracture. *Ann. Rheum. Dis.* **2015**, *74*, 533–534. [CrossRef]
40. Mirand, A.L.; Beehler, G.P.; Kuo, C.L.; Mahoney, M.C. Explaining the de-prioritization of primary prevention: Physicians' perceptions of their role in the delivery of primary care. *BMC Public Health* **2003**, *3*, 15. [CrossRef]
41. Leblanc, A.; Wang, A.T.; Wyatt, K.; Branda, M.E.; Shah, N.D.; Van Houten, H.; Pencille, L.; Wermers, R.; Montori, V.M. Encounter Decision Aid vs. Clinical Decision Support or Usual Care to Support Patient-Centered Treatment Decisions in Osteoporosis: The Osteoporosis Choice Randomized Trial II. *PLoS ONE* **2015**, *10*, e0128063. [CrossRef]
42. Smallwood, A.J.; Schapira, M.M.; Fedders, M.; Neuner, J.M. A pilot randomized controlled trial of a decision aid with tailored fracture risk tool delivered via a patient portal. *Osteoporos. Int.* **2016**, *28*, 567–576. [CrossRef] [PubMed]
43. Cornelissen, D.; de Kunder, S.; Si, L.; Reginster, J.-Y.; Evers, S.; Boonen, A.; Hiligsmann, M.; European Society for Clinical and Economic Aspect of Osteoporosis, Osteoarthritis and Musculoskeletal Diseases (ESCEO). Interventions to improve adherence to anti-osteoporosis medications: An updated systematic review. *Osteoporos. Int.* **2020**, *31*, 1645–1669. [CrossRef] [PubMed]
44. Majumdar, S.R.; Johnson, J.A.; Bellerose, D.; McAlister, F.A.; Russell, A.S.; Hanley, D.A.; Garg, S.; Lier, D.A.; Maksymowych, W.P.; Morrish, D.W.; et al. Nurse case-manager vs multifaceted intervention to improve quality of osteoporosis care after wrist fracture: Randomized controlled pilot study. *Osteoporos. Int.* **2010**, *22*, 223–230. [CrossRef] [PubMed]

Disclaimer/Publisher's Note: The statements, opinions and data contained in all publications are solely those of the individual author(s) and contributor(s) and not of MDPI and/or the editor(s). MDPI and/or the editor(s) disclaim responsibility for any injury to people or property resulting from any ideas, methods, instructions or products referred to in the content.

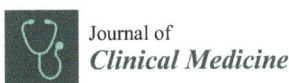

Article

Short and Middle Functional Outcome in the Static vs. Dynamic Fixation of Syndesmotic Injuries in Ankle Fractures: A Retrospective Case Series Study

Vito Pavone [1], Giacomo Papotto [2], Andrea Vescio [1], Gianfranco Longo [2], Salvatore D'Amato [1], Marco Ganci [2], Emanuele Marchese [1] and Gianluca Testa [1,*]

[1] Department of General Surgery and Medical-Surgical Specialties, Section of Orthopaedics and Traumatology, A.O.U. Policlinico Rodolico—San Marco, University of Catania, 95123 Catania, Italy; vitopavone@hotmail.com (V.P.)
[2] Department of Orthopedic Surgery, Trauma Center, Cannizzaro Hospital, 95100 Catania, Italy
* Correspondence: gianpavel@hotmail.com

Abstract: Background: Syndesmotic injuries are common lesions associated with ankle fractures. Static and dynamic fixation are frequently used in syndesmotic injury-associated ankle fractures. The purpose of this study is to compare short- and mid-term quality of life, clinical outcomes, and gait after static stabilization with a trans-syndesmotic screw or dynamic stabilization with a suture button device. Methods: Here, 230 patients were enrolled in a retrospective observational study. They were divided in two groups according to the fixation procedure (Arthrex TightRope®, Munich, Germany) synthesis vs. osteosynthesis with a 3.5 mm trans-syndesmotic tricortical screw). They then underwent clinical assessment using the American Foot and Ankle Score (AOFAS) at 1, 2, 6, 12, and 24 months after surgery. Quality of life was assessed according to the EuroQol-5 Dimension (EQ-5D) at 2 and 24 months after surgery in the follow-up; gait analysis was performed 2 and 24 months postoperatively. Results: Significant differences were found at a two-month follow-up according to the AOFAS ($p = 0.0001$) and EQ-5D ($p = 0.0208$) scores. No differences were noted in the other follow-ups ($p > 0.05$) or gait analysis. Conclusion: The dynamic and static fixation of syndesmotic injuries in ankle fracture are both efficacious and valid procedures for avoiding ankle instability. The suture button device was comparable to the screw fixation according to functional outcomes and gait analysis.

Keywords: ankle fractures; syndesmotic injury; dynamic fixation; trans-syndesmotic screw

Citation: Pavone, V.; Papotto, G.; Vescio, A.; Longo, G.; D'Amato, S.; Ganci, M.; Marchese, E.; Testa, G. Short and Middle Functional Outcome in the Static vs. Dynamic Fixation of Syndesmotic Injuries in Ankle Fractures: A Retrospective Case Series Study. *J. Clin. Med.* **2023**, *12*, 3637. https://doi.org/10.3390/jcm12113637

Academic Editor: Paul Alfred Grützner

Received: 7 March 2023
Revised: 16 May 2023
Accepted: 22 May 2023
Published: 24 May 2023

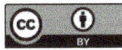

Copyright: © 2023 by the authors. Licensee MDPI, Basel, Switzerland. This article is an open access article distributed under the terms and conditions of the Creative Commons Attribution (CC BY) license (https:// creativecommons.org/licenses/by/ 4.0/).

1. Introduction

Ankle fractures are one of the most common injuries and often require surgical treatment to restore the anatomic congruity of the ankle mortise to provide stable load transmission and to ease rehabilitation [1–4]. In ankle fractures, syndesmotic injury occurs in approximately 50% of type Weber B and in all type Weber C fractures [5]. Thus, there are two common situations in which the syndesmosis is compromised according to the Lauge–Hansen classification: pronation external rotation (PER) fractures and supination external rotation fractures (SER) [5].

Syndesmosis injury could result in syndesmosis instability due to an SER fracture mechanism according to Stark and colleagues. Their study found that 39% of SER fractures with deltoid ligament rupture showed diastasis on stress testing [6]. Syndesmotic injuries can also be seen in 13% to 20% of ankle fracture patterns [7], Maisonneuve fracture [8,9], and posterior malleolar fractures [10]. Isolated syndesmosis injuries are common in the competitive athletic population [11,12]. The metallic trans-syndesmotic screw has been the gold standard for stabilizing unstable syndesmosis [13–15]. More recently, dynamic fixation such as the suture button device, especially the suture button device, has been reported with some potential advantages, including allowing physiological movement while retaining the required reduction. Flexible fixation also offers less risk of implant removal and recurrent syndesmotic diastasis as well as earlier rehabilitation [16–18].

Biomechanical investigations have demonstrated that the strength of the suture button device is comparable to that of a tricortical 3.5 mm syndesmotic screw [19,20]. However, the international literature has only a few high-quality studies that assess the quality of life and gait after syndesmosis fixation. Doll et al. [21] proposed a study protocol to assess the differences in gait analysis and clinical outcome after suture button device or screw fixation in acute syndesmosis rupture, but the trials have not yet been published. A pedobarographic analysis supports the nonsuperiority of a device when compared to the other tools [22,23]. The purpose of our study is to compare the short- and mid-term quality of life, clinical outcomes, and gait after static stabilization with a trans-syndesmotic screw or dynamic stabilization with a suture button fixation device (Arthrex TightRope®). It has been hypothesized that dynamic stabilization could thus reduce recovery time due to the removal surgery in trans-syndesmotic screws but not the patient's quality of life.

2. Materials and Methods
2.1. Demographic Data

Of the 312 patients in our study, 26.4% were lost to follow up. There are no differences between these patients and the remaining cohort. Thus, 230 patients with syndesmosis injury associated with bimalleolar and Maisonneuve fractures were treated and analyzed from December 2015 to December 2019 (Figure 1). The exclusion criteria were pediatric ankle fractures, isolated syndesmosis injuries, tibial plafond fractures, Weber type A fractures, trimalleolar fractures, open fractures, and pathological ankle fractures. Our cohort was aged 40.8 ± 13.2 years (range 18–63); 140 patients (60.9%) were male and 90 patients (39.1%) were female. In 129 patients (56.5% of cases), the right side was affected, and 101 patients (43.5%) had a left-side injury. The BMI average was 23.8 ± 4.7 (Table 1).

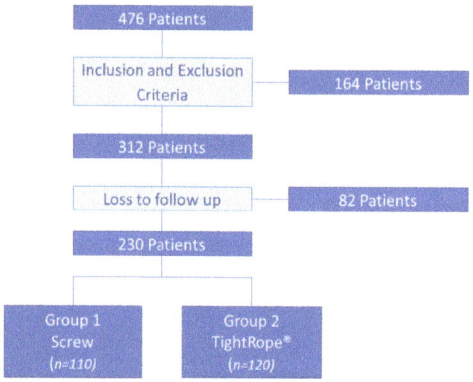

Figure 1. Study flowchart.

Table 1. Patient characteristics and baseline.

Characteristics	Group 1—Trans-Syndesmotic Screw (n = 110)	Group 2—TightRope (n = 120)	p-Value
Age (years)	41.2 ± 14.56	35.68 ± 11.57	0.34433
Gender (Male/Female)	64/46	76/44	0.66
Side (Left/Right)	44/66	57/63	0.08537
Weber (B/C)	57/53	62/58	0.74
Average BMI	24.2 ± 4.6	23.9 ± 4.6	0.72

2.2. Classification Systems

Danis–Weber classification divides fractures into three groups considering the peroneal fracture with respect to syndesmosis. In type A, the peroneal malleolus fracture is below the syndesmotic level and is due to SA. In type B, the fracture is at the syndesmosis and is due to SER or PA. The malleolar fracture is above the syndesmosis in type C and is due to PER [24]. According to Denis–Weber classification, 119 patients (51.7%) were type B, and 111 patients (48.3%) were type C.

2.3. Surgical Techniques

All of our patients were treated for lateral malleolus fixation with a 1/3 tubular plate with 3.5 mm screws as well as an interfragmentary screw. The tibial malleolus was synthesized with two 3.5 mm half-thread cannulated screws. In Weber B with small medial fragments, the synthesis was performed with two 2.5 mm half-thread cannulated screws. The syndesmosis was stabilized in all Weber type C (PER) cases. In the Weber type B (SER) fractures, the syndesmosis was synthesized after performing lateral and medial malleoli osteosynthesis and stress tests such as the Hook Test and the Cotton Test with positive results. The result was considered positive when there were 2 mm of diastasis of the syndesmosis during the stress tests assessed intraoperatively under fluoroscopy.

The syndesmosis was synthesized in GROUP 1 with a 3.5 mm trans-syndesmotic tricortical screw through the hole of the fibula's plate; the screw was removed after 45 days via outpatient surgical treatment. No weight-bearing was allowed until the screw removal. In GROUP 2, the syndesmosis was stabilized with a dynamic Tight-Rope synthesis without using a force calibrator. A cast immobilization was packed for 15 days post-operatively to facilitate the healing of the soft tissues. The two cohorts underwent the same post-operative protocol. The surgeries were performed by a four-surgeons team experienced in ankle trauma.

2.4. Outcomes Evaluation

Follow-ups were performed at 1, 2, 6, 12, and 24 months after the surgical treatment. At each follow-up, patients were studied with standard X-ray radiograms with antero-posterior, lateral, and Mortise views; they also underwent physical and clinical examinations using the American Foot and Ankle Score (AOFAS). Gait analysis was performed with the Oxford Foot Model (OFM) [25] that used multi-segment kinematics. A 12-camera VICON 612 system (Vicon Motion Systems Ltd., Oxford, UK) was used to collect the 3D kinematics of one foot as well as both lower limbs of each subject at 100 Hz. A static standing trial was performed to define the segment axes before three markers were removed for the walking trials. Subjects were asked to walk at their usual speed along a 10 m walkway. These trials were identified visually by looking at all traces from the session (average 20 trials). The following motions were determined: the hindfoot relative to the tibia (Hindfoot/Tibia), the forefoot relative to the hindfoot (Forefoot/Hindfoot), and the forefoot relative to the tibia (Forefoot/Tibia) [26]. Gait analysis was performed at 2 and 24 months after the surgery for GROUP 1 and GROUP 2.

The evaluation of the clinical and psychological conditions of the patients used the EuroQol-5 Dimension (EQ-5D) that was created as a generic measurement instrument for measuring the quality of life and its ease of use in self-administration. The EQ-5D consists of two separate sections: In the first one, there is a subjective assessment of five dimensions (mobility, self-care, daily activities, pain/anxiety, and anxiety/depression). Every item provides the possibility to choose a level of severity. Each item ranges from 1 to 3. Level 1 represents no problem, while level 3 indicates extreme limitations. The aggregation of answers forms a five-digit number, which represents the state of health of the respondent. The three levels of response for each of the five items offer a maximum of 243 possible descriptions of the health status and allow one to highlight the presence/absence of possible problems and their intensity. Finally, an algorithm can calculate a synthetic score (EQ-5D Index) of the perceived health status. The implementation of this algorithm provides that each dimension of the health status is associated with a specific weight, as calculated for the general population using techniques from cost-utility analyses [27]. The EuroQol-5 Dimension (EQ-5D) was performed at 2 and 24 months for every patient of GROUP 1 and GROUP 2. Clinical assessment data were electronically collected by the same authors (A.V. and S.D.A.).

2.5. Statistical Analysis

Continuous data are presented as the mean and standard deviation, as appropriate. The analysis of variance test and Tukey–Kramer method were used to compare the AOFAS, EQ-5D, and gait analysis parameters. The selected threshold for significance was $p < 0.05$. The estimated sample size for this study was obtained using the Bernoulli model with a z-score = 95%. All statistical analyses were performed using the 2016 GraphPad Software (GraphPad Inc., San Diego, CA, USA).

3. Results

The syndesmosis injuries were treated according to two different devices: one group was treated with a tricortical trans-syndesmotic screw (GROUP 1); the other group was treated with suture button fixation, TightRope (GROUP 2). The demographic characteristics of the sample are reported in Table 1. According to the demographics, no statistical differences were found between the cohorts ($p > 0.05$).

At a one-month follow-up, the Group 1 mean AOFAS score was 50.7 ± 6.4, while the corresponding Group 2 mean score was 51.7 ± 6.3 ($p > 0.05$). At two months, the average AOFAS score of Group 1 was 59.5 ± 11.01, while that of Group 2 was 66.7 ± 11.8 ($p = 0.0001$). At 24 months, the average AOFAS score of Group 1 was 94 ± 2.4, and that of Group 2 was 94.7 ± 1.5 (Table 2). The difference in mean EQ-5D scores was found to be significant at 2 months of follow-up; these scores were similar at 24 months of follow-up (Table 2).

Table 2. Group results according the AOFAS and EQ-5D scores.

	Trans-Syndesmotic Screw Group 1	Suture Button Device Group 2	*p*-Value
AOFAS 4 Weeks	50.7 ± 6.42	51.71 ± 6.30	0.9997
AOFAS 2 Months	59.5 ± 11.01	66.73 ± 11.76	0.0001
AOFAS 6 Months	84.6 ± 8.93	87.92 ± 8.38	0.4936
AOFAS 12 Months	89.1 ± 7.01	93.08 ± 5.06	0.2318
AOFAS 24 Months	94.0 ± 2.39	94.69 ± 1.46	1.00
EQ-5D 2 Months	0.0 ± 0.44	0.18 ± 0.41	0.0208
EQ-5D 24 Months	0.8 ± 0.06	0.87 ± 0.04	0.6701

At a two-month follow-up, significant differences were found for the following parameters: hindfoot/tibia dorsiflexion ($p = 0.03$), forefoot/tibia supination ($p = 0.03$), and forefoot/tibia adduction ($p = 0.03$). No other significant differences were found according to the gait analysis parameters ($p > 0.05$) at the two-month and 24-month follow-up (Tables 3 and 4).

In total, we reported 18 complications: 13 with wound dehiscence with superficial infection and 5 with wound necrosis. In the case of superficial infection, a second operation was performed with surgical wound debridement, biopsy samples, and targeted antibiotic therapy. In the second case, outpatient debridement and the placement of vacuum-assisted continuous-therapy (VAC-therapy) was performed (Table 5).

Table 3. Gait analysis results at two months.

	Trans-Syndesmotic Screw Group 1	Suture Button Device Group 2	*p*-Value
hindfoot/tibia inversion	3.2 ± 2.8	4.1 ± 1.6	0.0562
hindfoot/tibia dorsiflexion	6.2 ± 2.4	7.4 ± 2.9	0.0296
hindfoot/tibia rotation	10.6 ± 2.2	11.3 ± 2.9	0.1860
forefoot/hindfoot supination	10.4 ± 3.3	11.5 ± 2.4	0.0649
forefoot/hindfoot dorsiflexion	23.3 ± 4.1	24.2 ± 4.6	0.3142
forefoot/hindfoot adduction	7.8 ± 3.1	9.4 ± 4.8	0.0721
forefoot/tibia supination	7.2 ± 3.3	8.5 ± 2.4	0.0297
forefoot/tibia dorsiflexion	11.6 ± 3.1	11.8 ± 3.3	0.7603
forefoot/tibia adduction	8.8 ± 3.1	10.2 ± 3.2	0.0320

Table 4. Gait analysis results at 24 months.

	Trans-Syndesmotic Screw Group 1	Suture Button Device Group 2	*p*-Value
hindfoot/tibia inversion	4.9 ± 1.8	4.7 ± 1.6	1.00
hindfoot/tibia dorsiflexion	7.7 ± 3.0	8.2 ± 2.9	0.9998
hindfoot/tibia rotation	11.1 ± 4.2	12.0 ± 2.9	0.9847
forefoot/hindfoot supination	10.7 ± 4.3	12.7 ± 3.4	0.3039
forefoot/hindfoot dorsiflexion	24.3 ± 7.1	26.3 ± 5.6	0.3039
forefoot/hindfoot adduction	10.2 ± 4.7	10.7 ± 3.8	0.9965
forefoot/tibia supination	7.8 ± 2.3	9.1 ± 3.4	0.5786
forefoot/tibia dorsiflexion	13.6 ± 2.1	12.8 ± 2.3	0.9462
forefoot/tibia adduction	10.8 ± 3.6	11.2 ± 4.2	0.9992

Table 5. Postoperative complications.

	Trans-Syndesmotic Screw Group 1	Suture Button Device Group 2
wound necrosis	3	2
superficial infections	5	8

4. Discussion

Suture button device-treated patients at 2 months of follow-up had a faster recovery and higher foot dorsiflexion and forefoot supination and adduction than the trans-syndesmotic screw fixation cohort. The faster recovery in dynamic fixation was associated with a higher quality of life two months after the surgery. The procedures' functional outcomes were comparable six months after surgery. Syndesmotic lesions are widespread clinical conditions and can occur with concomitant ankle fractures or without fractures; however, the latter is extremely rare [28,29].

The treatment of the syndesmotic complex injury is necessary to avoid chronic instability [30]. Although the current gold standard for the treatment of syndesmotic lesions is the fixation of the syndesmotic screw, the use of the suture button technique has aroused interest and has increased rapidly over the last decade [31]. There is a strong debate in the literature about the screw placement and whether and when to remove it. Screw abandonment causes it to rupture because of the physiological movements of the syndesmosis between the tibia and fibula, although a low percentage of patients have experienced syndesmotic malreductions after it breaks. There are no absolute indications in the literature on the timing of trans-syndesmotic screw removal. Early removal of the syndesmotic screw before ligament healing can lead to instability and diastasis of the syndesmosis as well as an increase in complications related to the second surgery such as infection. This, in turn, could increase the recovery time and pain while harming the psychological state of the patients [32–35]. The use of a dynamic fixation such as a suture button device allows for physiological movements, and it does not require further intervention for its removal. In our study, a better functional outcome was recorded at two months of follow-up; in fact, the average AOFAS score of Group 1 was 59.5 ± 11.01, while that of Group 2 was 66.7 ± 11.8

(p = 0.0001). The weight bearing ban in patients treated with a tricortical screw has been assumed as the principal reason for the data. Moreover, the second surgery need for the screw removal could partially delay the physical recovery and provide a negative effect directly on the gait and indirectly on the quality of life.

Lubberts et al. [35] performed cadaver biomechanical studies and argued that the stabilization of the syndesmosis with a suture button device seems to stabilize the coronal plane but not the movement in the sagittal plane. This outcome can be explained considering that the suture button device is placed in dynamic compressions on the coronal plane, but the construct is installed through perforated channels that far exceed the diameter of the sutures of the suture button device [35]. This facilitates a considerable residual sagittal instability because of the persistence of diameter differences. LaMothe et al. [36] assessed fibular motion in a cadaveric model after fixation with a tetra-cortical 4.0 mm screw or a single suture-button construct using fluoroscopy, as validated by a four-camera motion-capture system. They found that the screw or suture-button fixations could constrain coronal plane fibular motion in response to an external rotation stress test. In contrast, Ebramzadeh et al. [37] and Forsythe et al. [38] observed that a single suture button construct could maintain syndesmotic stability in the coronal plane. Adding to these discrepancies, Soin et al. found that two suture button constructs provided similar syndesmotic stability in the coronal and sagittal planes compared to a single tetra-cortical syndesmotic screw, but neither restored native motion [39]. Teramoto et al. [36] found that one or two suture button constructs were not able to restore stability in both the coronal and sagittal planes compared to the intact syndesmosis or fixation with a tetra-cortical syndesmotic screw.

In our series, the ankle stability was intraoperatively clinically assessed, and malreductions or instabilities were recorded. At the same time, no further radiological or tomographic evaluations were performed; the literature includes studies of screw syndesmosis fixation using bilateral CT to evaluate the reduction in the syndesmosis. These studies have reported malreduction rates of 15–44% in 1.5–8.4 years of follow-up [40–42]. Most studies evaluating suture button device fixation for unstable syndesmosis reported malreduction rates of 0% but used only simple radiography to assess malreduction [17,43–48]. Only the study by Treon et al. [49] reported a syndesmotic malreduction rate of 11% when a suture button device was used. Naqvi et al. [47] compared the trans-syndesmotic screw and suture button device fixation with CT scans of both ankles to assess the reduction in the syndesmosis and found no malreduction with suture button device fixation in 23 patients after a follow-up of at least 18 months. Anand et al. published a multicenter case series consisting of 36 patients. They demonstrated that the ankle suture button device maintained satisfactory reduction in the ankle mortise in 97% of cases, with a mean follow-up of 14 months [50]. Sagi and colleagues [42] used CT and clinical follow-up at a minimum of two years from fracture fixation. They showed that this strategy produces significant improvements in terms of reducing syndesmosis. In conflict with this evidence, a recent study reported questionable advantages in assessing the quality of distal tibial-fibula joint reduction when a suture-button system is used due to a considerable rate of false-negatives [51].

The dynamic nature of the push-button suture device could theoretically allow for a certain degree of physiological micro-mobility of the syndesmosis, leading to an earlier return, full weight bearing, and a better objective range of motion measurements. Screw fixation does not allow for normal movement of the syndesmosis during healing; if stabilization is not achieved or if the load is early, the screw breaks or the implant is mobilized. Thornes et al. [47] noted that patients in the suture button group were maintained without weight bearing for a significantly shorter mean time than patients in the syndesmotic screw group (4.1 weeks versus 6.3 weeks, p = 0.01), with no patient in the suture button group requiring implant removal. Degroot et al. [45] reported an average lift time at full load of 5.7 weeks with TightRope, with no signs of implant failure or residual displacement in a follow-up of 20 months. Cottom et al. and Thornes et al. demonstrated that full and fast loading could lead to accelerated rehabilitation [52,53]. Interestingly, some included studies reported that patients in the dynamic fixation group appeared to have less pain and discomfort, which may also contribute to faster, full weight bearing [54–56]. It could be assumed that a faster recovery could improve the quality of life in ankle fracture patients treated with dynamic fixation. The functional limitation due to physical therapy interruption and the additional surgery in trans-syndesmotic screw patients could cause a negative interpretation of their clinical condition and backsliding during physical rehabilitation. To the best knowledge of the authors, no previous study aimed to assess the comparison between the two procedures according to the gait analysis performed. In 2020, Doll et al. [21] proposed a study protocol for a prospective randomized pilot study with the purpose of comparing the monitor ankle range of motion and maximum ankle power in gait as functional outcome parameters of instrumented gait analysis, as well as the clinical and radiographic outcome for assessing the stabilization of acute syndesmosis rupture. We strongly encourage the participation of these kinds of trials and study groups. The study accounts for different limits: the small sample size is the principal. Nodal irritation or secondary extension and radiologically visible osteolysis are the principal complications of suture button devices; due to the reduced number of participants, the study was not able to demonstrate this problem. Despite ankle fractures being common injuries and the fact that several trials are available, in our study, the midterm follow-up and the recurrent functional assessment in addition to gait analysis reduced the higher recruitment possibility. At the same time, the retrospective nature of the review could limit the proper evaluation. Prospective randomized clinical trials are strongly encouraged. The strengths of the study are the quality-of-life evaluation and gait analysis; both typologies of syndesmosis fixation are not common for this kind of lesion, and rarely were the measurements reported in the same trial. Moreover, our findings could help the surgeons and patients make an appropriate choice.

5. Conclusions

The dynamic and static fixation of syndesmotic injuries in ankle fracture are both efficacious and valid procedures for avoiding ankle instability. The suture button device was comparable to the screw fixation according to functional outcomes and gait analysis.

Author Contributions: Conceptualization, G.P.; methodology, G.T.; software, S.D.; validation, G.L.; formal analysis, A.V.; investigation, M.G.; resources, A.V.; data curation, G.P.; writing—original draft preparation, G.P.; writing—review and editing, G.T.; visualization, E.M.; supervision, G.L.; project administration, G.T.; funding acquisition, V.P. All authors have read and agreed to the published version of the manuscript.

Funding: This research received no external funding.

Institutional Review Board Statement: Ethical review and approval were waived for this study due to the retrospective nature.

Informed Consent Statement: Informed consent was obtained from all subjects involved in the study. Written informed consent has been obtained from the patients to publish this paper.

Data Availability Statement: The data presented in this study are available in text and in tables.

Conflicts of Interest: The authors declare no conflict of interest.

References

1. Zwieten, K.J.; Narain, F.; Munter, S.; Kosten, L.; Lamur, K.; Schmidt, K.; Lippens, P.; Zubova, I.; Piskùn, O.; Varzin, S. Analyzing pace frequencies in bipedal primates and primate "predecessors" reveals mechanisms that regulate foot inversion and thus ensure foot stability at touchdown. *UDK* **2015**, *10*, 820–822. [CrossRef]
2. Lobo, C.C.; Morales, C.R.; Sanz, D.R.; Corbalán, I.S.; Marín, A.G.; López, D.L. Ultrasonography Comparison of Peroneus Muscle Cross-sectional Area in Subjects with or Without Lateral Ankle Sprains. *J. Manip. Physiol. Ther.* **2016**, *39*, 635–644. [CrossRef] [PubMed]
3. Romero-Morales, C.; López-López, S.; Bravo-Aguilar, M.; Cerezo-Téllez, E.; Benito-de Pedro, M.; López López, D.; Lobo, C.C. Ultrasonography Comparison of the Plantar Fascia and Tibialis Anterior in People with and Without Lateral Ankle Sprain: A Case-Control Study. *J. Manip. Physiol. Ther.* **2020**, *43*, 799–805. [CrossRef] [PubMed]

4. Kazemi, K.; Arab, A.M.; Abdollahi, I.; López-López, D.; Calvo-Lobo, C. Electromiography comparison of distal and proximal lower limb muscle activity patterns during external perturbation in subjects with and without functional ankle instability. *Hum. Mov. Sci.* **2017**, *55*, 211–220. [CrossRef] [PubMed]
5. Hopkinson, W.J.; St Pierre, P.; Ryan, J.B.; Wheeler, J.H. Syndesmosis sprains of the ankle. *Foot Ankle* **1990**, *10*, 325–330. [CrossRef]
6. Andersen, M.R.; Frihagen, F.; Hellund, J.C.; Madsen, J.E.; Figved, W. Randomized trial comparing suture button with single syndesmotic screw for syndesmosis injury. *J. Bone Jt. Surg. Am.* **2018**, *100*, 2–12. [CrossRef]
7. Solan, M.C.; Davies, M.S.; Sakellariou, A. Syndesmosis Stabilisation: Screws Versus Flexible Fixation. *Foot Ankle Clin.* **2017**, *22*, 35–63. [CrossRef]
8. Pankovich, A.M. Maisonneuve fracture of the fibula. *J. Bone Joint Surg. Am.* **1976**, *58*, 337–342. [CrossRef]
9. Maisonneuve, J. Recherches sur la fracture du perone. *Arch. Gen. Med.* **1840**, *7*, 165.
10. Mason, L.W.; Marlow, W.J.; Widnall, J.; Molloy, A.P. Pathoanatomy and Associated Injuries of Posterior Malleolus Fracture of the Ankle. *Foot Ankle Int.* **2017**, *38*, 1229–1235. [CrossRef]
11. Mauntel, T.C.; Wikstrom, E.A.; Roos, K.G.; Djoko, A.; Dompier, T.P.; Kerr, Z.Y. The Epidemiology of High Ankle Sprains in National Collegiate Athletic Association Sports. *Am. J. Sports Med.* **2017**, *45*, 2156–2163. [CrossRef] [PubMed]
12. Mulcahey, M.K.; Bernhardson, A.S.; Murphy, C.P.; Chang, A.; Zajac, T.; Sanchez, G.; Sanchez, A.; Whalen, J.M.; Price, M.D.; Clanton, T.O.; et al. The Epidemiology of Ankle Injuries Identified at the National Football League Combine, 2009–2015. *Orthop. J. Sports Med.* **2018**, *6*, 2325967118786227. [CrossRef] [PubMed]
13. Van den Bekerom, M.P.; Raven, E.E. Current concepts review: Operative techniques for stabilizing the distal tibiofibular syndesmosis. *Foot Ankle Int.* **2007**, *28*, 1302–1308. [CrossRef]
14. Schepers, T. Acute distal tibiofibular syndesmosis injury: A systematic review of suture-button versus syndesmotic screw repair. *Int. Orthop.* **2012**, *36*, 1199–1206. [CrossRef]
15. Van Heest, T.J.; Lafferty, P.M. Injuries to the ankle syndesmosis. *J. Bone Joint Surg. Am.* **2014**, *96*, 603–613. [CrossRef]
16. Kortekangas, T.; Savola, O.; Flinkkilä, T.; Lepojärvi, S.; Nortunen, S.; Ohtonen, P.; Katisko, J.; Pakarinen, H. A prospective randomised study comparing TightRope and syndesmotic screw fixation for accuracy and maintenance of syndesmotic reduction assessed with bilateral computed tomography. *Injury* **2015**, *46*, 1119–1126. [CrossRef]
17. Laflamme, M.; Belzile, E.L.; Bedard, L.; van den Bekerom, M.P.; Glazebrook, M.; Pelet, S. A prospective randomized multicenter trial comparing clinical outcomes of patients treated surgically with a static or dynamic implant for acute ankle syndesmosis rupture. *J. Orthop. Trauma* **2015**, *29*, 216–223. [CrossRef]
18. Xu, G.; Chen, W.; Zhang, Q.; Wang, J.; Su, Y.; Zhang, Y. Flexible fixation of syndesmotic diastasis using the assembled bolt-tightrope system. *Scand. J. Trauma Res. Emerg. Med.* **2013**, *21*, 71.
19. Soin, S.P.; Knight, T.A.; Dinah, A.F.; Mears, S.C.; Swierstra, B.A.; Belkoff, S.M. Suturebutton versus screw fixation in a syndesmosis rupture model: A biomechanical comparison. *Foot Ankle Int.* **2009**, *30*, 346–352. [CrossRef]
20. Klitzman, R.; Zhao, H.; Zhang, L.Q.; Strohmeyer, G.; Vora, A. Suture-button versus screw fixation of the syndesmosis: A biomechanical analysis. *Foot Ankle Int.* **2010**, *31*, 69–75. [CrossRef]
21. Doll, J.; Waizenegger, S.; Bruckner, T.; Schmidmaier, G.; Wolf, S.I.; Fischer, C. Differences in gait analysis and clinical outcome after TightRope®or screw fixation in acute syndesmosis rupture: Study protocol for a prospective randomized pilot study. *Trials* **2020**, *21*, 606. [CrossRef] [PubMed]
22. Taskesen, A.; Okkaoglu, M.C.; Demirkale, I.; Haberal, B.; Yaradilmis, U.; Altay, M. Dynamic and Stabilometric Analysis After Syndesmosis Injuries. *J. Am. Podiatr. Med. Assoc.* **2020**, *110*, 9. [CrossRef] [PubMed]
23. Lauge-Hansen, N. Ligamentous ankle fractures; diagnosis and treatment. *Acta Chir. Scand.* **1949**, *97*, 544–550. [PubMed]
24. Fonseca, L.L.D.; Nunes, I.G.; Nogueira, R.R.; Martins, G.E.V.; Mesencio, A.C.; Kobata, S.I. Reproducibility of the Lauge-Hansen, Danis-Weber, and AO classifications for ankle fractures. *Rev. Bras. Ortop.* **2018**, *53*, 101–106. [CrossRef]
25. Stebbins, J.; Harrington, M.; Thompson, N.; Zavatsky, A.; Theologis, T. Repeatability of a model for measuring multisegment foot kinematics in children. *Gait Posture* **2006**, *23*, 401–410. [CrossRef]
26. Stebbins, J.; Harrington, M.; Thompson, N.; Zavatsky, A.; Theologis, T. Gait compensations caused by foot deformity in cerebral palsy. *Gait Posture* **2010**, *32*, 226–230. [CrossRef]
27. Balestroni, G.; Bertolotti, G. L'EuroQol-5D (EQ-5D), uno strumento per la misura della qualità della vita [EuroQol-5D (EQ-5D), an instrument for measuring quality of life]. *Monaldi Arch. Chest. Dis.* **2012**, *78*, 155–159.
28. Valkering, K.P.; Vergroesen, D.A.; Nolte, P.A. Isolated syndesmosis ankle injury. *Orthopedics* **2012**, *35*, e1705–e1710. [CrossRef]
29. Pakarinen, H. Stability-based classification for ankle fracture management and the syndesmosis injury in ankle fractures due to a supination external rotation mechanism of injury. *Acta Orthop.* **2012**, *83*, 1–31. [CrossRef] [PubMed]
30. Hunt, K.J. Syndesmosis injuries. *Curr. Rev. Musculoskelet Med.* **2013**, *6*, 304–312. [CrossRef]
31. Akoh, C.C.; Phisitkul, P. Anatomic Ligament Repairs of Syndesmotic Injuries. *Orthop. Clin. N. Am.* **2019**, *50*, 401–414. [CrossRef]
32. Andersen, M.R.; Frihagen, F.; Madsen, J.E.; Figved, W. High complication rate after syndesmotic screw removal. *Injury* **2015**, *46*, 2283–2387. [CrossRef] [PubMed]
33. Lalli, T.A.; Matthews, L.J.; Hanselman, A.E.; Hubbard, D.F.; Bramer, M.A.; Santrock, R.D. Economic impact of syndesmosis hardware removal. *Foot* **2015**, *25*, 131–133. [CrossRef]
34. Hsu, Y.T.; Wu, C.C.; Lee, W.C.; Fan, K.F.; Tseng, I.C.; Lee, P.C. Surgical treatment of syndesmotic diastasis, emphasis on effect of syndesmotic screw on ankle function. *Int. Orthop.* **2011**, *35*, 359–364. [CrossRef]

35. Schepers, T.; Van Lieshout, E.M.; de Vries, M.R.; Van der Elst, M. Complications of syndesmotic screw removal. *Foot Ankle Int.* **2011**, *32*, 1040–1044. [CrossRef]
36. Kostuj, T.; Stief, F.; Hartmann, K.A.; Schaper, K.; Arabmotlagh, M.; Baums, M.H.; Meurer, A.; Krummenauer, F.; Lieske, S. Using the Oxford Foot Model to determine the association between objective measures of foot function and results of the AOFAS Ankle-Hindfoot Scale and the Foot Function Index, a prospective gait analysis study in Germany. *BMJ Open* **2018**, *8*, e019872. [CrossRef]
37. LaMothe, J.M.; Baxter, J.R.; Murphy, C.; Gilbert, S.; DeSandis, B.; Drakos, M.C. Three-Dimensional Analysis of Fibular Motion After Fixation of Syndesmotic Injuries With a Screw or Suture-Button Construct. *Foot Ankle Int.* **2016**, *37*, 1350–1356. [CrossRef]
38. Ebramzadeh, E.; Knutsen, A.R.; Sangiorgio, S.N.; Brambila, M.; Harris, T.G. Biomechanical comparison of syndesmotic injury fixation methods using a cadaveric model. *Foot Ankle Int.* **2013**, *34*, 1710–1717. [CrossRef]
39. Forsythe, K.; Freedman, K.B.; Stover, M.D.; Patwardhan, A.G. Comparison of a novel FiberWire-button construct versus metallic screw fixation in a syndesmotic injury model. *Foot Ankle Int.* **2008**, *29*, 49–54. [CrossRef]
40. Teramoto, A.; Suzuki, D.; Kamiya, T.; Chikenji, T.; Watanabe, K.; Yamashita, T. Comparison of different fixation methods of the suture-button implant for tibiofibular syndesmosis injuries. *Am. J. Sports Med.* **2011**, *39*, 2226–2232. [CrossRef] [PubMed]
41. Wikeroy, A.K.; Hoiness, P.R.; Andreassen, G.S.; Hellund, J.C.; Madsen, J.E. No difference in functional and radiographic results 8.4 years after quadricortical compared with tricortical syndesmosis fixation in ankle fractures. *J. Orthop. Trauma* **2010**, *24*, 17–23. [CrossRef] [PubMed]
42. Sagi, H.C.; Shah, A.R.; Sanders, R.W. The functional consequence of syndesmotic joint malreduction at a minimum 2-year follow-up. *J. Orthop. Trauma* **2012**, *26*, 439–443. [CrossRef] [PubMed]
43. Naqvi, G.A.; Cunningham, P.; Lynch, B.; Galvin, R.; Awan, N. Fixation of ankle syndesmotic injuries, comparison of TightRope fixation and syndesmotic screw fixation for accuracy of syndesmotic reduction. *Am. J. Sports Med.* **2012**, *40*, 2828–2835. [CrossRef] [PubMed]
44. Cottom, J.M.; Hyer, C.F.; Philbin, T.M.; Berlet, G.C. Treatment of syndesmotic disruptions with the Arthrex TightRope, a report of 25 cases. *Foot Ankle Int.* **2008**, *29*, 773–780. [CrossRef]
45. Degroot, H.; Al-Omari, A.A.; El Ghazaly, S.A. Outcomes of suture button repair of the distal tibiofibular syndesmosis. *Foot Ankle Int.* **2011**, *32*, 250–256. [CrossRef]
46. Rigby, R.B.; Cottom, J.M. Does the Arthrex TightRope(R) provide maintenance of the distal tibiofibular syndesmosis? A 2-year follow-up of 64 TightRopes(R) in 37 patients. *J. Foot Ankle Surg.* **2013**, *52*, 563–567. [CrossRef]
47. Naqvi, G.A.; Shafqat, A.; Awan, N. TightRope fixation of ankle syndesmosis injuries, clinical outcome, complications and technique modification. *Injury* **2012**, *43*, 838–842. [CrossRef]
48. Cottom, J.M.; Hyer, C.F.; Philbin, T.M.; Berlet, G.C. Transosseous fixation of the distal tibiofibular syndesmosis, comparison of an interosseous suture and endobutton to traditional screw fixation in 50 cases. *J. Foot Ankle Surg.* **2009**, *48*, 620–630. [CrossRef]
49. Treon, K.; Beastell, J.; Kumar, K.; Hope, M. Complications of ankle syndesmosis stabilisation using a tightrope. *Orthop. Proc.* **2018**, *93-B*, 62.
50. Anand, A.; Wei, R.; Patel, A.; Vedi, V.; Allardice, G.; Anand, B.S. Tightrope fixation of syndesmotic injuries in Weber C ankle fractures, a multicenter case series. *Eur. J. Orthop. Surg. Traumatol.* **2017**, *27*, 461–467. [CrossRef]
51. Spindler, F.T.; Gaube, F.P.; Böcker, W.; Polzer, H.; Baumbach, S.F. Value of Intraoperative 3D Imaging on the Quality of Reduction of the Distal Tibiofibular Joint When Using a Suture-Button System. *Foot Ankle Int.* **2023**, *44*, 54–61. [CrossRef] [PubMed]
52. Thornes, B.; Shannon, F.; Guiney, A.M.; Hession, P.; Masterson, E. Suture-button syndesmosis fixation, accelerated rehabilitation and improved outcomes. *Clin. Orthop. Relat. Res.* **2005**, *431*, 207–212. [CrossRef]
53. Weening, B.; Bhandari, M. Predictors of functional outcome following transsyndesmotic screw fixation of ankle fractures. *J. Orthop. Trauma* **2005**, *19*, 102–108. [CrossRef] [PubMed]
54. Xenos, J.S.; Hopkinson, W.J.; Mulligan, M.E.; Olson, E.J.; Popovic, N.A. The tibiofibular syndesmosis. Evaluation of the ligamentous structures.; methods of fixation.; and radiographic assessment. *J. Bone Joint Surg. Am.* **1995**, *77*, 847–856. [CrossRef]
55. Bartoníček, J.; Rammelt, S.; Tuček, M.; Naňka, O. Posterior malleolar fractures of the ankle. *Eur. J. Trauma Emerg. Surg.* **2015**, *41*, 587–600. [CrossRef] [PubMed]
56. Testa, G.; Ganci, M.; Amico, M.; Papotto, G.; Giardina, S.M.C.; Sessa, G.; Pavone, V. Negative prognostic factors in surgical treatment for trimalleolar fractures. *Eur. J. Orthop. Surg. Traumatol.* **2019**, *29*, 1325–1330. [CrossRef]

Disclaimer/Publisher's Note: The statements, opinions and data contained in all publications are solely those of the individual author(s) and contributor(s) and not of MDPI and/or the editor(s). MDPI and/or the editor(s) disclaim responsibility for any injury to people or property resulting from any ideas, methods, instructions or products referred to in the content.

MDPI
St. Alban-Anlage 66
4052 Basel
Switzerland
www.mdpi.com

Journal of Clinical Medicine Editorial Office
E-mail: jcm@mdpi.com
www.mdpi.com/journal/jcm

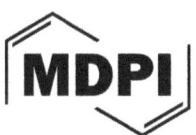

Disclaimer/Publisher's Note: The statements, opinions and data contained in all publications are solely those of the individual author(s) and contributor(s) and not of MDPI and/or the editor(s). MDPI and/or the editor(s) disclaim responsibility for any injury to people or property resulting from any ideas, methods, instructions or products referred to in the content.

www.ingramcontent.com/pod-product-compliance
Lightning Source LLC
LaVergne TN
LVHW070446100526
838202LV00014B/1680